Gestational Trophoblastic Disease

Current Clinical Pathology

Antonio Giordano, MD, PhD

Series Editor

For further volumes:
http://www.springer.com/series/7632

Pei Hui
Editor

Gestational Trophoblastic Disease

Diagnostic and Molecular Genetic Pathology

Humana Press

Editor
Pei Hui, MD, PhD
Department of Pathology
Yale University School of Medicine
New Haven, CT, USA
pei.hui@yale.edu

ISBN 978-1-61779-393-6 e-ISBN 978-1-61779-394-3
DOI 10.1007/978-1-61779-394-3
Springer New York Dordrecht Heidelberg London

Library of Congress Control Number: 2011941658

Printed on acid-free paper

Humana Press is part of Springer Science+Business Media (www.springer.com)

This book is dedicated to:

Professor Bingquan Wu, M.D.
An ultimate career mentor and a caring father-in-law

Foreword

In placental mammals, the trophoblast plays a critical role in the development of the embryo and fetus, and in normal circumstances is then discarded at the time of parturition, its functions fulfilled. Originating as the outer layer of the developing blastocyst, it ultimately differentiates into a diverse array of morphological phenotypes, each with highly specialized and differing functions: the cytotrophoblast functions as the stem cell component of the villous trophoblast, the syncytiotrophoblast as the terminally differentiated component that is of major importance in maternofetal exchange, and the intermediate trophoblast with multiple functions depending upon its location in villi, in the chorion laeve or in the implantation site. Not surprisingly, in diseases of the trophoblast, the different normal phenotypes are emulated to varying degrees, and the current classification of gestational trophoblastic disease is based on this structure.

In this volume, Dr Hui has brought together a comprehensive overview of gestational trophoblastic disease that includes all the currently recognized entities: complete and partial hydatidiform moles, placental site trophoblastic tumor, epithelioid trophoblastic tumor, gestational choriocarcinoma, persistent gestational trophoblastic neoplasia, placental site nodule, and exaggerated placental site reaction. Each entity is reviewed in detail, with emphasis on genetic background, clinical presentation, pathologic findings and ancillary studies, differential diagnosis, and clinicopathological correlations. Descriptions of the pathology are supported by numerous excellent photomicrographs. Recent advances in our understanding of the genetics of gestational trophoblastic diseases are stressed. Introductory chapters cover the developmental biology of the placenta and the genetic basis of gestational trophoblastic disease, and one chapter is devoted to the molecular diagnosis of gestational trophoblastic disease. This chapter includes a review of the use of short tandem repeat (STR) genotyping, which is of particular value in the diagnosis of hydatidiform moles. The final chapter covers clinical aspects of gestational trophoblastic disease, including treatment. The text throughout is current and thoroughly referenced.

Although written largely by a pathologist, Dr. Hui, with contributions from two other pathologists (Dr. Natalia Buza from Yale and Dr. Katja Gwin from the University of Chicago) and a chapter on clinical aspects of gestational trophoblastic disease by two gynecologists (Dr. Christine Richter and Dr. Peter Schwartz from Yale), this book will be of interest to anyone involved in the care of patients with gestational trophoblastic disease, including obstetricians and gynecologists as well as pathologists. It can serve as an up-to-date primer and reference source on the classification, clinical features, genetics and molecular diagnosis of gestational trophoblastic diseases, and as an aid to the histopathological diagnosis of these entities. Dr Hui is to be congratulated on making a valuable addition to the literature on these fascinating but complex entities.

New Haven, CT, USA A Brian West, MD, FRC Path

Preface

Gestational trophoblastic disease (GTD) deserves a special consideration in medicine. It encompasses a group of human disorders of reproduction resulting in significant morbidities in women, and is remarkable for its geographical distributions and varying frequencies in the different age and ethnic groups. In human pathology, these disorders are unique proliferative conditions with regard to their clinical setting, genetic compositions, and varying biological behaviors. Although as one of the earliest recognized human disorders in history, the biology, pathogenesis, diagnosis, and clinical management of the disease are still fascinating many of us either as a diagnostician or as a scientific investigator. My academic interest in GTD incurred at a morning pathology resident conference with Dr. Kurt Benirschke who was visiting Yale in 1997 as a grand rounds speaker. I was presenting him a placental site trophoblastic tumor, a uterine specimen processed by myself and diagnosed by my mentor, Dr. Maria Luisa Carcangiu, a few weeks earlier. Dr. Benirschke challenged me to prove that the lesion was indeed a clonal neoplastic lesion as opposed to a reactive process. His challenge eventually led to my first publication of the X chromosomal requirement by placental site trophoblastic tumor in 2000, and more importantly, opened many fascinating aspects of GTD in my academic career afterward.

With an intended broad spectrum of audience, the book starts with a general review of the medical history, epidemiology, and risk factors for GTD in Chapter 1. Chapter 2 provides a succinct review of developmental aspects of placenta with an emphasis on its early formation and molecular genetic regulation of implantation. Our current understanding of the genetic basis of GTD is given in Chapter 3. The following chapters provide a thorough review of diagnostic histopathology of the each entity of GTD. Although traditional histology is the foundation for morphological recognition, ancillary studies including immunohistochemistry and molecular genotyping have become an integral part of the routine diagnostic algorithm. Each diagnostic entity is richly illustrated histologically, often with multiple examples. Chapter 9 is written to cover the diagnostic entities under the category of persistent trophoblastic neoplasia by the WHO. Invasive mole is primarily discussed here. Chapter 11 provides a thorough review of the emerging molecular diagnostic applications in GTD. Finally, a comprehensive discussion of the clinical presentation and management of GTD is given in Chapter 12.

I can never express enough gratitude to my career mentors, present and past, at Peking University, SUNY at Buffalo, MSKCC and Yale. Their wisdom and training are the major source of knowledge and professional inspirations. Special thanks are owed to many colleagues who shared their insights and/or clinical cases in the past. Finally, this book is a product that represents not only an academic commitment but also the unfettered support and enduring love of my families.

New Haven, CT, USA Pei Hui, MD, PhD

Contents

Contributors

Natalia Buza, MD Department of Pathology, Yale University School of Medicine, 310 Cedar Street, PO Box 208023, New Haven, CT 06520-8023, USA
natalia.buza@yale.edu

Katja Gwin, MD, PhD Department of Pathology, University of Chicago Medical Center, 5841 S. Maryland Ave (MC6101), Chicago, IL 60637, USA
Katja.Gwin@uchospitals.edu

Pei Hui, MD, PhD Department of Pathology, Yale University School of Medicine, 310 Cedar Street, 254B New Haven, CT 06520-8023, USA
pei.hui@yale.edu

Christine E. Richter, MD Division of Gynecologic Oncology, Department of Obstetrics, Gynecology & Reproductive Sciences, Yale University School of Medicine, 333 Cedar Street, New Haven, CT 06510, USA
christine.richter@yale.edu

Peter E. Schwartz, MD Division of Gynecologic Oncology, Department of Obstetrics, Gynecology & Reproductive Sciences, Yale University School of Medicine, 333 Cedar Street, New Haven, CT 06510, USA
peter.schwartz@yale.edu

Gestational Trophoblastic Disease: General Aspects

1

Pei Hui

Keywords
Historical review • Epidemiology • Classification

Historical Remarks

As a major defining characteristic of eutherian mammals, the placenta is a transient organ of female reproduction that nourishes the developing fetus through nutrient supply, waste elimination, and gas exchange. In both Latin and Greek, the placenta means *flat cake*, in reference to its flat and round appearance in human. The placenta arises from the same fertilized egg that forms the fetus and is essentially a fetomaternal organ consisting of two components: the fetal part (chorion frondosum) and the maternal part (decidua basalis). It has been speculated that ancestral mammals might have evolved to attain the placenta, along with newly acquired retrotransposon-derived genes, or expression of endogenous version of the genes present in oviparous animals. This occurred sometime after the divergence of mammals and birds more than 90–130 million years ago [1].

P. Hui, MD, PhD (✉)
Department of Pathology, Yale University School of Medicine, 310 Cedar Street, 254B New Haven, CT 06520-8023, USA
e-mail: pei.hui@yale.edu

The major constituents of the placenta are trophoblasts of various types. Trophoblasts (from Greek *trephein*: to nourish, and *blastos*: budding) are cells forming the outer layer of a blastocyst, nourishing the embryo and developing into the ultimate placenta. Trophoblasts are formed during the first stage of pregnancy and are the first cells to differentiate from a fertilized egg. Trophoblasts play a dominant role in the early blastocyst implantation, placental formation, placental maturation, and maintenance of pregnancy, immunosurveillance, endocrine functions, and possibly placental delivery. Among various trophoblastic cell types, cytotrophoblasts likely possess the stem cell capability and differentiate into other types of trophoblast. Syncytiotrophoblasts are terminally matured cells with functions such as forming the syncytium during early implantation and hormonal secretions throughout gestation. Intermediate trophoblasts are functional cells involved in implantation, placental formation, and various placental functions.

One of the most common gestational trophoblastic diseases (GTDs) is the hydatidiform mole (HM). It is among the earliest recognized human diseases (Fig. 1.1). The etymology of HM is derived from *hydatisia* (Greek "a drop of water"), referring to the watery content of the

P. Hui (ed.), *Gestational Trophoblastic Disease: Diagnostic and Molecular Genetic Pathology*, Current Clinical Pathology, DOI 10.1007/978-1-61779-394-3_1,

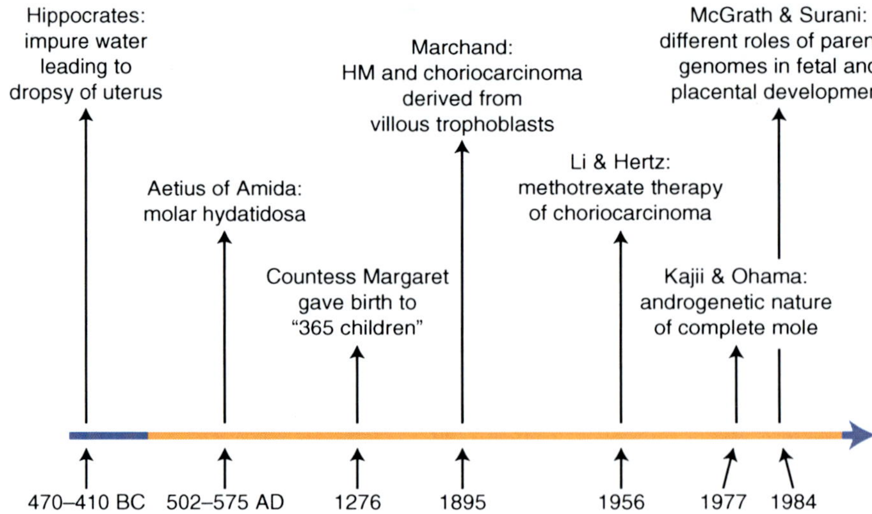

Fig. 1.1 Historical timeline: gestational trophoblastic disease (GTD)

cysts, and *mole* (from Latin *mola* = millstone/false conception) [2]. According to James Sands Elliott's "Outlines of Greek and Roman Medicine" [3], Hippocrates (470–410 bc), in the acclaimed treatise on "Airs, Water, and Places," described that drinking impure water will cause dropsy of the uterus. Aetius of Amida (502–575 ad), a doctor from Mesopotamia (modern day Iraq) who studied at Alexandria (the most famous medical school of the age), was the first to use the term "mola hydatidosa" in his work on Greek and Christian traditions of medicine [4]. He correctly described a woman with a molar pregnancy suffering from swollen breasts and suppressed menses. Aetius also developed a theory of molar pregnancy including "an inflammation or strenuous walking." The Dutch story of Countess Margaret of Henneberg giving birth to 365 children on Good Friday in 1276 at The Hague was considered as a punishment by God (Fig. 1.2). The Countess had insulted a poor beggar woman, who was carrying a twin. She accused the beggar of being promiscuous, believing that a twin must have two different fathers. The countess died soon after the delivery of her 365 "children," half males and half females according to the story (Fig. 1.2b) [5, 6]. It seems little doubt that Countess Margaret had a complete HM. Although the story was written more than 600 years ago [5], it has a striking relatedness to what we know genetically today about molar gestations. God's "punishment" on Countess Margaret (i.e., a complete HM) was a trophoblastic disease as a result of fertilization of an enucleated ovum by two copies of sperm (as opposed to two men in the case of the Countess's accusation against the poor beggar woman!).

In 1752, Smellie first related the terms "hydatid" and "mole" as "bunch of grapes of different sizes" [7]. Velpeau and Boivin in 1827 [2] recognized that the "grapes" of a HM were dilated hydropic chorionic villi. The cellular basis of HM was elucidated by Marchand in 1895 as a proliferation of syncytial and Langhan's (cytotrophoblast) cells. An excessive production of gonadotropic hormone in urine of patients with HM was identified by Rossler and Zondek in 1939 [8].

The earliest description of nowadays "gestational choriocarcinoma" dated back to 1889 when Sanger created the term *sarcoma uteri deciduocellulare* to describe a malignant tumor derived from the decidua of pregnancy [9]. Gottschalk in 1893 coined the term "deciduoma malignum" or "chorio-deciduo-cellular sarcoma" and "sarcoma of the chorial villi," believing that the tumor arose from the Langhan's cells

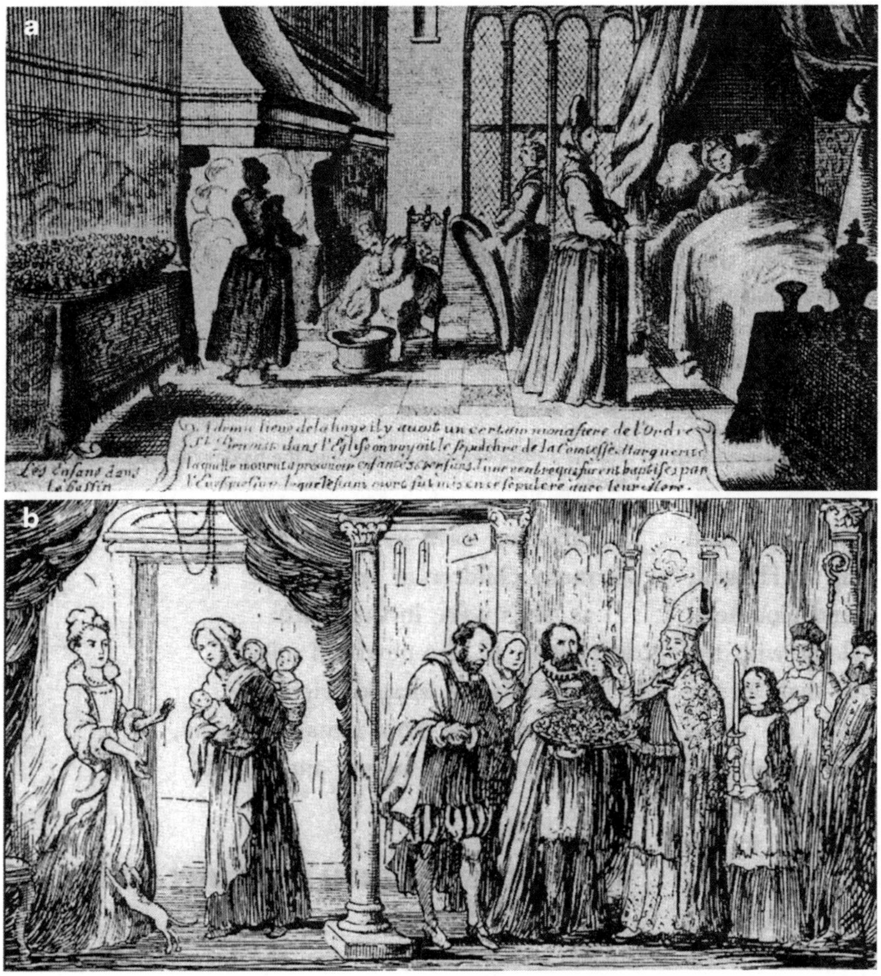

Fig. 1.2 (**a**) A French engraving of the Pieter Kaerius drawing of the legend of Countess Margaret of Henneberg in the seventeenth century. The Countess was lying on bed helped by midwives on the right, and her "365" children were displayed on table on the far left (Copyright permission obtained from J R Soc Med). (**b**) A copy by E van Offel of the paining of the legend by Michael Waginger displayed in the private chapel of the Castle Thierberg in Kufstein. On the left, Countess Margaret was insulting the poor beggar woman who was holding her twin, and on the right, the Countess's "365" children were baptized by the Bishop in the presence of noblemen and church dignitaries (Copyright permission obtained from J R Soc Med)

(cytotrophoblasts) and the stroma of chorionic villi [10, 11]. Beach described a choriocarcinoma in a 25-year-old woman, whom he took care of in 1894, and reported in the Annals of Surgery in 1895. He rightly concluded in his essay that "the nature of this tumor is very plain: it is a tumor composed of placental tissue" [10]. In the same year of 1895, Marchand demonstrated that the tumor was epithelial in nature arising exclusively from the syncytiotrophoblasts and cytotrophoblasts, and used the term "chorioepithelioma." He also illustrated that these tumors could be sequelae of pregnancy, abortion, or HM. In 1903, Teacher confirmed Marchand's work and disputed Sanger's theory of sarcomatous degeneration of the deciduas [9, 12]. The term "choriocarcinoma" was finally introduced by Ewing in 1910 [11, 13]. Ewing classified all trophoblastic lesions under the general term "chorioma" to include the common entities known today: HM, invasive mole (chorioadenoma destruens), and gestational choriocarcinoma (chorioepithelioma). He considered the term "syncytial endometritis" as equivalent to Marchand's atypical chorioepithelioma, an entity described as an infiltration of the uterus with syncytial wandering cells that occasionally might simulate a tumor "syncytioma," which could represent placental site trophoblastic tumor (PSTT) as we know it in modern pathology. A landmark in our understanding of the pathogenesis of HM at molecular/genetic level was made by Kajii in 1977 when he and his colleagues identified the androgenetic nature of complete HM [14]. Mouse pronuclear transfer experiments by McGrath and Surani in 1984 recognized different roles of the maternal and paternal genomes (genomic imprinting) in placental development [15, 16]. Abnormal genomic imprinting has been hypothesized as the fundamental basis for the development of GTD, particularly HM and choriocarcinoma [17–19].

The therapy of GTD carries a remarkably successful story in medicine [20, 21]. The once uniformly fatal choriocarcinoma could be cured by high dose of chemotherapeutic agent methotrexate in Li and Hertz's pioneering study in 1956. The success story was hailed as the beginning of a new era of cancer chemotherapy. While a 47% complete cure rate of choriocarcinoma was achieved in the early 1960s, Hertz subsequently introduced sequential regimes of actinomycin D and methotrexate, achieving a 74% remission rate [22, 23]. By 1965, over 95% cure rates were recorded for patients with the disease limited to the chest and pelvis after the sequential chemotherapy [24, 25]. In 1972, a specific antibody to the beta chain of human chorionic gonadotropin (hCG) was identified leading to the clinical radioimmunoassay of hCG with high sensitivity and specificity [26, 27]. The early diagnosis by ultrasound and other imaging studies combined with the highly sensitive hCG monitoring have resulted in a remarkable early intervention of HMs and choriocarcinoma. Over many years, significant contributions by Bagshawe, Acosta-Sison, Berkowitz, Goldstein, Lewis, Ross, Brewer, Kohorn, Lurain, Fisher, Seckl, and others were made to the advancement of clinical diagnosis and therapy of GTD. Hertig, Sheldon, Gore, Park, Ober, Benirschke, Scully, Young, Kurman, Fox, Sebire, Genest, Lage, Wells, Cheung, Shih, and many others contributed to modern wisdom in the pathology of GTD. Fukuyama and Fisher conceptually explored microsatellite markers by polymerase chain reaction in the diagnosis of HMs in the early 1990s [28, 29], although routine and cost-effective clinical applications of genotyping diagnosis of GTD did not occur until very recently [30–32].

Definition and Classification of GTDs

Although GTDs are composed of distinct entities in pathology, an assignment of all lesions under one common pathogenesis has been controversial and open to debate [33]. Gestational trophoblastic neoplasia (GTN) has been proposed to imply a clonal neoplastic nature of the disease. This is possibly incorrect as the most common HM has never been proven clonal, and in fact, some authors believe that molar pregnancies are degenerative processes with edema of the placenta [34]. Endorsed by the WHO, the term "GTD" appears to be acceptable by all parties [35]. It seems reasonable, however, to argue that GTDs are proliferative disorders of placental trophoblasts of either hyperplastic or neoplastic nature, a view put forward by Marchand more than a century ago [36]. GTDs are lesions of trophoblast with varying proliferative capacities, ranging from nonneoplastic HMs (complete HM, partial HM, and invasive mole) to bona fide neoplastic conditions (gestational choriocarcinoma, placental site trophoblastic tumor (PSTT), and epithelioid trophoblastic tumor (ETT)) [35, 37, 38]. Each of the entities has distinctive clinical behavior attributable to the proliferative capacity of its constituent trophoblast (Table 1.1). In addition, two tumor-like conditions of trophoblastic nature are also included in some textbooks, i.e., exaggerated placental site reaction and placental site nodule or plaque.

Recent investigations into biomarker expression have delineated cellular differentiation pathways for various trophoblastic diseases [39].

Table 1.1 Classification of Gestational Trophoblastic Disease

General Category	Subtypes
Hydatidiform Mole	Complete mole
	Partial mole
	Invasive mole
Trophoblastic Tumor	Gestational choriocarcinoma
	PSTT
	ETT
Tumor-like Condition	Exaggerated placental site reaction
	Placental site nodule/plaque

Hydatidiform moles are proliferative lesions of the villous trophoblasts. The most virulent choriocarcinoma is a fully malignant tumor of the trophoblasts recapitulating the primitive cells of the previllous stage of the placenta. The intermediate trophoblast at the implantation site is the putative cell type that gives rise to PSTT and exaggerated placental site reaction. On the other hand, the intermediate trophoblast in the chorion laeve is considered the cell type found in ETT and placental site nodule. A small subset of the disease does not fit into any established category and therefore, placed under the category, "trophoblastic disease, unclassifiable, in some textbooks."

Epidemiology and Risk Factors

The epidemiology of GTDs is unclear, and the statistics are at best inaccurate, primarily due to problems of diagnostic accuracy, inclusion criteria in a study cohort, data collection, and interpretation in the world literature. Nevertheless, HM is the most prevalent trophoblastic disease, of which only studies of complete mole have provided some reliable epidemiological data. Among plausible etiologies, maternal age, ethnicity, and genetic basis are the most convincing factors of HM. While a complete HM is significantly associated with the development of gestational choriocarcinoma, the etiology of gestational trophoblastic tumors following a normal gestation is largely unexplained in the literature.

Incidence

The incidence of GTD is generally recorded in relation to the total number of pregnancies in a study cohort, rather than the total population. Such an approach provides a direct comparison across a community, although significant limitations exist [40]. It should be kept in mind that epidemiological studies focusing on complete HM are likely more accurate than those including also partial HM, as significant diagnostic problems exist in the routine evaluation of the latter [41, 42]. Table 1.2 summarizes the incidence of GTD based on the world literature. The highest incidence of HM per 1,000 pregnancies is seen in South-East Asia with rates ranging from 13.0 in Indonesia, 8.0 in Taiwan, 5.0 in Philippines and China, and 3.8 in Japan [40, 43–49]. North America [50–54], Europe [55–61], and Oceania [62–66] have the lowest incidence with approximately 0.5–1.84/1,000 pregnancies. Nigeria and Uganda are the only African nations that have documentations in English of the incidence of the disease, averaged at 5.0/1,000 pregnancies [67–71]. Data from South America [72–74] are also limited with reported incidence ranging from 0.23 to 0.9/1,000 pregnancies. Possibly due to an improvement of general social economic status of the population, recent reports showed a significant reduction in the incidence of GTD in Korea [75–77] where the rate has fallen from 4.4/1,000 pregnancies in the 1960s to 2.3/1,000 pregnancies in the 1990s and in Japan where a reduction in the incidence of HM from 4.9 to 1.9/1,000 pregnancies for GTD was reported [78, 79]. Information from Saudi Arabia and Taiwan reports a similar trend [80, 81]. However, it is important to note that one recent thorough analysis in Japan indicates that the true incidence of molar pregnancy may be much higher (3.8/1,000 pregnancies), primarily due to an underdiagnosis of partial moles in general [82].

Reported incidence of gestational trophoblastic tumors varies significantly largely due to the diagnostic definitions and criteria used by pathologists. Gestational choriocarcinoma was the traditional bona fide malignant tumor, for which the

Table 1.2 World-wide incidence of GTD (incidence per 1,000 pregnancies)

Population	Hydatidiform Mole	Choriocarcinoma or aggressive GTD	References
Indonesia	13 (11.7[a])	5.4 (1.7[a])	[83, 87]
Philippine	5.0	0.7	[40, 132]
Taiwan	8.0[a]	2.0[a]	[43]
Korea	2.3(1.6[a]–4.1[a])	1.6[a]	[76, 77]
Hong Kong	1.8 (4.0[b])	0.7	[133–135]
Singapore	1.2	0.23	[91, 110]
India	2.0[b]		[136]
Mexico	1–6.3	0.11–1.5	[89, 137, 138]
Turkey	10.6[a]	2.35[a]	[108]
China	0.8–5.0		[45, 46]
Iran	3.2		[139]
Japan	1.9–3.8(3.0[a])	0.12	[47–49, 78, 82, 140]
Israel	0.42–1.1[a]	0.055[a]	[88, 99, 126]
USA	0.5–1.84 (3.9 for native Alaskans and 1.2[b] for Hawaii)	0.025–0.05	[40, 50–54, 86, 97, 104–106, 111]
Europe	0.6–1.0 (1.54[a])	0.02–0.05	[55–61, 97, 141, 142]
New Zealand	0.68		[62]
Australia	0.9–1.4 (0.7[a])	0.07	[63, 65, 66]
Samoa	0.9[a]		[64]
South America (Paraguay and Brazil)	0.23–0.9 (0.26[b])		[72–74]
Africa (Nagiria and Uganda)	2.6–8.2	1.2–1.9(1.5[b])	[67–71, 143]

[a] Per 1,000 live birth or deliveries
[b] Complete mole only

early epidemiology data were available. However, recent changes from the diagnosis of choriocarcinoma by pathology to the use of clinical parameters including radiological and biochemical diagnostic methods have blurred the boundaries between choriocarcinoma and invasive or persistent hydatidiform mole. Because of such a shift of clinical practice, the term "GTN" has been used recently to include all clinically aggressive lesions including gestational choriocarcinoma, persistent mole, invasive mole, and metastatic mole. Rare tumors of intermediate trophoblast such as PSTT and ETT are also included in the GTN category by the WHO. Since HMs, particularly complete moles, are strongly associated with the development of choriocarcinoma, the incidence of GTN generally reflects the geographical distributions of molar pregnancies (Table 1.2) with the highest rate in Indonesia, occurring in 5.4/1,000 pregnancies [83], lower in other parts of Asia [47, 84, 85] and the lowest in North America, Europe, and Oceania with figures between 0.02 and 0.07/1,000 pregnancies [60, 65, 86]. Concurrent with HMs, the incidence of GTN also dropped in Korea [76] from 4.4/1,000 births in the 1960s to 1.6/1,000 births in the 1990s. It was found in Indonesia that 76.4% of malignant trophoblastic diseases originated from HMs, 12.4% from abortions, 9.5% from normal deliveries, and 1.2% from ectopic pregnancies [87]. Reports from Japan [78] also showed a reduction in the incidence of choriocarcinoma from 1.6 to 0.3/1,000,000 of population, and the most common antecedent gestational event was a term pregnancy. In Israel, however, the incidence of gestational choriocarcinoma decreased significantly during 1960–1965 to one-third of the incidence during 1950–1954 [88]. Paradoxically, the incidence of HM continued to increase over the same period [89].

Risk Factors

Maternal Age

Maternal age is perhaps the most important risk factor for the development of HM and choriocarcinoma. Numerous studies have indicated that women over the age of 35 years and teenagers have a significantly increased risk of HM [50, 60, 73, 90–93] with a 1.5–2-fold increase in women under the age of 20 years [94], 2.5-fold increase in women over the age of 35 years [50, 95], and fivefold or more in women aged over 40 years [56, 86, 92, 95]. Such age-related risk is observed in different races and in different countries throughout the world. Interestingly, more than 100 cases of HM were reported in patients over 50 years of age [96, 97]. The oldest reported woman developed a complete mole at the age of 61 years [98].

Previous Pregnancies

Molar pregnancies are usually not recurrent. However, a previous HM is associated with an increased risk of having another [86, 89, 99, 100]. The estimated relative risks are 5–40 times that of the general population [99, 101]. The risk is even greater if a woman has had more than one. In a study from the United Kingdom, it was reported that 1 in 76 pregnancies after a mole would result in another mole but in women who had already had two consecutive molar pregnancies the risk increased to 1 in 6.5 pregnancies [56]. The risk appears to be diminished, however, if there are one or more normal pregnancies following a prior HM.

A previous complete HM also predisposes the patient to the development of GTN with the risk estimated to be 1,000 times higher than that after a term pregnancy [102].

Ethnicity

There is little doubt that the geographical distribution of HM reflexes the distribution of different ethnic groups rather than environmental or climatic factors. A study from Malaysia [103] reported an incidence for Malays, Chinese, and Indians at 2.43, 2.66, and 3.29/1,000 pregnancies, respectively. Hawaiian studies [104, 105] reported that the incidences of HM were highest in Japanese and Filipinos, low in Chinese, and lowest in whites and native Hawaiians. Another study in Hawaii found that Orientals had a higher incidence than Europeans of the same socioeconomic class and native Hawaiians of a lower status [106]. Yet another study in early 1980s found that Hawaiians of Filipino origin had five times higher risk of complete mole than Caucasians [107]. An earlier report from Singapore showed no real difference in the incidence in these groups, although the trend was found to be highest in Indians and lowest in Malays [91]. Studies from the United States across the racial groups have not produced consistent results [106]. Various studies have shown that black women have a higher, lower, or similar incidence to that of white women [50, 104, 108]. A study of Alaskan natives has, however, shown that their incidence rate is 3–4 times higher than that of the white population [86]. The clear ethnic differences in the incidence of molar pregnancy suggest a genetic basis either for a high incidence of abnormal fertilization or an increased capacity to permit implantation of a genetically abnormal pregnancy [109].

Because of the strong association of choriocarcinoma with a prior complete mole, it is not a surprise that the disease incidence is higher in those populations with a high incidence of HM. In a study from Singapore [110], the incidence of choriocarcinoma was highest in Malays at 1.0/1,000 pregnancies, intermediate in Chinese at 0.63/1,000 pregnancies, and lowest in Indians at 0.13/1,000 pregnancies. Interestingly, this does not quite mirror the rate of HM in these groups, where it is highest in Indians, intermediate in Chinese, and lowest in Malays [110], suggesting that some other factor(s) are involved in initiating the malignant transformation.

Genetics

Increased risk of GTD in patients with prior HM suggests that genetic factors may play a role in the development of the disease. The high frequency of HM per delivery in the native Alaskan was suspected due to genetic factors [111]. The existence of recurrent and familial biparental complete moles further attests to a genetic role. Recent findings of various mutations involving NALP7 on chromosome 19q13.4 are likely the fundamental molecular events leading to the development of familial biparental moles, likely through an alteration of genomic imprinting, see Chap. 3 for details [112].

Diet or Socioeconomic Factors

The data on dietary and socioeconomic factors as risk factors for GTD have been conflicting. The original suggestion was that a deficiency of first class protein predisposed patients to the development of GTD [44]. A joint project for the study of choriocarcinoma and HM in Asia in 1959 also suggested that socioeconomic factors played an important role in the development of HMs [113]. This idea was postulated at a time when the general nutrition in South-East Asian countries was poor. Studies of patients with HMs found that serum creatinine and urea were comparably higher than those in normal individuals [114] although, at the same time, total protein and serum albumin concentrations were significantly decreased. It was suggested that these findings were indicative of catabolism due to dietary inadequacies. Berkowitz and others implied that vitamin A deficiency might be related to molar pregnancy [115, 116]. However, an association of dietary factors with molar gestation was not found in Hawaii and the United States by other studies [86, 106]. The high frequency of HM per delivery in the native Alaskan was found not associated with protein deficiency as an etiologic factor, instead genetic contribution may be involved [111]. In another study from Mexico [89], food histories of women with HM and a control group of pregnant women were taken and no difference was detected in the intake of proteins, carbohydrates, and fats. African Americans had a similar incidence as whites [117]. However, recent reports from Korea, Japan, and Taiwan showed a significant reduction in the incidence of GTD [75–78, 80], arguing for a causal relationship linked to an improvement of socioeconomic status of the populations.

Factors not Found Etiologically Associated with GTD

Although some earlier data suggested an association between oral contraceptive intake and the development of HM [118], studies looking at the association with past use of an intrauterine device have produced conflicting results [104, 115, 119]. Similarly, despite earlier reports suggesting an association between oral contraceptive intake after a molar gestation and an increased incidence of post molar choriocarcinoma [120, 121], the findings could not be reproduced in subsequent studies [122, 123]. Extensive follow-up studies also failed to confirm an association between the use of postmolar oral contraception and the development of GTN [124].

Gravidity, parity, smoking, exposure to herbicides, paternal age, viral infection, and blood types are not significantly associated with the development of HM [86, 125–127].

Overview of Diagnosis

The introduction of diagnostic ultrasound following the development of gray scale and Doppler made initial significant inroads in the early detection and diagnosis of GTD. As such equipments became simpler and cheaper, their availability has become more widespread in the world. In developed countries, any patient presenting during early pregnancy with abnormal bleeding or severe vomiting will be recommended to have ultrasound examination specifically to exclude GTD. Ultrasound findings of mixed echogenic patterns in combination with elevated serum hCG above that expected for gestational age are highly suggestive of molar pregnancy. Moreover, GTD is often diagnosed much earlier in pregnancy than was previously possible. In current practice GTD patients presenting with a large uterus and compound theca luteum cysts in the ovaries are very rare in developed countries. The earlier evacuation of abnormal pregnancies now presents diagnostic challenges for pathologists due to the less developed morphological features that frequently overlap with those of more common non-molar gestations.

The development of assays for urinary and then subsequent serum pregnancy associated hormones has significantly changed the diagnosis and management of GTD. Assays for luteinizing hormone (because of its cross-reactivity with the hCG molecule) were followed by the development of specific assays for the βhCG molecule. These tests have become increasingly simpler and easier to perform and resulted in a major improvement in the accuracy of diagnosis and follow-up of patients with GTD. This is particularly significant in the detection of neoplastic transformation into choriocarcinoma following evacuation of HM, leading to much earlier introduction of chemotherapy prior to the development of metastases.

Histopathological examination of gestational tissue samples remains a fundamental diagnostic procedure. Immunohistochemistry for p57 and DNA ploidy analysis are useful ancillary tests to help resolve some difficult cases. However, there are important confounding issues in the current diagnostic pathology, particularly when dealing with partial HMs. An estimated 50% of true partial moles cannot be accurately diagnosed by routine histology [41], and significant inter- and intra-observer variability exists among even expert pathologists [128]. Overdiagnosis of partial molar pregnancy occurs not infrequently due to interpretation errors of ploidy data and the presence of non-molar triploidy, and undoubtedly leads to going through unnecessary and costly HM surveillance program and long-term contraception of the patient. Misinterpretation of an early complete mole as hydropic abortus or partial mole should not be made as it carries a similar prognosis as a well-developed one in the development of persistent trophoblastic neoplasia. Applications of more accurate diagnostic methods, such as DNA genotyping, should be advocated.

Overview of Clinical Management

Advances in gynecological care in the last five decades have reduced the incidence of GTD. The introduction of termination of pregnancy and the commencement in the 1960s and 1970s of its widespread availability, along with analytical improvements and safety of the technique, resulted in reducing a large number of conceptions of high-risk age groups for the development of GTD, particularly among the teenage patients [109]. Similarly, the development and availability of reliable oral contraception in the past three decades have enabled women to avoid conception, especially at the extremes of reproductive age, further reducing their chances of developing GTD. Improved contraception with intrauterine contraceptive devices has also had a similar effect, and this combined with the availability of termination of pregnancy would explain the falling birth rate in those countries where a significant reduction in the incidence of GTD has been reported. The development and improvement of suction curettage equipment and techniques for the termination of pregnancy have also simplified the management of HM. Trophoblastic embolism associated with syntocinon (oxytocin) infusion or hysterectomy is rarely observed in patients where evacuation is performed by suction curettage.

One of the most significant changes in the management of GTD in the last four decades has been the introduction of clinical surveillance program for patients with GTD using assays for hCG. As an integral component in the molar surveillance program, serial serum hCG determinations are performed after uterine curettage evacuation of the molar tissue. The hCG monitoring starts 2 days after the evacuation, followed by once every 1–2 weeks when above normal, and then once every 1–2 months after normalization for the following 6–12 months. During the hCG monitoring, effective contraception should be in place to avoid misdiagnosis of persistent GTD as normal pregnancy [42, 129]. Aggressive GTDs (invasive mole and choriocarcinoma) are generally classified into low- and high-risk groups based on clinical, pathological, and imaging studies (CT, spiral tomography, and MRI) and serum hCG levels. Currently, the International Federation of Gynecology and Obstetrics (FIGO) Risk Scoring System [130, 131] is the standard classification used in clinics to stratify patients with aggressive GTD into low- and high-risk categories for management. In contrast to gestational choriocarcinoma, PSTT and ETT are chemoresistant. Recently combined chemotherapeutic regimen has resulted in some significant response in treating these rare trophoblastic tumors.

Perspectives

The availability of diagnostic ultrasound and highly sensitive serum hCG measurement has led to the early diagnosis and management of HMs and thus has caused a reduction in the incidence of malignant trophoblastic transformation, that is, gestational choriocarcinoma. Development of suction curettage for the termination of pregnancy has enabled easier and safer molar evacuation. Improved contraceptive techniques have further reduced the incidence of molar pregnancy at the extremes of childbearing ages. As a result, the birth rate in many countries has fallen concurrent with a decline in the incidence of GTD. Improved medical imaging and biochemical testing have enabled the development of organized follow-up of patients with earlier intervention and improved clinical outcomes. However, there are important medical issues with regard to the accuracy of the diagnosis. Histological diagnosis of HM, particularly partial mole, is far from being accurate, compounded by a high percentage of so-called genetic partial moles that are clinically unrecognized as missed abortion. On the contrary, significant percentages of gestations are over-diagnosed as partial HMs. Moreover, because of such diagnostic inaccuracy, the epidemiology of GTD cannot be accurately assessed with currently available data. The most recent development of cost-effective DNA genotyping has drawn greater attention as a highly practical and accurate method of diagnosis, particularly for subtyping of HMs that will likely overcome many of the current diagnostic problems.

References

1. Hedges SB. The origin and evolution of model organisms. Nat Rev Genet. 2002;3(11):838–49.
2. Sebastian A. A dictionary of the history of medicine. NY: The Parthenon Publishing Group Inc; 1999.
3. Elliott JS. Outlines of greek and roman medicine. Boston: Milford House Inc; 1971.
4. Ricci J. The genealogy of gynaecology: history of the development of gynaecology throughout the ages 2000 BC - 1800 AD, with excerpts from the many authors who have contributed to the various phases of the subject. 2nd ed. Philadelphia: The Blakston Company; 1950.
5. Bondeson J, Molenkamp A. The countess margaret of henneberg and her 365 children. J R Soc Med. 1996;89(12):711–6. PMCID: 1296041.
6. Rather LJ, Ambroise Pare. The countess margaret, multiple births, and hydatidiform mole. Bull N Y Acad Med. 1971;47(5):508–15. PMCID: 1749900.
7. Brews A. Hydatidiform mole and chorion-epithelioma. J Obstet Gynaecol Br Commonw. 1939; 46(5):22.
8. Brews A. Hydatidiform mole and chorion-epithelioma. J Obstet Gynaecol Br Emp. 1939;46(5): 813–35.
9. Stewart CJ. History of gynecological pathology. VIII. John Hammond teacher. Int J Gynecol Pathol. 2000;19(3):284–92.
10. Beach GW. IV. The deciduoma malignum. Ann Surg. 1895;21(5):525–42. PMCID: 1494170.
11. Ober WB, Fass RO. The early history of choriocarcinoma. J Hist Med Allied Sci. 1961;16:49–73.
12. Dallenbach-Hellweg G, Schmidt D. History of gynecological pathology. VI. Jacob Felix Marchand. Int J Gynecol Pathol. 1999;18(3):281–7.
13. Ewing J. Chorioma: a clinical pathological study. Surg Gynecol Obstet. 1910;10:26.
14. Kajii T, Ohama K. Androgenetic origin of hydatidiform mole. Nature. 1977;268(5621):633–4.
15. McGrath J, Solter D. Completion of mouse embryogenesis requires both the maternal and paternal genomes. Cell. 1984;37(1):179–83.
16. Surani MA, Barton SC, Norris ML. Development of reconstituted mouse eggs suggests imprinting of the genome during gametogenesis. Nature. 1984; 308(5959):548–50.
17. Mutter GL, Stewart CL, Chaponot ML, Pomponio RJ. Oppositely imprinted genes H19 and insulin-like growth factor 2 are coexpressed in human androgenetic trophoblast. Am J Hum Genet. 1993;53(5): 1096–102. PMCID: 1682317.
18. Wake N, Arima T, Matsuda T. Involvement of IGF2 and H19 imprinting in choriocarcinoma development. Int J Gynaecol Obstet. 1998;60 Suppl 1:S1–8.
19. Arima T, Matsuda T, Takagi N, Wake N. Association of IGF2 and H19 imprinting with choriocarcinoma development. Cancer Genet Cytogenet. 1997;93(1):39–47.
20. Lewis Jr JL. Chemotherapy of gestational choriocarcinoma. Cancer. 1972;30(6):1517–21.
21. Li MC, Hertz R, Spencer DB. Effect of methotrexate therapy upon choriocarcinoma and chorioadenoma. Proc Soc Exp Biol Med. 1956;93:5.
22. Hertz R, Lewis Jr J, Lipsett MB. Five year's experience with the chemotherapy of metastatic choriocarcinoma and related trophoblastic tumors in women. Am J Obstet Gynecol. 1961;82:631–40.
23. Ross GT, Stolbach LL, Hertz R. Actinomycin D in the treatment of methotrexate-resistant trophoblastic disease in women. Cancer Res. 1962;22:1015–7.
24. Ross GT, Goldstein DP, Hertz R, Lipsett MB, Odell WD. Sequential Use of Methotrexate and Actinomycin D in the Treatment of Metastatic Choriocarcinoma and Related Trophoblastic Diseases in Women. Am J Obstet Gynecol. 1965;93:223–9.
25. Goldstein DP. The chemotherapy of gestational trophoblastic disease: principles of clinical management. JAMA. 1972;220(2):209–13.
26. Vaitukaitis JL, Braunstein GD, Ross GT. A radioimmunoassay which specifically measures human chorionic gonadotropin in the presence of human

luteinizing hormone. Am J Obstet Gynecol. 1972; 113(6):751–8.

27. Rayford PL, Vaitukaitis JL, Ross GT, Morgan FJ, Canfield RE. Use of specific antisera to characterize biologic activity of hCG-beta subunit preparations. Endocrinology. 1972;91(1):144–6.
28. Fukuyama R, Takata M, Kudoh J, Sakai K, Tamura S, Shimizu N. DNA diagnosis of hydatidiform mole using the polymerase chain reaction. Hum Genet. 1991;87(2):216–8.
29. Fisher RA, Newlands ES. Rapid diagnosis and classification of hydatidiform moles with polymerase chain reaction. Am J Obstet Gynecol. 1993;168(2):563–9.
30. Bifulco C, Johnson C, Hao L, Kermalli H, Bell S, Hui P. Genotypic analysis of hydatidiform mole: an accurate and practical method of diagnosis. Am J Surg Pathol. 2008;32(3):445–51.
31. McConnell TG, Murphy KM, Hafez M, Vang R, Ronnett BM. Diagnosis and subclassification of hydatidiform moles using p57 immunohistochemistry and molecular genotyping: validation and prospective analysis in routine and consultation practice settings with development of an algorithmic approach. Am J Surg Pathol. 2009;33(6):805–17.
32. Lipata F, Parkash V, Talmor M, Bell S, Chen S, Maric V, et al. Precise DNA genotyping diagnosis of hydatidiform mole. Obstet Gynecol. 2010;115(4):784–94.
33. Benirschke K, Kaufmann P, Baergen RN. Pathology of the human placenta. 5th ed. NY: Springer; 2006.
34. Benirschke K. What's new in gestational trophoblastic disease? Gen Diagn Pathol. 1997;143(2–3):85–6.
35. Tavassoli F, Peter D. World Health Organization: tumours of the breast and female genital organs. Lyon: IARC PRESS; 2004.
36. Marchand F. Uber den Bau der Blasenmole. Z Geburtshilfe Gynakol. 1898;32:67.
37. Tham KF, Ratnam SS. The classification of gestational trophoblastic disease: a critical review. Int J Gynaecol Obstet. 1998;60 Suppl 1:S39–49.
38. Hancock BW. Staging and classification of gestational trophoblastic disease. Best Pract Res Clin Obstet Gynaecol. 2003;17(6):869–83.
39. Shih IM, Kurman RJ. The pathology of intermediate trophoblastic tumors and tumor-like lesions. Int J Gynecol Pathol. 2001;20(1):31–47.
40. Buckley JD. The epidemiology of molar pregnancy and choriocarcinoma. Clin Obstet Gynecol. 1984; 27(1):153–9.
41. Genest DR. Partial hydatidiform mole: clinicopathological features, differential diagnosis, ploidy and molecular studies, and gold standards for diagnosis. Int J Gynecol Pathol. 2001;20(4):315–22.
42. Berkowitz RS, Goldstein DP. Clinical practice. Molar pregnancy. N Engl J Med. 2009;360(16):1639–45.
43. Wei PY, Ouyang PC. Trophoblastic diseases in Taiwan. A review of 157 cases in a 10 year period. Am J Obstet Gynecol. 1963;85:844–9.
44. Acosta-Sison H. Observations which may indicate the etiology of hydatidiform mole and explain its high incidence in the Philippines and Asiatic countries. Philipp J Surg Surg Spec. 1959;14:290–3.
45. Shang ER. A retrospective investigation on the incidence of hydatidiform mole in 20,548 fertile women. Zhonghua Yi Xue Za Zhi. 1982;62(5):282–5.
46. Song HZ, Wu PC. Hydatidiform mole in China: a preliminary survey of incidence on more than three million women. Bull World Health Organ. 1987;65(4): 507–11. PMCID: 2491037.
47. Nakano R, Sasaki K, Yamoto M, Hata H. Trophoblastic disease: analysis of 342 patients. Gynecol Obstet Invest. 1980;11(4):237–42.
48. Honda J, Yanagida K, Sato E, Sugawara N, Munakata S, Fukushima T. Incidence of hydatidiform mole and aging of mothers (author's transl). Nippon Sanka Fujinka Gakkai Zasshi. 1982;34(7):915–9.
49. Takeuchi S. Incidence of gestational trophoblastic disease by regional registration in Japan. Hum Reprod. 1987;2(8):729–34.
50. Hayashi K, Bracken MB, Freeman Jr DH, Hellenbrand K. Hydatidiform mole in the United States (1970-1977): a statistical and theoretical analysis. Am J Epidemiol. 1982;115(1):67–77.
51. Atrash HK, Hogue CJ, Grimes DA. Epidemiology of hydatidiform mole during early gestation. Am J Obstet Gynecol. 1986;154(4):906–9.
52. Hertig AT, Sheldon WH. Hydatidiform mole; a pathologico-clinical correlation of 200 cases. Am J Obstet Gynecol. 1947;53(1):1–36.
53. Slocumb JC, Lund CJ. Incidence of trophoblastic disease: increased rate in youngest age group. Am J Obstet Gynecol. 1969;104(3):421–3.
54. Douglas GW. The diagnosis and management of hydatidiform mole. Surg Clin North Am. 1957;37(2): 379–92.
55. Womack C, Elston CW. Hydatidiform mole in Nottingham: a 12-year retrospective epidemiological and morphological study. Placenta. 1985;6(2): 93–105.
56. Bagshawe KD, Dent J, Webb J. Hydatidiform mole in England and Wales 1973-83. Lancet. 1986;2(8508): 673–7.
57. Mazzanti P, La Vecchia C, Parazzini F, Bolis G. Frequency of hydatidiform mole in Lombardy, Northern Italy. Gynecol Oncol. 1986;24(3):337–42.
58. Franke HR, Risse EK, Kenemans P, Vooijs GP, Stolk JG. Epidemiologic features of hydatidiform mole in the Netherlands. Obstet Gynecol. 1983;62(5):613–6.
59. Flam F, Lundstrom-Lindstedt V, Rutqvist LE. Incidence of gestational trophoblastic disease in Stockholm County, 1975-1988. Eur J Epidemiol. 1992;8(2):173–7.
60. Ringertz N. Hydatidiform mole, invasive mole and choriocarcinoma in Sweden 1958-1965. Acta Obstet Gynecol Scand. 1970;49(2):195–203.
61. Stevenson AC, Dudgeon MY, Mc CH. Observations on the results of pregnancies in women resident in Belfast. II. Abortions, hydatidiform moles and ectopic pregnancies. Ann Hum Genet. 1959;23: 395–414.
62. Duff GB. Gestational trophoblastic disease in New Zealand, 1980-1986. Aust N Z J Obstet Gynaecol. 1989;29(2):139–42.

63. Olesnicky G, Long AR, Quinn MA, Pepperell RJ, Fortune DW, Kneale BL. Hydatidiform mole in Victoria: aetiology and natural history. Aust N Z J Obstet Gynaecol. 1985;25(1):1–7.
64. Paksoy N, Reich B. The occurrence of trophoblastic disease in Western Samoa. N Z Med J. 1989; 102(865):162–3.
65. Steigrad SJ. The incidence of neoplastic trophoblastic disease in Australia. Aust N Z J Obstet Gynaecol. 1969;9(2):100–2.
66. Beischer NA, Bettinger HF, Fortune DW, Pepperell R. Hydatidiform mole and its complications in the state of Victoria. J Obstet Gynaecol Br Commonw. 1970;77(3):263–76.
67. Ogunbode O. Benign hydatidiform mole in Ibadan, Nigeria. Int J Gynaecol Obstet. 1978;15(5):387–90.
68. Agboola A. Trophoblastic neoplasia in an african urban population. J Natl Med Assoc. 1979;71(10): 935–7. PMCID: 2537523.
69. Ayangade O. Gestational trophoblastic disease in Nigeria – A 10 year review. East Afr Med J. 1979; 56(6):278–82.
70. Diejomaoh FM, Omu AE, Okpere EE, Ezimokhai M, Tabowei O, Ajabor LN. The problems of management of gestational trophoblastic neoplasms at the University of Benin Teaching Hospital, Benin City, Nigeria. Adv Exp Med Biol. 1984;176:417–28.
71. Egwuatu VE, Ozumba BC. Observations on molar pregnancy in Enugu, Nigeria. Int J Gynaecol Obstet. 1989;29(3):219–25.
72. Rolon PA, Hochsztajn B, Llamosas F. Epidemiology of complete hydatidiform mole in Paraguay. J Reprod Med. 1990;35(1):15–8.
73. Rolon PA, de Lopez BH. Epidemiological aspects of hydatidiform mole in the Republic of Paraguay (South America). Br J Obstet Gynaecol. 1977;84(11): 862–4.
74. Aguero O, Kizer S, Pinedo G. Hydatidiform mole in concepcion palacios maternity hospital. Am J Obstet Gynecol. 1973;116(8):1117–20.
75. Martin BH, Kim JH. Changing face of gestational trophoblastic tumor. Int J Gynaecol Obstet. 1998;60 Suppl 1:S111–20.
76. Martin BH, Kim JH. Changes in gestational trophoblastic tumors over four decades. A Korean experience. J Reprod Med. 1998;43(1):60–8.
77. Kim SJ, Bae SN, Kim JH, Kim CJ, Han KT, Chung JK, et al. Epidemiology and time trends of gestational trophoblastic disease in Korea. Int J Gynaecol Obstet. 1998;60 Suppl 1:S33–8.
78. Hando T, Ohno M, Kurose T. Recent aspects of gestational trophoblastic disease in Japan. Int J Gynaecol Obstet. 1998;60 Suppl 1:S71–6.
79. Kanazawa K. Trophoblastic disease: twenty years' experience at Niigata University. Int J Gynaecol Obstet. 1998;60 Suppl 1:S97–103.
80. Wang JC, Wang PH, Yuan CC. Review of trophoblastic disease at Taipei Veterans General Hospital. Zhonghua Yi Xue Za Zhi (Taipei). 2000;63(5): 399–406.
81. Khashoggi TY. Prevalence of gestational trophoblastic disease. A single institution experience. Saudi Med J. 2003;24(12):1329–33.
82. Fukunaga M, Ushigome S, Endo Y. Incidence of hydatidiform mole in a Tokyo hospital: a 5-year (1989 to 1993) prospective, morphological, and flow cytometric study. Hum Pathol. 1995;26(7):758–64.
83. Poen HT, Djojopranoto M. The possible etiologic factors of hydatidiform mole and choriocarcinoma: preliminary report. Am J Obstet Gynecol. 1965;92:510–3.
84. Chan DP. Treatment of chorionepithelioma with methotrexate. Br Med J. 1962;2(5310):957–61. PMCID: 1926395.
85. Brewer JI, Gerbie AB. Early development of choriocarcinoma. In: Holland JF, Hreshchyshyn MM, editors. Choriocarcinoma: transactions of a conference of the international union against cancer. Berlin: Springer; 1967. p. 8.
86. Yen S, MacMahon B. Epidemiologic features of trophoblastic disease. Am J Obstet Gynecol. 1968; 101(1):126–32.
87. Aziz MF, Kampono N, Moegni EM, Sjamsuddin S, Barnas B, Samil RS. Epidemiology of gestational trophoblastic neoplasm at the Dr. Cipto Mangunkusumo Hospital, Jakarta, Indonesia. Adv Exp Med Biol. 1984;176:165–75.
88. Matalon M, Paz B, Modan M, Modan B. Malignant trophoblastic disorders. Epidemiologic aspects and relationship to hydatidiform mole. Am J Obstet Gynecol. 1972;112(1):101–6.
89. MacGregor C, Ontiveros E, Vargas E, Valenzuela S. Hydatidiform mole. Analysis of 145 patients. Obstet Gynecol. 1969;33(3):343–51.
90. Nielsen NH, Hansen JP. Trophoblastic tumors in Greenland. J Cancer Res Clin Oncol. 1979;95(2):177–86.
91. Teoh ES, Dawood MY, Ratnam SS. Epidemiology of hydatidiform mole in Singapore. Am J Obstet Gynecol. 1971;110(3):415–20.
92. Bandy LC, Clarke-Pearson DL, Hammond CB. Malignant potential of gestational trophoblastic disease at the extreme ages of reproductive life. Obstet Gynecol. 1984;64(3):395–9.
93. Sebire NJ, Foskett M, Fisher RA, Rees H, Seckl M, Newlands E. Risk of partial and complete hydatidiform molar pregnancy in relation to maternal age. BJOG. 2002;109(1):99–102.
94. Bayatpour MRJ. Gestational trophoblastic disease among adolescents. Adolesc and Pediatr Gynecol. 1993;6:3.
95. La Vecchia C, Franceschi S, Parazzini F, Fasoli M, Decarli A, Gallus G, et al. Risk factors for gestational trophoblastic disease in Italy. Am J Epidemiol. 1985;121(3):457–64.
96. Maudsley RF, Robertson EM. Hydatidiform mole in a woman over 52 years old. Report of a case. Obstet Gynecol. 1965;26(4):542–3.
97. Di Cintio E, Parazzini F, Rosa C, Chatenoud L, Benzi G. The epidemiology of gestational trophoblastic disease. Gen Diagn Pathol. 1997;143(2–3): 103–8.

98. Garcia M, Romaguera RL, Romaguera C. A hydatidiform mole in a postmenopausal woman. A case report and review of the literature. Arch Pathol Lab Med. 2004;128(9):1039–42.
99. Matalon M, Modan B. Epidemiologic aspects of hydatidiform mole in Israel. Am J Obstet Gynecol. 1972;112(1):107–12.
100. Sand PK, Lurain JR, Brewer JI. Repeat gestational trophoblastic disease. Obstet Gynecol. 1984;63(2):140–4.
101. Matsui H, Iitsuka Y, Suzuka K, Seki K, Sekiya S. Subsequent pregnancy outcome in patients with spontaneous resolution of HCG after evacuation of hydatidiform mole: comparison between complete and partial mole. Hum Reprod. 2001;16(6):1274–7.
102. Bagshawe KD. Recent observations related to the chemotherapy and immunology of gestational choriocarcinoma. Adv Cancer Res. 1973;18:231–63.
103. Cheah PL, Looi LM, Sivanesaratnam V. Hydatidiform molar pregnancy in malaysian women: a histopathological study from the University Hospital, Kuala Lumpur. Malays J Pathol. 1993;15(1):59–63.
104. Matsuura J, Chiu D, Jacobs PA, Szulman AE. Complete hydatidiform mole in Hawaii: an epidemiological study. Genet Epidemiol. 1984;1(3):271–84.
105. Natoli WJ, Rashad MN. Hawaiian moles. Am J Roentgenol Radium Ther Nucl Med. 1972;114(1):142–4.
106. McCorriston CC. Racial incidence of hydatidiform mole. A study in a contained polyracial community. Am J Obstet Gynecol. 1968;101(3):377–82.
107. Jacobs PA, Hunt PA, Matsuura JS, Wilson CC, Szulman AE. Complete and partial hydatidiform mole in Hawaii: cytogenetics, morphology and epidemiology. Br J Obstet Gynaecol. 1982;89(4):258–66.
108. Gul T, Yilmazturk A, Erden AC. A review of trophoblastic diseases at the medical school of Dicle University. Eur J Obstet Gynecol Reprod Biol. 1997;74(1):37–40.
109. Steigrad SJ. Epidemiology of gestational trophoblastic diseases. Best Pract Res Clin Obstet Gynaecol. 2003;17(6):837–47.
110. Teoh ES, Dawood MY, Ratnam SS. Observations on choriocarcinoma in Singapore. Obstet Gynecol. 1972;40(4):519–24.
111. Martin PM. High frequency of hydatidiform mole in native Alaskans. Int J Gynaecol Obstet. 1978;15(5):395–6.
112. Slim R, Mehio A. The genetics of hydatidiform moles: new lights on an ancient disease. Clin Genet. 2007;71(1):25–34.
113. The Joint Project for Study of Choriocarcinoma and Hydatidiform Mole in Asia. Geographic variation in the occurrence of hydatidiform mole and choriocarcinoma. Ann N Y Acad Sci. 1959;80:178–95.
114. Pour-Reza M, Agheli N, Vaghefi SB. Serum creatinine, urea, and protein level changes in hydatidiform mole. JAMA. 1974;230(4):580–1.
115. Berkowitz RS, Cramer DW, Bernstein MR, Cassells S, Driscoll SG, Goldstein DP. Risk factors for complete molar pregnancy from a case-control study. Am J Obstet Gynecol. 1985;152(8):1016–20.
116. Parazzini F, La Vecchia C, Mangili G, Caminiti C, Negri E, Cecchetti G, et al. Dietary factors and risk of trophoblastic disease. Am J Obstet Gynecol. 1988;158(1):93–9.
117. Bracken MB. Incidence of hydatidiform mole. Am J Obstet Gynecol. 1988;158(4):1016–7.
118. Palmer JR, Driscoll SG, Rosenberg L, Berkowitz RS, Lurain JR, Soper J, et al. Oral contraceptive use and risk of gestational trophoblastic tumors. J Natl Cancer Inst. 1999;91(7):635–40.
119. Brinton LA, Wu BZ, Wang W, Ershow AG, Song HZ, Li JY, et al. Gestational trophoblastic disease: a case-control study from the People's Republic of China. Am J Obstet Gynecol. 1989;161(1):121–7.
120. Baltazar JC. Epidemiological features of choriocarcinoma. Bull World Health Organ. 1976;54(5):523–32. PMCID: 2366480
121. Curry SL, Schlaerth JB, Kohorn EI, Boyce JB, Gore H, Twiggs LB, et al. Hormonal contraception and trophoblastic sequelae after hydatidiform mole (a gynecologic oncology group study). Am J Obstet Gynecol. 1989;160(4):805–9; discussion 9–11.
122. Deicas RE, Miller DS, Rademaker AW, Lurain JR. The role of contraception in the development of postmolar gestational trophoblastic tumor. Obstet Gynecol. 1991;78(2):221–6.
123. Morrow P, Nakamura R, Schlaerth J, Gaddis Jr O, Eddy G. The influence of oral contraceptives on the postmolar human chorionic gonadotropin regression curve. Am J Obstet Gynecol. 1985;151(7):906–14.
124. Rosenberg L, Palmer JR, Shapiro S. Gestational trophoblastic disease and use of oral contraceptives. Am J Obstet Gynecol. 1989;161(4):1087–8.
125. Palmer JR. Advances in the epidemiology of gestational trophoblastic disease. J Reprod Med. 1994;39(3):155–62.
126. Matalon M, Modan M, Paz B, Modan B. Trophoblastic disorders in Istael. Harefuah. 1972;83(12):566–8.
127. Bracken MB, Brinton LA, Hayashi K. Epidemiology of hydatidiform mole and choriocarcinoma. Epidemiol Rev. 1984;6:52–75.
128. Fukunaga M, Katabuchi H, Nagasaka T, Mikami Y, Minamiguchi S, Lage JM. Interobserver and intraobserver variability in the diagnosis of hydatidiform mole. Am J Surg Pathol. 2005;29(7):942–7.
129. Soper JT. Gestational trophoblastic disease. Obstet Gynecol. 2006;108(1):176–87.
130. Kohorn EI. The new FIGO 2000 staging and risk factor scoring system for gestational trophoblastic disease: description and critical assessment. Int J Gynecol Cancer. 2001;11(1):73–7.
131. Ngan HY, Bender H, Benedet JL, Jones H, Montruccoli GC, Pecorelli S. Gestational trophoblastic neoplasia, FIGO 2000 staging and classification. Int J Gynaecol Obstet. 2003;83 Suppl 1:175–7.
132. Acosta-Sison H. Trophoblastic or chorionic tumours as observed in the Philippines. In: Hollander JF,

Hreshchyshyn MM, editors. Choriocarcinoma: transactions of a conference of the international union against cancer. Berlin: Springer; 1967.

133. Chun D, Braga C, Chow C, Lok L. Clinical observations on some aspects of hydatidiform moles. J Obstet Gynaecol Br Commonw. 1964;71:180–4.
134. Chan DP. Chorionepithelioma: a study of 41 cases. Br Med J. 1962;2(5310):953–7. PMCID: 1926430.
135. King G. Hydatidiform mole and chorion-epithelioma–the problem of the borderline case. Proc R Soc Med. 1956;49(7):381–90. PMCID: 1889150.
136. Das PC. Hydatidiform mole: a statistical and clinical study. J Obstet Gynaecol. 1938;45:6.
137. Marquez-Monter H, de la Vega GA, de la Vega GA, Robles M, Robles M, Bolio-Cicero A, et al. Epidemiology and pathology of hydatidiform mole in the general hospital in Mexico. Am J Obstet Gynecol. 1963;85:8.
138. Lara FM, Alvarado AM, Candelaria M, Arce CS. Gestational trophoblastic disease. Experience at National Institute of Cancerology. Ginecol Obstet Mex. 2005;73(6):308–14.
139. Javey H, Sajadi H. Hydatidiform mole in southern Iran: a statistical survey of 113 cases. Int J Gynaecol Obstet. 1978;15(5):390–5.
140. Ishizuka N. Studies on trophoblastic neoplasia. Gann Monogr. 1976;18:14.
141. Mills W. Chorion-Carcinoma in the Midlands. Clin Radiol. 1964;15:260–2.
142. Kolstad P, Hognestad J. Trophoblastic tumours in Norway. Acta Obstet Gynecol Scand. 1965;44:80–8.
143. Leighton PC. Trophoblastic disease in Uganda. Am J Obstet Gynecol. 1973;117(3):341–4.

Developmental Biology of the Placenta

2

Pei Hui

Keywords
Placental development • Implantation • Trophoblastic cells • Genomic imprinting and placental evolution

Introduction

The placenta is a transient organ consisting of cell types that are unique to eutherian mammals. It is fetal in origin and shares just half of the genome with that of the maternal uterus. Although existing for only 9 months, there are constant morphological and biological fluctuations within the placenta proper and at the interface between the placenta and the maternal endomyometrium. It is at the latter interface that unique fetomaternal tissue remodeling, hormonal regulation, and immunological interactions are regulated in such a delicate balance, so that appropriate maternal support can be delivered to the embryo and the mother does not elicit an immunologic rejection response to the growing gestational structures. Proliferative disorders including tumors arising from the placenta have distinct genetic, biological, and immunological properties that are drastically different from those of the maternal neoplasms. Recent findings of genomic imprinting including imprinted X chromosome inactivation in the placenta and its implication in the pathogenesis of gestational trophoblastic diseases raise some fundamental questions in mammalian biology and oncology.

P. Hui, MD, PhD (✉)
Department of Pathology, Yale University
School of Medicine, 310 Cedar Street, 254B New Haven, CT 06520-8023, USA
e-mail: pei.hui@yale.edu

Placenta Formation

Upon fertilization, the ovum rapidly grows within the fallopian tube into a 16-cell morula and then a 32-cell blastocyst, reaching the endometrial cavity by day 3 after fertilization. The blastocyst is covered by the zona pellucida that acts as a protective chaperone during the transportation from the fallopian tube to the uterine cavity. The blastocyst then loses its covering zona pellucida and implants into the receptive gestational endometrium by day 7 [1]. During the implantation, the outer cell layer of the blastocyst differentiates into the trophoblastic shell, and the inner cell mass ultimately develops into the embryo (Fig. 2.1) [2, 3]. The trophoblastic shell grows circumferentially, and peripheral trophoblasts invade the stroma of endometrium at the implantation site. Then, the trophoblasts closer to the

P. Hui (ed.), *Gestational Trophoblastic Disease: Diagnostic and Molecular Genetic Pathology*, Current Clinical Pathology, DOI 10.1007/978-1-61779-394-3_2,

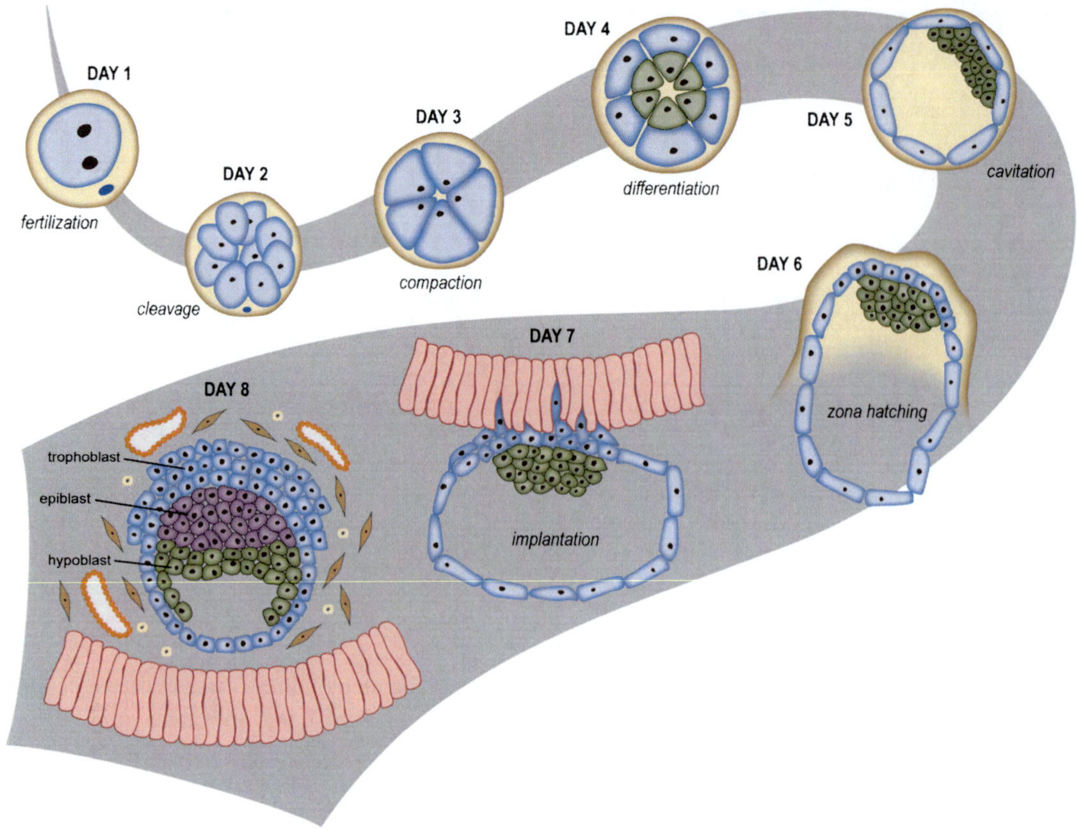

Fig. 2.1 Schematic presentation of the early phases of embryogenesis and implantation

endometrium proliferate and differentiate into two layers: the inner cytotrophoblastic layer and the outer overlying syncytiotrophoblastic layer. Cytotrophoblast likely possesses the stem cell properties in the placenta and is mitotically active. Syncytiotrophoblast is multinucleated cell forming a continuous syncytium that wraps the entire surface of the growing placenta. It forms as a result of fusion of the differentiated cytotrophoblast, a process that continues throughout placental development. The syncytiotrophoblastic syncytium thereby contributes to the barrier function of the placenta.

By day 13, lacunae form within the previllous trophoblast (Fig. 2.2). Trophoblastic columns are formed with blood-filled spaces in between and covered by a syncytiotrophoblastic outer layer and an immature cytotrophoblastic inner layer. Thereafter, extraembryonic mesenchyme invades trophoblastic columns leading to the appearance of primary chorionic villi along with the formation of fetal vascular channels (Fig. 2.3), which eventually connect with each other and with channels of the body stalk/allantois to establish fetoplacental circulation. Early formed chorionic villi appear primitive with smaller sizes, cellular myxoid stroma, and marked proliferative activities (Fig. 2.4). Solid trophoblastic columns remain at the periphery of the stem villi anchoring them to the basal plate (Fig. 2.5) to eventually form a complete shell that continues to grow and expand. At the implantation site of the developing placenta, a dense stratum of fibroid material forms as "Nitabuch's fibrin" to separate the gestational sac from the underlying decidua (Fig. 2.6a and b). Through the Nitabuch's fibrin, the so-called intermediate trophoblast invades into the underlying endometrium and its vasculatures (Fig. 2.6c). Their invasion of the endometrial spiral arteries leads to the release of maternal

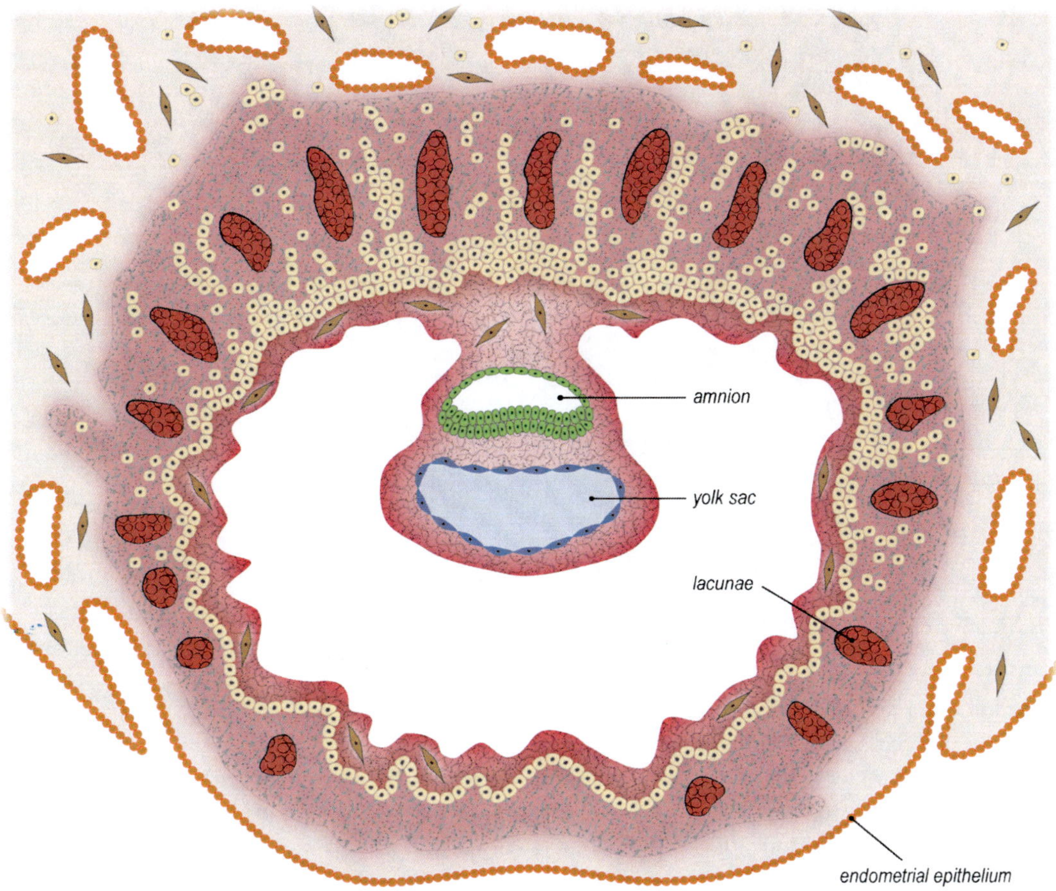

Fig. 2.2 Schematic presentation of implantation at the previllous stage

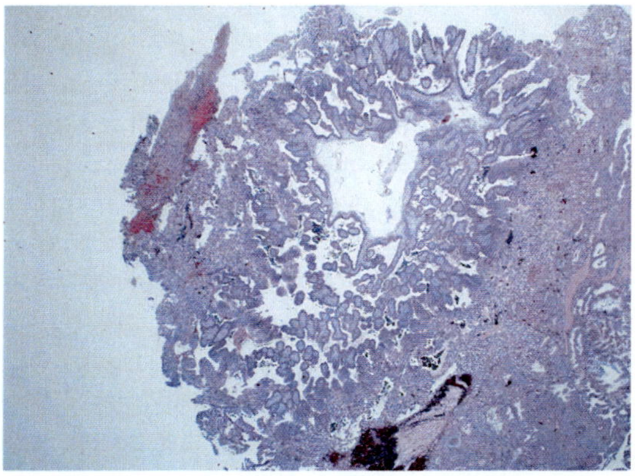

Fig. 2.3 Early villous stage of placental development. Implantation and placental formation with extraembryonic mesenchymal invasion into trophoblastic columns, forming primitive chorionic villi

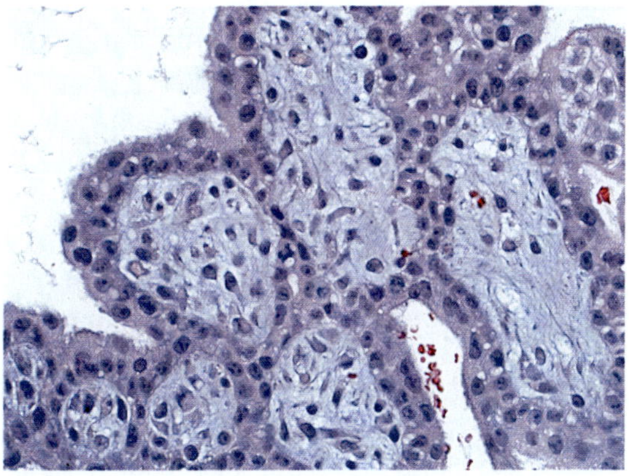

Fig. 2.4 Primitive chorionic villi. There is a presence of bilayer of trophoblastic cells covering the surface of villi: cytotrophoblast as an inner layer and syncytiotrophoblast as an outer layer. The villous stroma of these early formed villi demonstrates cellular and myxoid appearance with primitive stromal cells

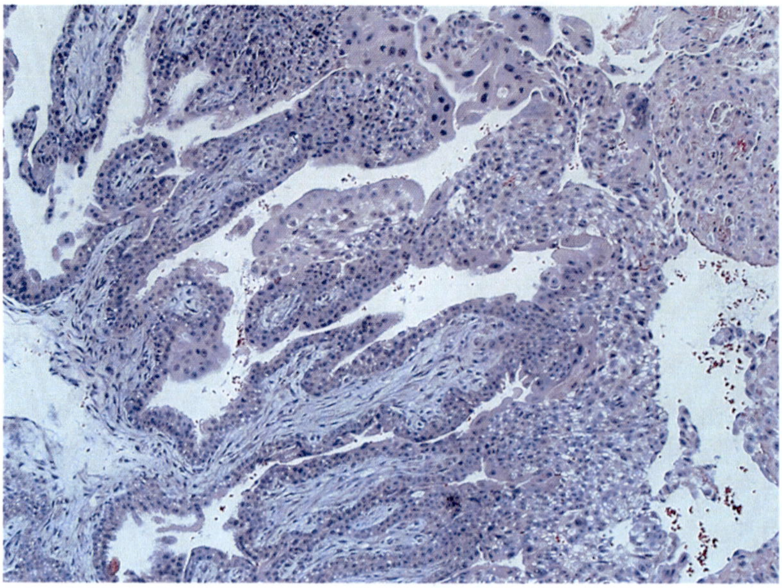

Fig. 2.5 Trophoblastic column at the tips of anchoring chorionic villi

blood into the previllous trophoblastic lacunae to form the precursor of intervillous spaces. However, the ultimate fetal–maternal circulation is not established until the 12th week of gestation. As the chorion protrudes into the endometrial cavity, the villi toward the uterine surface undergo regression to form chorionic laeve or fetal membranes with eventual obliteration of the uterine cavity. Meanwhile, the villi on the embryonic site continue to proliferate and mature with additional septa formation and structural modification to form the ultimate placenta.

In human, the term placenta has a disc shape with an average diameter of 22 cm and a thickness of 2–2.5 cm at the center. At this point, the placenta typically weighs approximately 550 g and has a dark reddish-blue color. It is linked to the fetus by an umbilical cord of approximately 55–60 cm in length and containing two arteries and one vein. The umbilical cord inserts into the chorionic plate generally in an eccentric fashion. Vessels branch out over the surface of the placenta and divide further to form a network visible on the chorionic plate. On the maternal side, the chorionic villous structures are partitioned into 15 to 20 lobulated cotyledons, which are in direct contact with the maternal decidua.

Stages of Implantation

Predecidualization and Decidualization of the Endometrium

The hormonally regulated cyclic changes of the endometrium are divided into proliferative, secretory, and menstrual phases. The proliferative phase involves both endometrial glands and stroma, corresponding to the level of estrogen production by the growing follicle in the ovary. The transition between the proliferative to the secretory phase marks the ovulation of the ovary occurring at day 14 of a 28-day menstrual cycle. During the secretory phase, the endometrium increases in its glandular complexity, secretion, vascularization, and stromal edema, reaching its peak at day 23. Endometrial predecidualization occurs around day 25 marked by stromal cell changes including increased cell size, cytoplasmic eosinophilia, rounding of the nuclei, and overall confluent epithelioid appearance. During the so-called implantation window, the endometrial epithelial cells are characterized by the presence of apical cytoplasmic projections.

The blastocyst spends approximately 3 days in the uterine cavity before its implantation into the

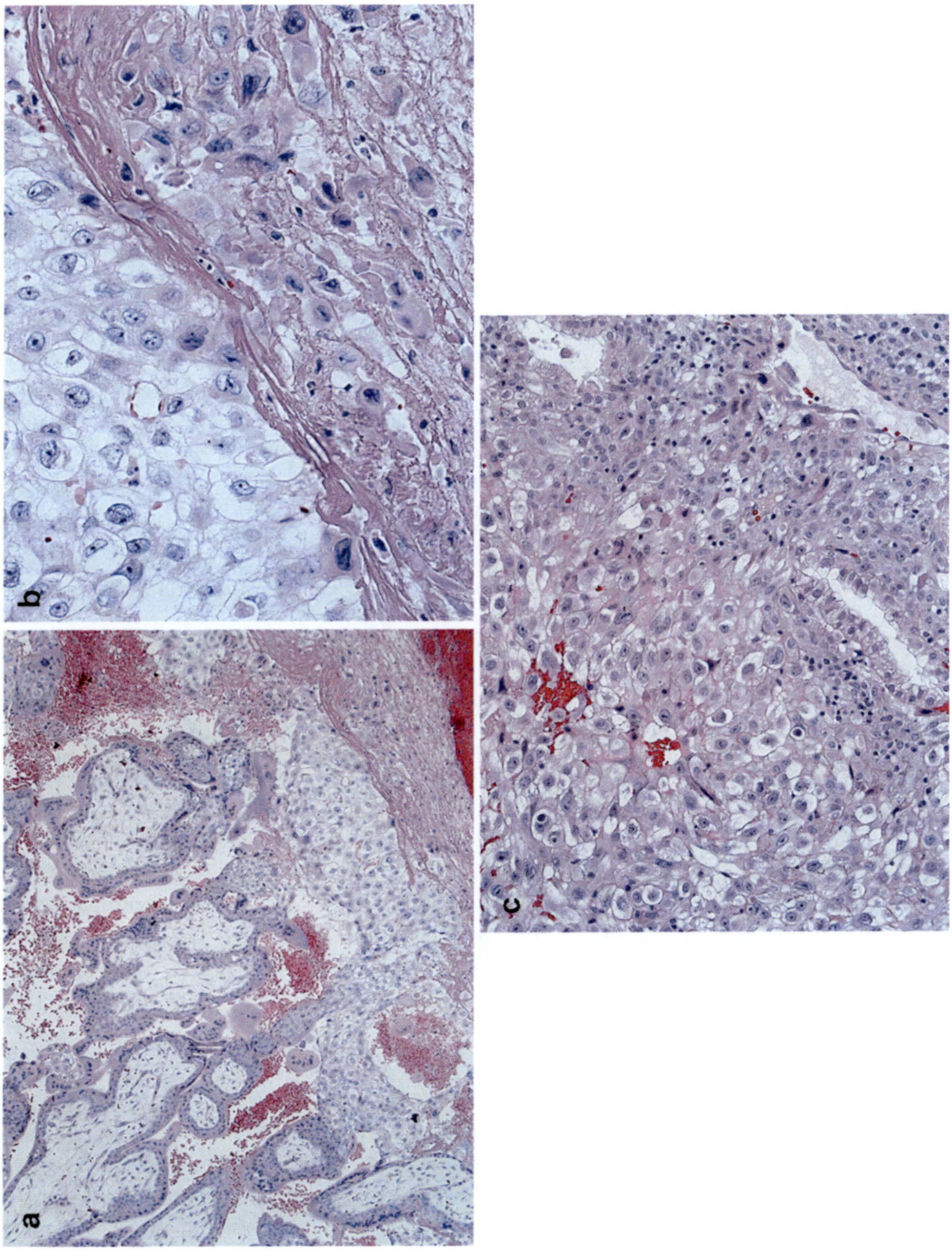

Fig. 2.6 Early placenta formation. At the implantation site, a dense stratum of eosinophilic fibrin material forms to separate the gestational sac from the underlying endometrial decidua as Nitabuch's fibrin (**a** and **b**). Intermediate trophoblastic cells at the implantation site invade the underlying decidualized endometrium (**c**)

receptive endometrium. In addition to iron and vitamins, the endometrium secretes several steroid-dependent proteins [4, 5] and cholesterol [6] that are important for blastocyst growth and implantation. Implantation is further facilitated by synthesis of matrix substances [7, 8], adhesion molecules [9–11], and surface receptors for the matrix substances. Decidua capsularis grows over the blastocyst, enclosing it within the endometrium. After implantation, the decidua and endometrial glandular secretions remain during the first trimester, but their function as a surrounding tissue is replaced by the developing placenta. Some glands remain hypersecretory and manifest as Arias-Stella phenomenon under the microscope throughout the pregnancy [12, 13].

Phases of Implantation

Implantation is initiated when the blastocyst comes to contact with the uterine endometrial cavity and follows a highly orchestrated process involving extensive cell–cell interactions between blastocyst and endometrium. Highly coordinated expression and secretion of growth factors, cytokines, and adhesion molecules at both local and systemic levels are essential for implantation [14–19]. Three stages of implantation have been proposed [3, 20, 21].

Stage 1: Apposition

The human placenta begins to develop once the blastocyst establishes contact (apposition) with the receptive endometrial mucosa [21]. Around day 5 after fertilization, the blastocyst escapes or hatches from its outer zona pellucida. Protein enzymes (hatching enzymes) in the fluid of the endometrial cavity are responsible for the dissolution of the zona pellucida. The hatching enzymes of vertebrates have been identified in a variety of organisms ranging from fish to birds to mammals [19, 22–24]. It is generally believed that serine proteases/metalloproteases are responsible for the process of hatching [25, 26]. It has been shown that in bovine embryos, one important enzyme is plasmin, which is the product of blastocyst factor-mediated conversion of its precursor, plasminogen [23, 27]. Two serine protease (ISP1 and 2) genes that are expressed during the implantation period are involved in the dissolution of the zona pellucida. The ISP1 gene encodes the embryo-derived enzyme strypsin, which is necessary for blastocyst hatching in vitro and initiation of invasion. ISP2 is a related tryptase but is expressed in endometrial glands during the peri-implantation period [25, 26]. Two hatching enzyme genes identified in *Oryzias latipes*, HCE and LCE, were found to be able to cleave the homologous glycoproteins present in the zona pellucida [22]. Without zona pellucida, the blastocyst physically contacts the underlying decidua of the endometrium. Although the contact may occur at any region of the exposed blastocyst, the inner cell mass appears to guide itself during the implantation window, to the apposition site for ultimate attachment through the preferential expression of EGF receptor of the inner cell mass and the trophoblast only at the embryonic pole of blastocyst [21, 28, 29].

Stage 2: Attachment/Adhesion

Implantation occurs by the attachment of cytoplasmic membrane of the blastocyst trophectoderm to the apical surface of endometrial epithelial cells. Preimplantation embryos prepare the endometrium for reception by secreting chorionic gonadotropin (CG). CG modulates the endometrial environment and stimulates various trophoblastic activities [30, 31]. Apical adhesiveness between endometrial epithelium and microvilli on the surface of the outermost trophoblasts apparently exists for only a short, specific period. Such a receptive state exits within a narrow window or "window of implantation" for less than 3 days in human, after which the endometrium becomes resistant to implantation [32, 33]. A cross communication via various glycoproteins/adhesion molecules between the implantation-competent blastocyst and the uterine luminal epithelial/stromal cells are all essential to the process of implantation [18, 34]. This cross communication involves numerous signaling pathways, such as integrin, trophinin–tastin, progranulin, ezrin/radixin/moesin (ERM) proteins, and ERM-associated cytoskeletal cross-linker proteins CD43, CD44, ICAM-1, and ICAM-2, interferon gamma-induced protein 10 kDa, PECAM-1 (CD31), and Fas ligand [9, 18, 35–39]. The blastocyst instructs the endometrium to adapt further to its presence, through likely changes in the cytoskeleton of decidual cells [36, 40]. This, in turn, leads to dissolution of decidual cells from their connection to the underlying basal lamina, which enables the blastocyst to perform the subsequent invasion. This communication is accomplished by receptor–ligand interactions. Both the integrin–matrix [39] and the ligand–receptor system involved in adhesion are mediated by proteoglycan receptors found on the surface of the decidua [41, 42]. Their corresponding ligands, the proteoglycans, are found around the trophoblastic cells of blastocyst. Both are expressed only during the implantation window. Trophoblasts were also found to express integrins, L-selection, and other cell surface proteins [43–45]. Genes that regulate immune response may also play a significant role through upregulating decay accelerating factor (DAF), IL-15, interferon regulatory factor-1, and others [46].

Stage 3: Invasion

Trophoblasts at the implantation site invade the decidualized endometrium [47]. Invasion continues with syncytiotrophoblast reaching the basal membrane beneath the surface endometrial epithelium, penetrating it and further invading into the uterine stroma. Finally, the whole embryo is embedded in the endometrium. Eventually, the syncytiotrophoblasts come into contact with maternal blood and initiate the formation of the placenta marked by the appearance of chorionic villi. It is possible that oxygen tension dictates the direction of invasion, thereby regulating placental growth and cellular architecture [48]. An oxygen tension is present in the placental bed with increase in O_2 tension toward the maternal side [49]. The role of O_2 tension has been implied to negatively regulate PIGF gene expression [50].

In addition to maternal systemic hormonal factors that stimulate trophoblastic invasion [31], local tissue remodeling molecules produced by the trophoblasts degrade the extracellular matrix of the endometrium and thereby facilitate invasion. These remodeling molecules are serine endopeptidases and metalloproteinases, including collagenases, gelatinases, and stromelysins [51–54]. Cell adhesion molecules are degraded by syncytiotrophoblast secretion of TNF-alpha, leading to an inhibition of expression of cadherins and beta-catenin. Cadherins are cell adhesion molecules and beta-catenin helps to anchor them to the cell membrane. Inhibited expression of these molecules thus loosens the connection between decidual cells, permitting the syncytiotrophoblasts and the whole embryo to invade into the endometrium. It is important that there is a simultaneous synthesis of matrix metalloproteinases (MMPs) and their specific tissue inhibitors (TIMPs) in both human trophoblast and decidual membranes. This suggests that their balanced expression is crucial for rapid matrix remodeling and controlled blastocyst invasion during early pregnancy [54–56]. IGFBP-1 and IFG-II promote migration of the trophoblasts through paracrine and/or autocrine fashion, likely by the activation of MAPK [57–59]. Coordinated expression of certain cellular receptors for various growth factors of endometrium and their binding proteins in trophoblasts play an important role in guiding appropriate invasion and/or confinement of the invasion. Mel-CAM, an adhesion molecule produced by implantation site intermediate trophoblasts, interacts with its ligand on the myometrial smooth muscle. This appears to control the extent of trophoblast invasion [60]. TGF-beta has been shown to negatively regulate the invasion [61]. MTOR mediates human trophoblast invasion through the regulation of matrix-remodeling enzymes and is associated with serine phosphorylation of STAT3 [62].

Syncytiotrophoblasts do not express any HLA suggesting their ability to escape from the maternal immune surveillance. Differentiated intermediate trophoblasts express HLA-G, a trophoblast-specific HLA class I molecule that is likely important in avoiding rejection of the conceptus by the maternal immune system [63–65]. Cytotrophoblasts produce the immunoinhibitory cytokine, IL-10. In normal pregnancy, invading intermediate trophoblasts differentiate to mimic the cell surface properties of vascular cells, a process called pseudovasculogenesis. This process involves various adhesion molecules. Intermediate trophoblasts also produce many chemokines or regulatory proteins. Gene expression profiling revealed upregulation and downregulation of various cytokines, chemokines, and angiogenic factors of endometrial stromal cells in response to secretions of trophoblasts [66]. Downregulation of E-cadherin is important for the migration of intermediate trophoblasts at the placentomaternal interface [67–69]. VE-cadherin, a major endothelial-specific molecule, is upregulated in intermediate trophoblasts that invade the distal columns of anchoring villi [70]. Integrin β3, an angiogenesis-related endothelial adhesion molecule, is upregulated by the invasive and endovascular intermediate trophoblasts [71–73]. Modulation of NK cells and other immune cells may play also important roles in the fetoplacental tolerance and implantation [74–76].

Placental Trophoblastic Cells

Trophoblasts are functional cells of the placenta and play an important role in embryonic implantation and placenta–maternal interactions during pregnancy. Once the primitive chorionic villi are formed and throughout the pregnancy, distinct subtypes of the trophoblast can be recognized (Fig. 2.7). Chorionic villi are composed of mesenchymal and trophoblastic components. The mesenchyme of chorionic villi contains stromal cells and blood vessels that are directly connected to the fetal circulation via the umbilical cord. The surface of chorionic villi is covered by two layers of trophoblast: an inner mononuclear cytotrophoblast and an outer multinucleated syncytiotrophoblast. In addition, cytotrophoblast at the apices of anchoring villi can differentiate into another type of trophoblast called the extravillous intermediate trophoblast. Extravillous trophoblast grows out

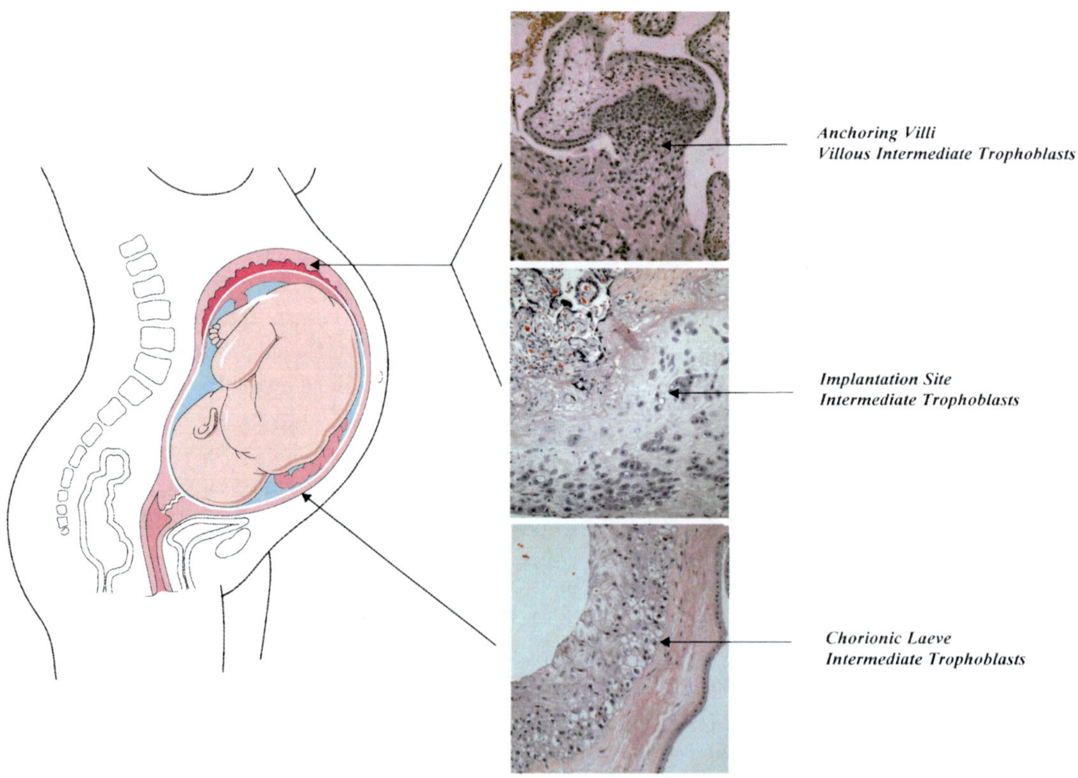

Fig. 2.7 Classification of various extraembryonic trophoblastic cells in relation to their anatomic locations

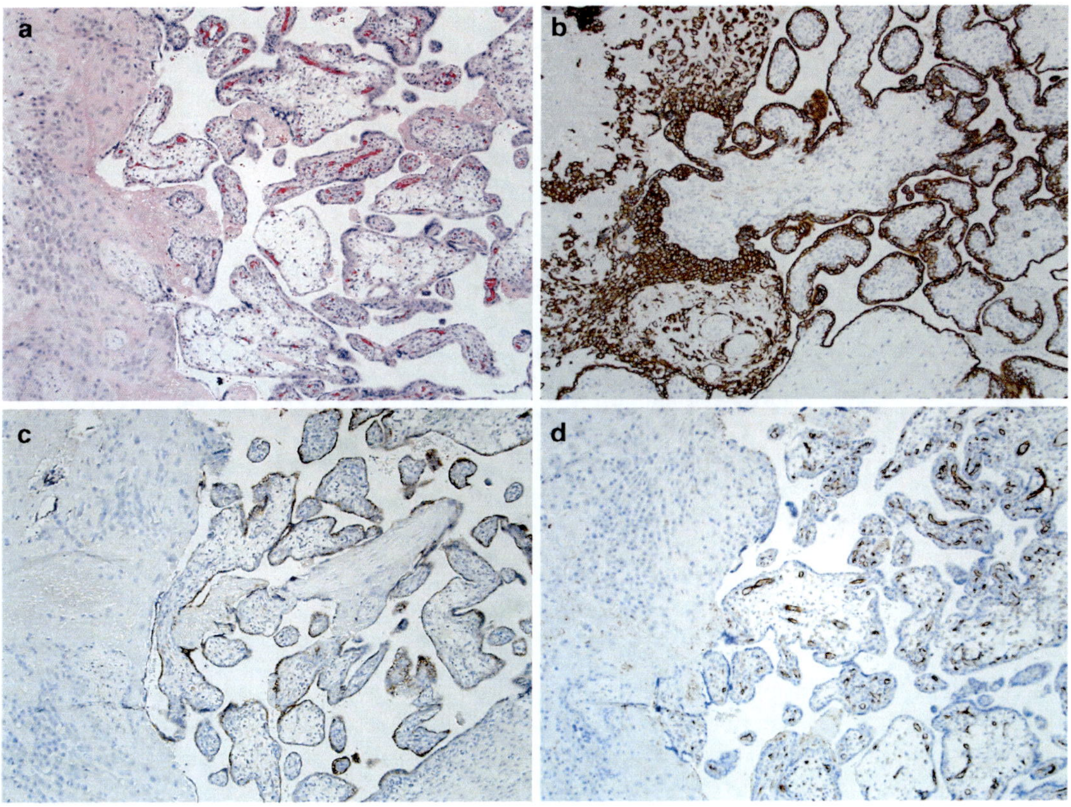

Fig. 2.8 Immunohistochemical profiles of villous trophoblasts. (**a**) H&E. stain of chorionic villi attaching to the maternal decidua. (**b**) Strong cytokeratin (AE1/3) expression in villous trophoblasts (cytotrophoblast and syncytiotrophoblast), villous intermediate trophoblast, and implantation intermediate trophoblast. (**c**) HCG expression is only present in the syncytiotrophoblast. (**d**) CD31 immunohistochemical stain demonstrates capillary vasculatures with the chorionic villous stroma

from the anchoring villi and invades into the decidualized endometrium (Fig. 2.6c, b). This process is crucial for physically attaching the placenta to the and maternal vascular remodeling to provide an adequate blood supply to the rapidly growing fetus. The implantation trophoblasts may even replace the endothelial cells of maternal vessels into wide open structures that are independent of maternal vasoconstriction. As a result, the fetus receives a steady supply of blood.

Morphological features of various trophoblasts have been well characterized [77, 78]. Cytotrophoblastic cells are a primitive cell type and likely have a stem cell profile in the placenta. They differentiate into functional syncytiotrophoblasts and intermediate trophoblasts [77]. Cytotrophoblasts are present at the inner layer of the chorionic villous epithelium, interior to the syncytiotrophoblasts (Fig. 2.8a). They are mitotically active, medium-sized cells in polygonal to oval shapes. However, they are not hormonally functional. Syncytiotrophoblasts are fully matured cells that are in direct contact with the maternal circulation and produce most of the placental hormones. They can be found to produce hCG and hPL as early as 12 days of gestation (Fig. 2.8c). Syncytiotrophoblasts are multinuclear with a large amount of cytoplasm and are located external to the cytotrophoblasts on the surface of the chorionic villi (Fig. 2.8a). They do not have detectable proliferative activity or mitoses and are formed likely by fusion of differentiated

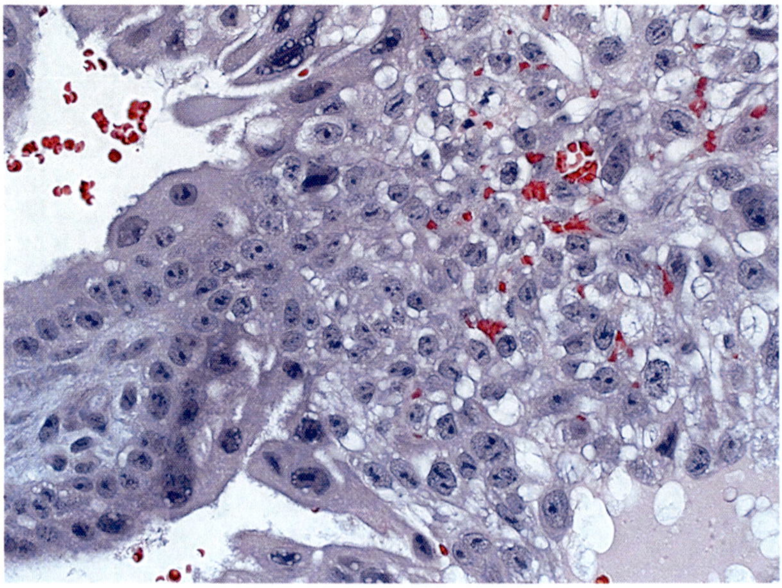

Fig. 2.9 Villous intermediate trophoblast at the tip of an anchoring villus

trophoblasts mediated by the function of syncytin, a captive retroviral envelope protein involved in cell fusion [79]. Intermediate trophoblasts are of various subtypes and have been traditionally referred to as extravillous trophoblast, X-cells, or interstitial cytotrophoblasts. These are generally large mononuclear cells with abundant cytoplasm and may exsit as individual cells or in sheets. Three types of intermediate trophoblasts have been proposed [78, 80, 81]: villous intermediate trophoblast, implantation site intermediate trophoblast, and chorionic laeve intermediate trophoblast (Fig. 2.7).

Arising from cytotrophoblasts at the anchoring villi and forming the trophoblastic columns, villous intermediate trophoblastic cells are mononuclear and larger than cytotrophoblasts. They are relatively uniform with a distinct cell border and abundant eosinophilic to clear cytoplasm (Fig. 2.9). From the base of the trophoblastic column, a subset of intermediate trophoblasts (implantation site intermediate trophoblasts) infiltrate into the placental bed and interact with the maternal endometrium with the main function of establishing fetal–maternal circulation (Fig. 2.6). Present as individual cells or in sheets at the implantation site, implantation site intermediate trophoblasts are large cells ranging from 15 to 30 μm with pleomorphic and hyperchromatic nuclei, convoluted nuclear membranes, and pseudonuclear inclusions [82]. They are generally polygonal, but spindle forms can be found infiltrating the myometrium (Fig. 2.10). While most are mononucleate [82], multinucleation of the cells is common (Fig. 2.10). The growth pattern of implantation site intermediate trophoblast is infiltrative. One characteristic feature of these cells is the replacement of smooth muscle component of the maternal vasculature while keeping the overall vascular structure open for blood circulation (Fig. 2.11). Occasionally, the endothelial cells may be replaced as well. Chorionic laeve intermediate trophoblasts are found within the chorion membrane (chorion frondosum). They are uniformly medium-sized cells with eosinophilic or clear cytoplasm, forming a monolayer in the chorion laeve (Fig. 2.12). Table 2.1 summarizes common immunohistochemical marker expression in various placental trophoblasts [60, 69, 78, 80, 83–85].

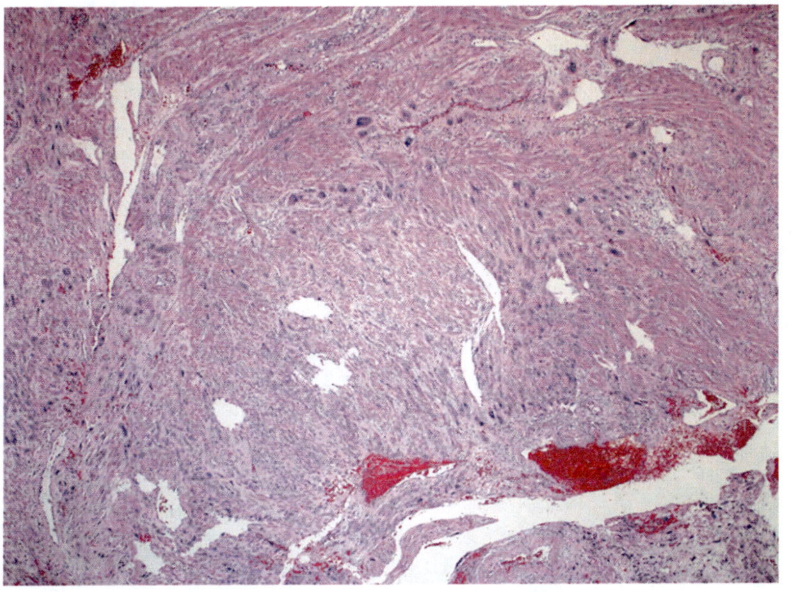

Fig. 2.10 Implantation site intermediate trophoblast involving myometrium

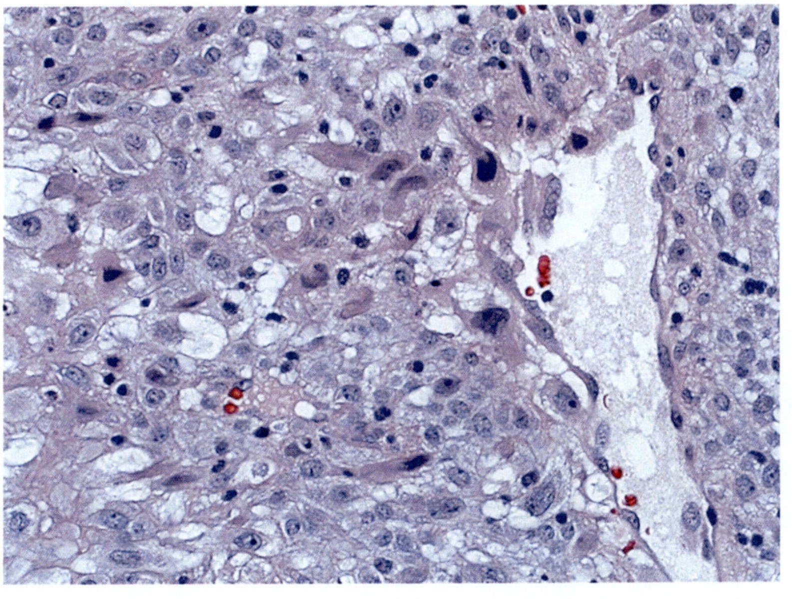

Fig. 2.11 Implantation site intermediate trophoblast replacing structures of maternal vasculature

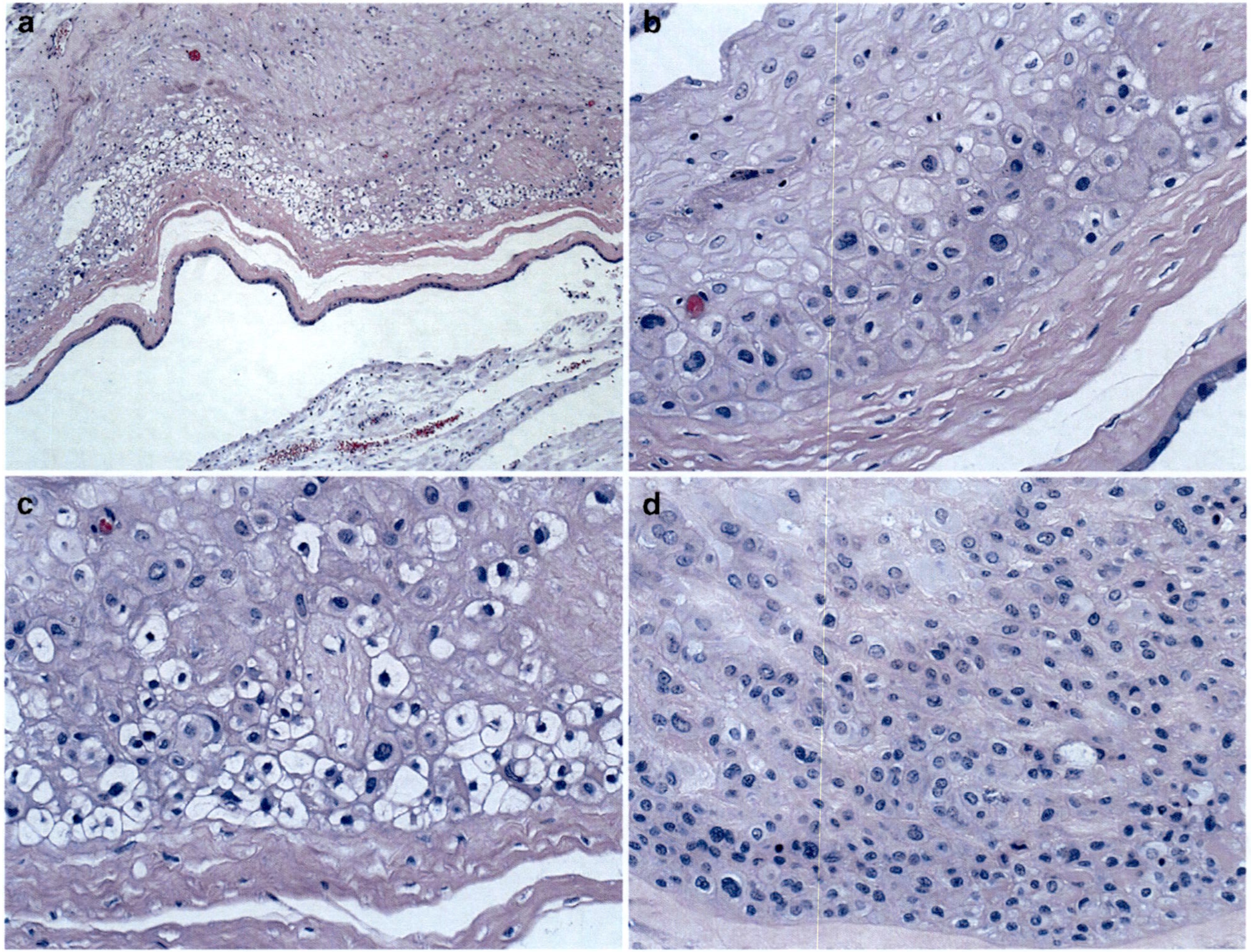

Fig. 2.12 Chorionic laeve intermediate trophoblast. A layer of intermediate trophoblast is present in the chorionic laeve in the form of continuous sheet between the fetal membrane and endometrial decidua (**a**). They are medium in size and with abundant amphophilic (**b**) or clear cytoplasm (**c**), sometimes even forming cords and nests with an epithelioid appearance (**d**)

Table 2.1 Protein biomarkers for various trophoblastic cells [78, 160, 161]

	β-Catenin	GPC3	hCG	hPL	p63	CK18	CD146	Cyclin E	HLA-G	MUC-4	HSD3B	KI-67
Cytotrophoblast	+++ (nuclear)	+	–	–	++++	+++	–	++	–	–	–	++
Syncitiotrophoblast	–	++++	++++	++++	–	+++	–	–	–	+	++++	–
Villous intermediate trophoblast	+++ (membrane)	?	–	+	–	?	++	+++	++++	++++	±	++
Implantation intermediate trophoblast	+	++	±	+++	–	+++	++++	++++	+++	++++	++++	–
Chorionic laeve intermediate trophoblast	+	++	±	+	++++	+++	+	+	++++	–	++++	+

Genomic Imprinting and Placental Development

During evolution, the acquisition of the placenta in oviparous animals led to the first time that the fetal tissue came in direct contact with maternal endomyometrial structures. Not only did such contact create a safer, nourishing "house" – the placenta – for the development of the offspring, but it also brought in a spectrum of complex biological interactions between the fetus and the mother. In biology and genetics, the placental tissue is unique in that it is fetal in origin and shares half of the genome with that of the maternal uterus. Despite a short life span, there are constant morphological and biological fluctuations within the placenta proper and at the interface with the maternal gestational endomyometrium. Therefore, highly sophisticated cellular and molecular interactions are expected.

While detailed molecular regulations of placental development are still emerging, epigenetic imprinting, the selective suppression of various genes derived from one parent or the other has been proposed to have an important regulatory function in the development of the placenta of eutherian mammals. Among mammalian organs, the placenta is remarkably famous for its prolific expression of imprinted genes. A significant body of work has demonstrated that, among different species, the emergence of genomic imprinting during evolution is linked to the placental development and function [86–90]. The most informative data have been found in mice, in which many imprinted genes are present in extraembryonic tissue (i.e., placenta). Many of these genes are subject to imprinting only in the placental tissue (Table 2.2) [91–96]. Some of the imprinted genes important for placental development are highly conserved in eutherian mammals [97]. It has been speculated that ancestral mammals might have evolved with the placenta from newly acquired, retrotransposon-derived genes, or modified endogenous versions of the genes present in oviparous animals, via so-called exaptation. This likely occurred sometime after the divergence of mammals and birds, more than 90–130 million years ago [98, 99] (Fig. 2.13).

Approximately half of the known 100 or so imprinted genes are related to cellular proliferation and growth, many of which are involved in placental development and function [90, 100, 101]. A significant number of these genes are expressed and imprinted only in the placenta (Table 2.2). Moreover and remarkably, in mice, almost all imprinted genes known to be specific to the placenta are paternally imprinted and functionally expressed only from the maternal alleles (Table 2.2) [102]. In the human placenta, a limited number of studies have also shown that the pattern of genomic imprinting is similar to that of the mouse. Human PHLDA2 gene is expressed only from the maternal allele and is not expressed in unidisomy complete hydatidiform mole [103]. P57kip1 is another paternally imprinted gene that is expressed only from the maternal allele in the cytotrophoblastic cells and villous stromal cells of the human placenta [91, 104]. Placenta-specific imprinted genes such as CTNNA3/alpha3 catenin, HERC4/ubiquitin ligase, MAWBP/MAP activator, STOX1, and KCNKMA1/calcium-activated potassium channel alpha subunit are all maternally expressed and paternally imprinted genes in the human placenta [105, 106]. Regulatory non-protein encoding microRNA genes have also been found imprinted in the human placenta [107]. It should be noted that there are genes imprinted only in mice but not in humans. The lack of imprinting conservation between the two species may be linked to their respective placental anatomy and physiology. For example, in contrast to the accommodation of multiple paternities and multiple offsprings in a litter of mice, human pregnancy generally involves singletons.

Imprinted genes are frequently clustered in the genome. At the DNA level, the maintenance of genomic imprinting in extraembryonic tissue is mainly dependant on non-DNA methylation mechanisms including histone deacetylation and methylation. This is, however, not the case for the imprinting genes found in somatic embryonic tissues [102, 108]. Convincing molecular data confirm that in the mouse placenta, the mechanism of initiation and maintenance of imprinting involves an imprinting initiation center, from which a noncoding RNA is produced to coat the

Table 2.2 Selected imprinted genes involved in placenta development and function

Gene name	Gene location	Functional aspect or gene product	Imprinted expression	Species	Imprint alleles	References
Esx 1	X	X-linked homeobox gene	Placenta, testis	Mouse	Paternal	Li 1997,
Pem	X	X-linked homeobox gene	Placenta	Mouse	Paternal	Lin 1994
Xist	X	X dosage counting	Placenta	Mouse	Paternal	Mak 2004, Nolen 2005
BEX1(REX3)/ Bex1(Rex 3)	Xq22	X-linked	Blasstocyst, placenta	Human, mouse	Paternal	Brown 1999, Williams 2002
Eed	X	X-linked polycomb group gene	Fetus, placenta	Mouse	Paternal	Wang 2001, Monk 2008
Tsix	X	Regulating Xist	Fetus, placenta	Mouse	Paternal	Lee 2000
TFPI2	7q21/6	Tissue factor pathway inhibitor	Placenta	Human/mouse	Paternal	Monk 2008
Rtl1/Peg11	Distal 12	Aspartyl protease motif/ maintennace of fetal capillaries	Fetus, placenta	Mouse	Maternal	Seitz 2003
IGF-II/Igf-2	11p15.5	Growth factor	Fetus, placenta	Human/mouse	Maternal	Constancia 2002, Tilghman 1999, Ferguson-Smith 2000
H19/H19	11p15.5	Encoding regulatory nontranslated RNA	Fetuas placenta	Human/mouse	Paternal	Tilghman 1999, Ferguson-Smith 2000
PEG10/Peg10	7q216	DNA/RNA binding/cell cycle regulator	Embryo, placenta	Human/mouse	Matenal	Ono 2006
IGF2/Igf2-r	11p15.5/Distal 7	Growth promoting	Fetus, placenta	Mouse	Paternal	Wutz 1998, Sleutels 2002
INS/Ins	11p15.5	Encodes proinsulin	Fetus, placenta	Human/mouse/ marsupia	Maternal	Ager 2007
PEG1(MEST)/ Peg1(mest)	7q32.2	Hydrolase enzyme/Angiogenesis	Fetus, placenta	Human, mouse	Maternal	Mayer 2000,Kaneko-Ishino 1995, McMinn 2006
Gatm	Central 2	L-arginie:glycine amidinotranserase	Placenta	Mouse	Paternal	Sandell 2003
Ppp1r9a	Proximal 6	Neural tissue-specfic F-actin binding protein	Placenta	Mouse	Paternal	Ono 2003
Pon 2 and 3	Proximal 6	Paraoxonases	Placenta	Mouse	Paternal	Ono 2003
Osbpl5	Distal 7	Oxysterol binding protein-like 5	Placenta	Mouse	Paternal	Engemann 2000
Tssc4	Distal 7	Tumor suppressor	Placenta	Mouse	Paternal	Paulsen 2000
Tspan32	Distal 7	AML1 regulated tranmembrance protein	Placenta	Mouse	paternal	Umlauf 2004
Ascl2	Distal 7	Achaet-scute homolog 2	Placenta	Mouse	Paternal	Guillemot 1995
Cd81	Distal 7	Cd81 antigen	Placenta	Mouse	Paternal	Umlauf 2004

(continued)

Table 2.2 (continued)

Gene name	Gene location	Functional aspect or gene product	Imprinted expression	Species	Imprint alleles	References
Dcn	Distal 10	Decorin	Placenta	Mouse	Paternal	Mizuno 2002
Slc22a2/Slc22a3	Proximal 17	Solure carrier family 22	Placenta	Mouse	Paternal	Sleutels 2002, Zwart 2001.
CTNNA3	10q21	Catenin, alpha3	Placenta	Human	Paternal	Van Dijk 2004
HERC4	10q21	Ubiquitin ligase domain	Placenta	Human	Paternal	Oudejans 2004
MAWBP	10q21	MAP Activator	Placenta	Human	Paternal	Oudejans 2004
STOX1	10q22	Storkead Box 1	Placenta	Human	Paternal	Van Dijk 2005
KCNMA1	10q22	Calcium-activted potassium channel alpha subunit 1	Placenta	Human	Paternal	Oudejans 2004
OSBPL5	11p15	Oxysterol binding protein-like	Placenta	Human	Paternal	Higashimoto 2002
P57kip2(CDKN1C)	11p15	G1 cyclin inhibitor/tumor suppressor	Fetus, placenta	Human	Paternal	Takahashi 2000
KCNQ1OT1/ Kcnq1ot1	11p15	Imprinting control	Fetus, placenta	Human/mouse	Paternal	Mancini-DiNardo D 2003, Lewis 2004, Umlauf D 2004
Mash2	Distal 7	Helix-turn-helix transcription factor	Placenta, fetus	Mouse	Paternal	Guillemot 1995.
PHLDA2/Phlda2	11p15	Tumor suppressor	Placenta	Human/mouse	Paternal	Hu RJ. Genomics 1998 46:9–17; Qian N. Hum Mol Genet 1997. 6:2021–2029.
GRB10/Grb10	7p12	Insulin receptor-binding protein	Placenta	Human/mouse	Paternal	Monk D. Hum Mol Genet 2009;18:3066–3074

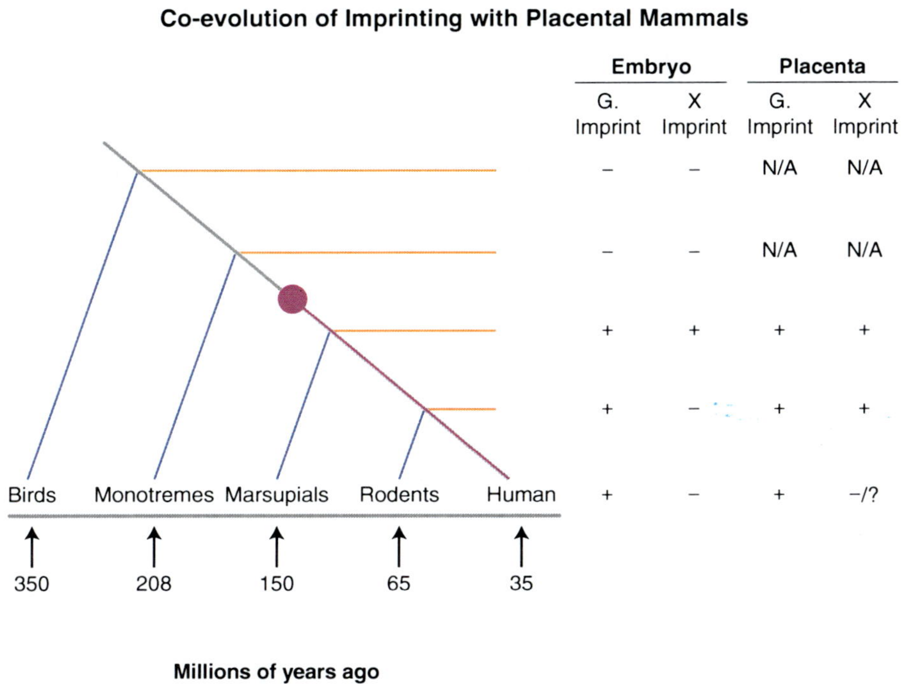

Fig. 2.13 Co-evolution of genomic imprinting and imprinted X chromosomal inactivation. It is speculated that ancestral mammals evolved with the placenta from newly acquired retrotransposon-derived genes some time after the divergence of mammals and birds, about 150 million years ago (purple dot). While the genomic imprinting is conserved in both embryonic and placental tissues, placental imprinted X chromosome inactivation is conserved only in marsupials and rodents. Human placenta appears to have a random X chromosome inactivation based on available data. Adapted from Reik and Lewis [89]

imprinting cluster in-cis. Subsequently, histone H3 deacetylation at K4 and acquisition of H3-K9 and K27 methylation occur (Fig. 2.14), and eventually lead to the recruitment of polycomb complex proteins to the repressed paternal chromosome regions [109–113]. A similar molecular mechanism has been recently established for the imprinted X chromosome inactivation in mouse placenta (see the following section).

Imprinted X Chromosome Inactivation and Placental Development

X chromosome inactivation plays a central role in balancing the gene dosage in a female cell. Among various X dosage compensation schemes, X inactivation occurs only in placental mammals including eutherians (rodents and primates), and such sex chromosomal imprinting occurs only in the extraembryonic tissue (imprinted X chromosomal inactivation). In marsupial mammals, the imprinted paternal X chromosome is preferentially inactivated in both embryonic and extraembryonic tissues [114, 115]. The paternal X chromosome is preferentially imprinted and silent in mouse trophectoderm, and genes on the X chromosome are expressed only from the maternal alleles [116, 117]. Therefore, in mouse and marsupial placenta, X chromosome inactivation represents a special form of genomic imprinting, that is, imprinted X chromosome inactivation. Such imprinted X inactivation is established early during preimplantation development in all cells of the embryo. However, the imprinting is maintained only in the extraembryonic tissue. The embryonic tissues switch the X imprinting pattern to random X inactivation later during the development [118, 119]. The imprinted X inacti-

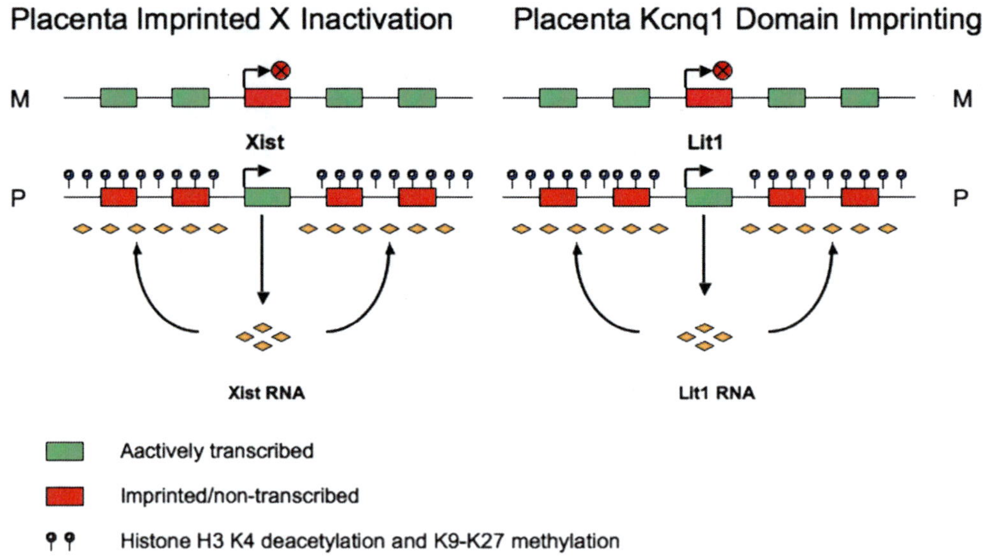

Fig. 2.14 Co-evolution of genomic imprinting and imprinted X chromosomal inactivation, sharing similar molecular and epigenetic mechanisms of DNA silencing (M: maternal allele; P: paternal allele). In mouse placenta, both Kcnq1 genomic imprinting domain and Xist X inactivation center involve a nontranscribed RNA molecule that is expressed from the to-be imprinted paternal allele. The nontranscribed RNA, Lit1 from Kcnq1 domain or Xist from X inactivation center, coats the neighborhood DNA regions or the entire X chromosome in-cis, leading to imprinting silencing through the induction of various histone modifications including deacetylation and loss of H3-K4 methylation in addition to H3-K9 and K27 methylation. Adapted from Wagschal and Feil [116]

vation is independent of DNA methylation [108, 120] and involves a non-translated RNA gene, Xist expressed only from the paternal X chromosome. The paternally expressed Xist RNA carpets the entire paternal X chromosome in-cis, followed by the recruitment of various chromatin-modifying molecules (Fig. 2.14) [121, 122]. In a sharp contrast, DNA methylation is the main mechanism involved in random X inactivation in embryo proper [120, 123]. At genetic regulatory level, there are ontogenetic similarities of imprinting between autosomal genes and those of the X chromosome (see the next section).

Co-evolution of Genomic Imprinting and Imprinted X Chromosome Inactivation

Paternal imprinting expression of autosomal genes and imprinted paternal X inactivation in mouse placenta raise an important biological question: were they co-evolutionarily established in placental animals [89, 115, 124, 125]? A growing body of evidence has supported this hypothesis [89, 102]. Of studied species, all female somatic cells reserve certain mechanisms of dosage compensation of the X chromosome. Recent evidence has argued that imprinted X inactivation and genomic imprinting may have co-evolved under similar adaptive pressures during evolution (Fig. 2.13) [89]. Molecular evidence clearly demonstrated that in the placenta, both processes involve paternally transcribed noncoding RNA to initiate silencing of the neighborhood paternal genes (Fig. 2.14) [102]. The Xist on the X chromosome is expressed only from the paternal alleles in female placental cells. The resultant nontranscribed Xist RNA coats the paternal X chromosome in-cis and shuts down the entire chromosome through induction of various modifications of histone molecules, including histone deacetylation and loss of H3-K4 methylation, and H3-K9 and K27 methylation. Similarly, for autosomal imprinting in placenta, the Kcnq1 domain in control of IC2 cluster imprinting genes expresses Kcnq1 ot1 or Lit1 nontranscribed RNA that coats the neighborhood DNA regions leading to imprinting silencing, also likely through histone H3 methylation at K9 and K27, and histone deacetylation and loss of H3-K4 methylation (Fig. 2.14). It appears that both Xist and Kcnq1 imprinting silencing occur independent of DNA methylation [102]. Figure 2.13 summarizes current available evidence of co-evolution of genomic imprinting and imprinted X inactivation during evolution.

It is reasonable to argue that in primates including humans, as in mice [126–129], an imprinted X chromosomal inactivation is possible in extraembryonic trophoblasts, the cells that give rise to various gestational trophoblastic diseases, such as placental site trophoblastic tumor and hydatidiform moles. Unexpectedly, the mode of X chromosomal inactivation appears random in human placental tissue according to recent data [130–133], although not without controversies [128, 134–137]. In human placental tissue, reversal of inactivated X or global X reactivation is inducible in chorionic villous cells only from first-trimester spontaneous abortions but not from first-trimester elective terminations. These differences in inducibility are not associated with detectable variation in histone H4 acetylation, DNA methylation, or XIST expression – hallmarks of the inactivation process [138]. Therefore, it is important to consider that the maintenance of the X imprinting pattern in the placenta is largely dependent on histone deacetylation and methylation pathways as opposed to direct DNA methylation. Additionally, imprinting patterns of some autosomal genes appear cell type specific among various placental cells (Fig. 2.15). Therefore, it is still possible that a heterogeneity of X inactivation exists among various cell populations in the human placenta.

"Parental Conflict of Interest" Theory of Genomic Imprinting

The "parental conflict hypothesis" is the prevailing theory of genomic imprinting in placental biology [139–141]. It views that parents of opposite sex have conflicting interests in allocating resources to their offspring by the mother

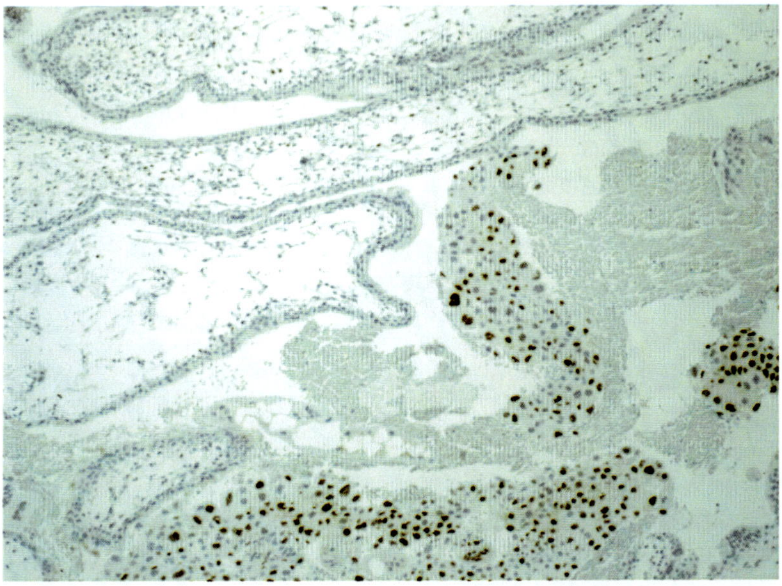

Fig. 2.15 Heterogeneous imprinting expression of P57 gene among various placental trophoblasts. In the absence of maternal genome in this diandric complete mole, the paternally imprinted p57 is not expressed in villous cytotrophoblast (upper left chorionic villi). However, such paternal imprinting silencing is not homogenous as there is an apparent expression or relaxation of imprinting of p57 among other types of trophoblast, that is, villous intermediate trophoblast (lower right strong nuclear staining of p57), suggesting that the paternal imprinting in human placenta is heterogeneous, in contrast to an absolute paternal imprinting in mouse placenta

[140, 142–144]. The intent of the paternal genome would be to maximize resources for the father's own progeny. In contrast, the interest of the maternal genome would be to distribute resources equally among her offspring. This implies that growth-promoting genes are mainly expressed from the paternally inherited genome and are silent in the maternally inherited counterpart. Analyses of many imprinted genes in mammals support this theory [145, 146], and many known imprinted genes are involved in the regulation of cellular proliferation and growth (Table 2.2) and are important for the placental development and function [101]. Pronuclear transfer experiments showed that unipaternal disomy (androgenote) in mice led to placental overgrowth plus early fetal lethality while unimaternal disomy (gynogenote) resulted in hypoplasia of the placenta [147, 148]. Many mouse imprinted genes (Table 2.2) are exclusively found in the placenta and are paternally silenced, although the functions of many of these genes are yet to be elucidated. Among a few studied, paternally expressed Igf2 gene is a growth-promoting factor, and inappropriate expression in a mouse model led to abnormal growth [149]. Biallelic expression of Igf2 resulted in overgrowth [150]. Similar function of the human IGF2 gene has also been observed [151]. The receptor of Igf2 is a maternally expressed imprinted gene, Igf2r, and has the opposite effect on the growth in mouse studies [152]. Phlda2 (Ipl/Tssc3) is a maternally expressed and paternally imprinted gene in the placenta. Homozygous knockout mouse conceptuses lacking the active maternal allele had markedly enlarged placentas [103, 153]. Phlda2, a paternally imprinted gene, leads to a marked reduction of the placenta size [103]. Human study of the gene resulted in a similar conclusion [154]. P57Kip2/CDKN1C is a paternally imprinted gene in human and mouse placenta. Loss of its expression is associated with trophoblastic hypertrophy and placentomegaly in mice [91, 104] and hyperplasia of trophoblasts in human diandric hydatidiform mole [155, 156]. GRB10 is another paternally imprinted gene in the placenta, and its maternal allelic expression appears specific to cytotrophoblasts. Silencing of the maternal allele resulted in embryonic overgrowth accompanied by a disproportionate size of the placenta [157–159].

References

1. Aplin JD. The cell biology of human implantation. Placenta. 1996;17(5–6):269–75.
2. Fox H. Pathology of the placenta. Clin Obstet Gynaecol. 1986;13(3):501–19.
3. Carson DD, Bagchi I, Dey SK, Enders AC, Fazleabas AT, Lessey BA, et al. Embryo implantation. Dev Biol. 2000;223(2):217–37.
4. Bagchi IC, Li Q, Cheon YP. Role of steroid hormone-regulated genes in implantation. Ann N Y Acad Sci. 2001;943:68–76.
5. Cheng JG, Rodriguez CI, Stewart CL. Control of uterine receptivity and embryo implantation by steroid hormone regulation of LIF production and LIF receptor activity: towards a molecular understanding of "the window of implantation". Rev Endocr Metab Disord. 2002;3(2):119–26.
6. Momoeda M, Taketani Y, Mizuno M, Iwamori M, Nagai Y. Characteristic expression of cholesterol sulfate in rabbit endometrium during the implantation period. Biochem Biophys Res Commun. 1991;178(1):145–50.
7. Abulencia A, Acosta D, Adelman J, Affolder T, Akimoto T, Albrow MG, et al. Measurement of the tt production cross section in pp collisions at square root of s = 1.96 TeV. Phys Rev Lett. 2006;97(8):082004.
8. Nardo LG, Nikas G, Makrigiannakis A. Molecules in blastocyst implantation. Role of matrix metalloproteinases, cytokines and growth factors. J Reprod Med. 2003;48(3):137–47.
9. Wang J, Mayernik L, Armant DR. Trophoblast adhesion of the peri-implantation mouse blastocyst is regulated by integrin signaling that targets phospholipase C. Dev Biol. 2007;302(1):143–53.
10. Shimomura Y, Ando H, Furugori K, Kajiyama H, Suzuki M, Iwase A, et al. Possible involvement of crosstalk cell-adhesion mechanism by endometrial CD26/dipeptidyl peptidase IV and embryonal fibronectin in human blastocyst implantation. Mol Hum Reprod. 2006;12(8):491–5.
11. Kimber SJ. Molecular interactions at the maternal-embryonic interface during the early phase of implantation. Semin Reprod Med. 2000;18(3):237–53.
12. Charles D. The Arias Stella reaction. J Obstet Gynaecol Br Emp. 1962;69:1006–10.
13. Arias-Stella J. The Arias-Stella reaction: facts and fancies four decades after. Adv Anat Pathol. 2002;9(1):12–23.
14. Achen MG, Gad JM, Stacker SA, Wilks AF. Placenta growth factor and vascular endothelial growth factor are co-expressed during early embryonic development. Growth Factors. 1997;15(1):69–80.
15. Cross JC, Werb Z, Fisher SJ. Implantation and the placenta: key pieces of the development puzzle. Science. 1994;266(5190):1508–18.
16. Damsky CH, Fitzgerald ML, Fisher SJ. Distribution patterns of extracellular matrix components and adhesion receptors are intricately modulated during first tri-

mester cytotrophoblast differentiation along the invasive pathway, in vivo. J Clin Invest. 1992;89(1):210–22.
17. Simon C, Moreno C, Remohi J, Pellicer A. Molecular interactions between embryo and uterus in the adhesion phase of human implantation. Hum Reprod. 1998;13 Suppl 3:219–32. discussion 33-6.
18. Kimber SJ, Spanswick C. Blastocyst implantation: the adhesion cascade. Semin Cell Dev Biol. 2000; 11(2):77–92.
19. Yoshinaga K. Research on blastocyst implantation essential factors (BIEFs). Am J Reprod Immunol. 2010;63(6):413–24.
20. Carlson BM. Human Embryology and Developmental Biology. St.Louis: Mosby; 1994.
21. Enders AC, Schlafke S. Cytological aspects of trophoblast-uterine interaction in early implantation. Am J Anat. 1969;125(1):1–29.
22. Yasumasu S, Kawaguchi M, Ouchi S, Sano K, Murata K, Sugiyama H, et al. Mechanism of egg envelope digestion by hatching enzymes, HCE and LCE in medaka, *Oryzias latipes*. J Biochem. 2010;148(4):439–48.
23. Cannon MJ, Menino Jr AR. Changes in the bovine zona pellucida induced by plasmin or embryonic plasminogen activator. Mol Reprod Dev. 1998;51(3): 330–8.
24. Quesada V, Sanchez LM, Alvarez J, Lopez-Otin C. Identification and characterization of human and mouse ovastacin: a novel metalloproteinase similar to hatching enzymes from arthropods, birds, amphibians, and fish. J Biol Chem. 2004;279(25):26627–34.
25. O'Sullivan CM, Liu SY, Karpinka JB, Rancourt DE. Embryonic hatching enzyme strypsin/ISP1 is expressed with ISP2 in endometrial glands during implantation. Mol Reprod Dev. 2002;62(3):328–34.
26. Sharma N, Liu S, Tang L, Irwin J, Meng G, Rancourt DE. Implantation Serine Proteinases heterodimerize and are critical in hatching and implantation. BMC Dev Biol. 2006;6:61.
27. Coates AA, Menino Jr AR. Effects of blastocoelic expansion and plasminogen activator activity on hatching and zona pellucida solubility in bovine embryos in vitro. J Anim Sci. 1994;72(11):2936–42.
28. Wu TC, Wan YJ, Damjanov I. Positioning of inner cell mass determines the development of mouse blastocysts in vitro. J Embryol Exp Morphol. 1981;65: 105–17.
29. Copp AJ. Interaction between inner cell mass and trophectoderm of the mouse blastocyst. II. The fate of the polar trophectoderm. J Embryol Exp Morphol. 1979;51:109–20.
30. Jones CJ, Fazleabas AT. Ultrastructure of epithelial plaque formation and stromal cell transformation by post-ovulatory chorionic gonadotrophin treatment in the baboon (Papio anubis). Hum Reprod. 2001;16(12): 2680–90.
31. Zygmunt M, Hahn D, Munstedt K, Bischof P, Lang U. Invasion of cytotrophoblastic JEG-3 cells is stimulated by hCG in vitro. Placenta. 1998;19(8): 587–93.
32. Wilcox AJ, Baird DD, Weinberg CR. Time of implantation of the conceptus and loss of pregnancy. N Engl J Med. 1999;340(23):1796–9.
33. Edwards RG. Human uterine endocrinology and the implantation window. Ann N Y Acad Sci. 1988; 541:445–54.
34. Grewal S, Carver JG, Ridley AJ, Mardon HJ. Implantation of the human embryo requires Rac1-dependent endometrial stromal cell migration. Proc Natl Acad Sci USA. 2008;105(42):16189–94.
35. Qin J, Diaz-Cueto L, Schwarze JE, Takahashi Y, Imai M, Isuzugawa K, et al. Effects of progranulin on blastocyst hatching and subsequent adhesion and outgrowth in the mouse. Biol Reprod. 2005;73(3): 434–42.
36. Matsumoto H, Daikoku T, Wang H, Sato E, Dey SK. Differential expression of ezrin/radixin/moesin (ERM) and ERM-associated adhesion molecules in the blastocyst and uterus suggests their functions during implantation. Biol Reprod. 2004;70(3):729–36.
37. Nagaoka K, Nojima H, Watanabe F, Chang KT, Christenson RK, Sakai S, et al. Regulation of blastocyst migration, apposition, and initial adhesion by a chemokine, interferon gamma-inducible protein 10 kDa (IP-10), during early gestation. J Biol Chem. 2003;278(31):29048–56.
38. Robson P, Stein P, Zhou B, Schultz RM, Baldwin HS. Inner cell mass-specific expression of a cell adhesion molecule (PECAM-1/CD31) in the mouse blastocyst. Dev Biol. 2001;234(2):317–29.
39. Galan A, O'Connor JE, Valbuena D, Herrer R, Remohi J, Pampfer S, et al. The human blastocyst regulates endometrial epithelial apoptosis in embryonic adhesion. Biol Reprod. 2000;63(2):430–9.
40. Grewal S, Carver J, Ridley AJ, Mardon HJ. Human endometrial stromal cell rho GTPases have opposing roles in regulating focal adhesion turnover and embryo invasion in vitro. Biol Reprod. 2010;83(1):75–82.
41. Carson DD, DeSouza MM, Regisford EG. Mucin and proteoglycan functions in embryo implantation. Bioessays. 1998;20(7):577–83.
42. Smith SE, French MM, Julian J, Paria BC, Dey SK, Carson DD. Expression of heparan sulfate proteoglycan (perlecan) in the mouse blastocyst is regulated during normal and delayed implantation. Dev Biol. 1997;184(1):38–47.
43. Carson DD, Tang JP, Julian J. Heparan sulfate proteoglycan (perlecan) expression by mouse embryos during acquisition of attachment competence. Dev Biol. 1993;155(1):97–106.
44. Lessey BA, Castelbaum AJ, Sawin SW, Sun J. Integrins as markers of uterine receptivity in women with primary unexplained infertility. Fertil Steril. 1995;63(3):535–42.
45. Genbacev OD, Prakobphol A, Foulk RA, Krtolica AR, Ilic D, Singer MS, et al. Trophoblast L-selectin-mediated adhesion at the maternal-fetal interface. Science. 2003;299(5605):405–8.
46. Lobo SC, Huang ST, Germeyer A, Dosiou C, Vo KC, Tulac S, et al. The immune environment in human

endometrium during the window of implantation. Am J Reprod Immunol. 2004;52(4):244–51.
47. Pijnenborg R, Robertson WB, Brosens I, Dixon G. Review article: trophoblast invasion and the establishment of haemochorial placentation in man and laboratory animals. Placenta. 1981;2(1):71–91.
48. Genbacev O, Joslin R, Damsky CH, Polliotti BM, Fisher SJ. Hypoxia alters early gestation human cytotrophoblast differentiation/invasion in vitro and models the placental defects that occur in preeclampsia. J Clin Invest. 1996;97(2):540–50.
49. Genbacev O, Zhou Y, Ludlow JW, Fisher SJ. Regulation of human placental development by oxygen tension. Science. 1997;277(5332):1669–72.
50. Gobble RM, Groesch KA, Chang M, Torry RJ, Torry DS. Differential regulation of human PlGF gene expression in trophoblast and nontrophoblast cells by oxygen tension. Placenta. 2009;30(10):869–75.
51. Hurskainen T, Seiki M, Apte SS, Syrjakallio-Ylitalo M, Sorsa T, Oikarinen A, et al. Production of membrane-type matrix metalloproteinase-1 (MT-MMP-1) in early human placenta. A possible role in placental implantation? J Histochem Cytochem. 1998;46(2):221–9.
52. Liu G, Zhang X, Lin H, Wang H, Li Q, Ni J, et al. Effects of E-cadherin on mouse embryo implantation and expression of matrix metalloproteinase-2 and -9. Biochem Biophys Res Commun. 2006;343(3):832–8.
53. Gao F, Chen XL, Wei P, Gao HJ, Liu YX. Expression of matrix metalloproteinase-2, tissue inhibitors of metalloproteinase-1, -3 at the implantation site of rhesus monkey during the early stage of pregnancy. Endocrine. 2001;16(1):47–54.
54. Li L, Chen S, Xing F. Expression of matrix metalloproteinase-9 and tissue inhibitor of metalloproteinase-3 protein in the implantation window phase of endometrium. Zhonghua Fu Chan Ke Za Zhi. 2000; 35(9):544–6.
55. Raga F, Casan EM, Wen Y, Huang HY, Bonilla-Musoles F, Polan ML. Independent regulation of matrix metalloproteinase-9, tissue inhibitor of metalloproteinase-1 (TIMP-1), and TIMP-3 in human endometrial stromal cells by gonadotropin-releasing hormone: implications in early human implantation. J Clin Endocrinol Metab. 1999;84(2):636–42.
56. Irwin JC, Suen LF, Faessen GH, Popovici RM, Giudice LC. Insulin-like growth factor (IGF)-II inhibition of endometrial stromal cell tissue inhibitor of metalloproteinase-3 and IGF-binding protein-1 suggests paracrine interactions at the decidua:trophoblast interface during human implantation. J Clin Endocrinol Metab. 2001;86(5):2060–4.
57. Klemke RL, Cai S, Giannini AL, Gallagher PJ, de Lanerolle P, Cheresh DA. Regulation of cell motility by mitogen-activated protein kinase. J Cell Biol. 1997;137(2):481–92.
58. McKinnon T, Chakraborty C, Gleeson LM, Chidiac P, Lala PK. Stimulation of human extravillous trophoblast migration by IGF-II is mediated by IGF type 2 receptor involving inhibitory G protein(s) and phosphorylation of MAPK. J Clin Endocrinol Metab. 2001;86(8):3665–74.
59. Gleeson LM, Chakraborty C, McKinnon T, Lala PK. Insulin-like growth factor-binding protein 1 stimulates human trophoblast migration by signaling through alpha 5 beta 1 integrin via mitogen-activated protein Kinase pathway. J Clin Endocrinol Metab. 2001;86(6):2484–93.
60. Shih I, Wang T, Wu T, Kurman RJ, Gearhart JD. Expression of Mel-CAM in implantation site intermediate trophoblastic cell line, IST-1, limits its migration on uterine smooth muscle cells. J Cell Sci. 1998;111(Pt 17):2655–64.
61. Graham CH, Lala PK. Mechanisms of placental invasion of the uterus and their control. Biochem Cell Biol. 1992;70(10–11):867–74.
62. Busch S, Renaud SJ, Schleussner E, Graham CH, Markert UR. mTOR mediates human trophoblast invasion through regulation of matrix-remodeling enzymes and is associated with serine phosphorylation of STAT3. Exp Cell Res. 2009;315(10):1724–33.
63. Kovats S, Main EK, Librach C, Stubblebine M, Fisher SJ, DeMars R. A class I antigen, HLA-G, expressed in human trophoblasts. Science. 1990; 248(4952):220–3.
64. McMaster MT, Librach CL, Zhou Y, Lim KH, Janatpour MJ, DeMars R, et al. Human placental HLA-G expression is restricted to differentiated cytotrophoblasts. J Immunol. 1995;154(8):3771–8.
65. Bondarenko GI, Burleigh DW, Durning M, Breburda EE, Grendell RL, Golos TG. Passive immunization against the MHC class I molecule Mamu-AG disrupts rhesus placental development and endometrial responses. J Immunol. 2007;179(12):8042–50.
66. Hess AP, Hamilton AE, Talbi S, Dosiou C, Nyegaard M, Nayak N, et al. Decidual stromal cell response to paracrine signals from the trophoblast: amplification of immune and angiogenic modulators. Biol Reprod. 2007;76(1):102–17.
67. Arimoto-Ishida E, Sakata M, Sawada K, Nakayama M, Nishimoto F, Mabuchi S, et al. Up-regulation of alpha5-integrin by E-cadherin loss in hypoxia and its key role in the migration of extravillous trophoblast cells during early implantation. Endocrinology. 2009;150(9):4306–15.
68. Li Q, Wang J, Armant DR, Bagchi MK, Bagchi IC. Calcitonin down-regulates E-cadherin expression in rodent uterine epithelium during implantation. J Biol Chem. 2002;277(48):46447–55.
69. Shih Ie M, Hsu MY, Oldt 3rd RJ, Herlyn M, Gearhart JD, Kurman RJ. The role of E-cadherin in the motility and invasion of implantation site intermediate trophoblast. Placenta. 2002;23(10):706–15.
70. Bulla R, Villa A, Bossi F, Cassetti A, Radillo O, Spessotto P, et al. VE-cadherin is a critical molecule for trophoblast-endothelial cell interaction in decidual spiral arteries. Exp Cell Res. 2005;303(1):101–13.
71. Garcia P, Nieto A, Sanchez MA, Pizarro M, Flores JM. Expression of alphav, alpha4, alpha5 and beta3 integrin subunits, fibronectin and vitronectin in goat peri-implantation. Anim Reprod Sci. 2004;80(1–2): 91–100.

72. Ruan HC, Huang HF, Jin F. The expression of integrin beta3 in mice's endometrium during the implantation window based on different ovarian stimulation protocols. Zhonghua Yi Xue Za Zhi. 2004;84(10): 857–60.
73. von Wolff M, Strowitzki T, Becker V, Zepf C, Tabibzadeh S, Thaler CJ. Endometrial osteopontin, a ligand of beta3-integrin, is maximally expressed around the time of the "implantation window". Fertil Steril. 2001;76(4):775–81.
74. Saito S, Nakashima A, Myojo-Higuma S, Shiozaki A. The balance between cytotoxic NK cells and regulatory NK cells in human pregnancy. J Reprod Immunol. 2008;77(1):14–22.
75. Saito S, Shiozaki A, Sasaki Y, Nakashima A, Shima T, Ito M. Regulatory T cells and regulatory natural killer (NK) cells play important roles in feto-maternal tolerance. Semin Immunopathol. 2007;29(2):115–22.
76. King A, Allan DS, Bowen M, Powis SJ, Joseph S, Verma S, et al. HLA-E is expressed on trophoblast and interacts with CD94/NKG2 receptors on decidual NK cells. Eur J Immunol. 2000;30(6):1623–31.
77. Shih IM, Kurman RJ. New concepts in trophoblastic growth and differentiation with practical application for the diagnosis of gestational trophoblastic disease. Verh Dtsch Ges Pathol. 1997;81:266–72.
78. Shih Ie M. Gestational trophoblastic tumors and related tumor-like lesions. In: Kurman R, editor. Blaustein's Pathology of the Female Genital Tract. 6th ed. New York: Springer; 2010.
79. Mi S, Lee X, Li X, Veldman GM, Finnerty H, Racie L, et al. Syncytin is a captive retroviral envelope protein involved in human placental morphogenesis. Nature. 2000;403(6771):785–9.
80. Shih IM, Kurman RJ. The pathology of intermediate trophoblastic tumors and tumor-like lesions. Int J Gynecol Pathol. 2001;20(1):31–47.
81. Yeh IT, O'Connor DM, Kurman RJ. Vacuolated cytotrophoblast: a subpopulation of trophoblast in the chorion laeve. Placenta. 1989;10(5):429–38.
82. Wan SK, Lam PW, Pau MY, Chan JK. Multiclefted nuclei. A helpful feature for identification of intermediate trophoblastic cells in uterine curetting specimens. Am J Surg Pathol. 1992;16(12):1226–32.
83. Shih Ie M. Trophogram, an immunohistochemistry-based algorithmic approach, in the differential diagnosis of trophoblastic tumors and tumorlike lesions. Ann Diagn Pathol. 2007;11(3):228–34.
84. Mao TL, Seidman JD, Kurman RJ, Shih Ie M. Cyclin E and p16 immunoreactivity in epithelioid trophoblastic tumor–an aid in differential diagnosis. Am J Surg Pathol. 2006;30(9):1105–10.
85. Shih IM, Kurman RJ. Ki-67 labeling index in the differential diagnosis of exaggerated placental site, placental site trophoblastic tumor, and choriocarcinoma: a double immunohistochemical staining technique using Ki-67 and Mel-CAM antibodies. Hum Pathol. 1998;29(1):27–33.
86. Ferguson-Smith AC, Surani MA. Imprinting and the epigenetic asymmetry between parental genomes. Science. 2001;293(5532):1086–9.
87. Coan PM, Burton GJ, Ferguson-Smith AC. Imprinted genes in the placenta–a review. Placenta. 2005; 26(Suppl A):S10–20.
88. Morison IM, Ramsay JP, Spencer HG. A census of mammalian imprinting. Trends Genet. 2005;21(8): 457–65.
89. Reik W, Lewis A. Co-evolution of X-chromosome inactivation and imprinting in mammals. Nat Rev Genet. 2005;6(5):403–10.
90. Frost JM, Moore GE. The importance of imprinting in the human placenta. PLoS Genet. 2010;6:e1001015.
91. Caspary T, Cleary MA, Baker CC, Guan XJ, Tilghman SM. Multiple mechanisms regulate imprinting of the mouse distal chromosome 7 gene cluster. Mol Cell Biol. 1998;18(6):3466–74.
92. Zwart R, Sleutels F, Wutz A, Schinkel AH, Barlow DP. Bidirectional action of the Igf2r imprint control element on upstream and downstream imprinted genes. Genes Dev. 2001;15(18):2361–6.
93. Higashimoto K, Soejima H, Yatsuki H, Joh K, Uchiyama M, Obata Y, et al. Characterization and imprinting status of OBPH1/Obph1 gene: implications for an extended imprinting domain in human and mouse. Genomics. 2002;80(6):575–84.
94. Mizuno Y, Sotomaru Y, Katsuzawa Y, Kono T, Meguro M, Oshimura M, et al. Asb4, Ata3, and Dcn are novel imprinted genes identified by high-throughput screening using RIKEN cDNA microarray. Biochem Biophys Res Commun. 2002;290(5):1499–505.
95. Ono R, Shiura H, Aburatani H, Kohda T, Kaneko-Ishino T, Ishino F. Identification of a large novel imprinted gene cluster on mouse proximal chromosome 6. Genome Res. 2003;13(7):1696–705.
96. Sandell LL, Guan XJ, Ingram R, Tilghman SM. Gatm, a creatine synthesis enzyme, is imprinted in mouse placenta. Proc Natl Acad Sci USA. 2003;100(8): 4622–7.
97. Ono R, Nakamura K, Inoue K, Naruse M, Usami T, Wakisaka-Saito N, et al. Deletion of Peg10, an imprinted gene acquired from a retrotransposon, causes early embryonic lethality. Nat Genet. 2006; 38(1):101–6.
98. Hedges SB. The origin and evolution of model organisms. Nat Rev Genet. 2002;3(11):838–49.
99. Kaneko-Ishino T, Ishino F. Retrotransposon silencing by DNA methylation contributed to the evolution of placentation and genomic imprinting in mammals. Dev Growth Differ. 2010;52(6):533–43.
100. Tycko B, Efstratiadis A. Genomic imprinting: piece of cake. Nature. 2002;417(6892):913–4.
101. Tycko B, Morison IM. Physiological functions of imprinted genes. J Cell Physiol. 2002;192(3):245–58.
102. Feil R, Berger F. Convergent evolution of genomic imprinting in plants and mammals. Trends Genet. 2007;23(4):192–9.
103. Salas M, John R, Saxena A, Barton S, Frank D, Fitzpatrick G, et al. Placental growth retardation due to loss of imprinting of Phlda2. Mech Dev. 2004; 121(10):1199–210.
104. Takahashi K, Kobayashi T, Kanayama N. p57(Kip2) regulates the proper development of labyrinthine and

spongiotrophoblasts. Mol Hum Reprod. 2000;6(11): 1019–25.

105. Oudejans CB, Mulders J, Lachmeijer AM, van Dijk M, Konst AA, Westerman BA, et al. The parent-of-origin effect of 10q22 in pre-eclamptic females coincides with two regions clustered for genes with down-regulated expression in androgenetic placentas. Mol Hum Reprod. 2004;10(8):589–98.
106. van Dijk M, Mulders J, Konst A, Janssens B, van Roy F, Blankenstein M, et al. Differential downregulation of alphaT-catenin expression in placenta: trophoblast cell type-dependent imprinting of the CTNNA3 gene. Gene Expr Patterns. 2004;5(1):61–5.
107. Noguer-Dance M, Abu-Amero S, Al-Khtib M, Lefevre A, Coullin P, Moore GE, et al. The primate-specific microRNA gene cluster (C19MC) is imprinted in the placenta. Hum Mol Genet. 2010;19(18):3566–82.
108. Lewis A, Mitsuya K, Umlauf D, Smith P, Dean W, Walter J, et al. Imprinting on distal chromosome 7 in the placenta involves repressive histone methylation independent of DNA methylation. Nat Genet. 2004;36(12):1291–5.
109. Mager J, Montgomery ND, de Villena FP, Magnuson T. Genome imprinting regulated by the mouse Polycomb group protein Eed. Nat Genet. 2003;33(4): 502–7.
110. Silva J, Mak W, Zvetkova I, Appanah R, Nesterova TB, Webster Z, et al. Establishment of histone h3 methylation on the inactive X chromosome requires transient recruitment of Eed-Enx1 polycomb group complexes. Dev Cell. 2003;4(4):481–95.
111. Cao R, Zhang Y. The functions of E(Z)/EZH2-mediated methylation of lysine 27 in histone H3. Curr Opin Genet Dev. 2004;14(2):155–64.
112. Umlauf D, Goto Y, Cao R, Cerqueira F, Wagschal A, Zhang Y, et al. Imprinting along the Kcnq1 domain on mouse chromosome 7 involves repressive histone methylation and recruitment of Polycomb group complexes. Nat Genet. 2004;36(12):1296–300.
113. Montgomery ND, Yee D, Chen A, Kalantry S, Chamberlain SJ, Otte AP, et al. The murine polycomb group protein Eed is required for global histone H3 lysine-27 methylation. Curr Biol. 2005;15(10): 942–7.
114. Cooper DW, VandeBerg JL, Sharman GB, Poole WE. Phosphoglycerate kinase polymorphism in kangaroos provides further evidence for paternal X inactivation. Nat New Biol. 1971;230(13):155–7.
115. Graves JA. Review: sex chromosome evolution and the expression of sex-specific genes in the placenta. Placenta. 2010;31(Suppl):S27–32.
116. Wagschal A, Feil R. Genomic imprinting in the placenta. Cytogenet Genome Res. 2006;113(1–4):90–8.
117. Hemberger M. Epigenetic landscape required for placental development. Cell Mol Life Sci. 2007; 64(18):2422–36.
118. Mak W, Nesterova TB, de Napoles M, Appanah R, Yamanaka S, Otte AP, et al. Reactivation of the paternal X chromosome in early mouse embryos. Science. 2004;303(5658):666–9.
119. Okamoto I, Otte AP, Allis CD, Reinberg D, Heard E. Epigenetic dynamics of imprinted X inactivation during early mouse development. Science. 2004; 303(5658):644–9.
120. Sado T, Fenner MH, Tan SS, Tam P, Shioda T, Li E. X inactivation in the mouse embryo deficient for Dnmt1: distinct effect of hypomethylation on imprinted and random X inactivation. Dev Biol. 2000;225(2):294–303.
121. Avner P, Heard E. X-chromosome inactivation: counting, choice and initiation. Nat Rev Genet. 2001;2(1):59–67.
122. Brockdorff N. X-chromosome inactivation: closing in on proteins that bind Xist RNA. Trends Genet. 2002;18(7):352–8.
123. Li E, Beard C, Forster AC, Bestor TH, Jaenisch R. DNA methylation, genomic imprinting, and mammalian development. Cold Spring Harb Symp Quant Biol. 1993;58:297–305.
124. Lee JT. Molecular links between X-inactivation and autosomal imprinting: X-inactivation as a driving force for the evolution of imprinting? Curr Biol. 2003;13(6):R242–54.
125. Reik W, Ferguson-Smith AC. Developmental biology: the X-inactivation yo-yo. Nature. 2005;438(7066): 297–8.
126. Li Y, Lemaire P, Behringer RR. Esx1, a novel X chromosome-linked homeobox gene expressed in mouse extraembryonic tissues and male germ cells. Dev Biol. 1997;188(1):85–95.
127. Lin TP, Labosky PA, Grabel LB, Kozak CA, Pitman JL, Kleeman J, et al. The Pem homeobox gene is X-linked and exclusively expressed in extraembryonic tissues during early murine development. Dev Biol. 1994;166(1):170–9.
128. Huynh KD, Lee JT. Inheritance of a pre-inactivated paternal X chromosome in early mouse embryos. Nature. 2003;426(6968):857–62.
129. Sado T, Ferguson-Smith AC. Imprinted X inactivation and reprogramming in the preimplantation mouse embryo. Hum Mol Genet. 2005;14(Spec No 1): R59–64.
130. Migeon BR, Do TT. In search of nonrandom X inactivation: studies of the placenta from newborns heterozygous for glucose-6-phosphate dehydrogenase. Basic Life Sci. 1978;12:379–91.
131. Looijenga LH, Gillis AJ, Verkerk AJ, van Putten WL, Oosterhuis JW. Heterogeneous X inactivation in trophoblastic cells of human full-term female placentas. Am J Hum Genet. 1999;64(5):1445–52.
132. Lee JT. Is X-chromosome inactivation a homology effect? Adv Genet. 2002;46:25–48.
133. Moreira de Mello JC, de Araujo ES, Stebellini R, Fraga AM, de Souza JE, Sumita DR, et al. Random X inactivation and extensive mosaicism in human placental revealed by analysis of allele-specific gene expression along the X chromosome. PLoS One. 2010;5(6):e10947.
134. Ropers HH, Wolff G, Hitzeroth HW. Preferential X inactivation in human placenta membranes: is the

paternal X inactive in early embryonic development of female mammals? Hum Genet. 1978;43(3):265–73.
135. Harrison KB, Warburton D. Preferential X-chromosome activity in human female placental tissues. Cytogenet Cell Genet. 1986;41(3):163–8.
136. Goto T, Wright E, Monk M. Paternal X-chromosome inactivation in human trophoblastic cells. Mol Hum Reprod. 1997;3(1):77–80.
137. Uehara S, Tamura M, Nata M, Ji G, Yaegashi N, Okamura K, et al. X-chromosome inactivation in the human trophoblast of early pregnancy. J Hum Genet. 2000;45(3):119–26.
138. Migeon BR, Axelman J, Jeppesen P. Differential X reactivation in human placental cells: implications for reversal of X inactivation. Am J Hum Genet. 2005;77(3):355–64.
139. Haig D, Graham C. Genomic imprinting and the strange case of the insulin-like growth factor II receptor. Cell. 1991;64(6):1045–6.
140. Moore T, Haig D. Genomic imprinting in mammalian development: a parental tug-of-war. Trends Genet. 1991;7(2):45–9.
141. Haig D, Westoby M. An earlier formulation of the genetic conflict hypothesis of genomic imprinting. Nat Genet. 2006;38(3):271.
142. Solter D. Imprinting. Int J Dev Biol. 1998;42(7):951–4.
143. Abu-Amero S, Monk D, Apostolidou S, Stanier P, Moore G. Imprinted genes and their role in human fetal growth. Cytogenet Genome Res. 2006;113(1–4):262–70.
144. Barlow DP. Gametic imprinting in mammals. Science. 1995;270(5242):1610–3.
145. Tilghman SM. The sins of the fathers and mothers: genomic imprinting in mammalian development. Cell. 1999;96(2):185–93.
146. Constancia M, Kelsey G, Reik W. Resourceful imprinting. Nature. 2004;432(7013):53–7.
147. McGrath J, Solter D. Completion of mouse embryogenesis requires both the maternal and paternal genomes. Cell. 1984;37(1):179–83.
148. Surani MA, Barton SC, Norris ML. Development of reconstituted mouse eggs suggests imprinting of the genome during gametogenesis. Nature. 1984;308(5959):548–50.
149. Ferguson-Smith AC, Cattanach BM, Barton SC, Beechey CV, Surani MA. Embryological and molecular investigations of parental imprinting on mouse chromosome 7. Nature. 1991;351(6328):667–70.
150. Leighton PA, Ingram RS, Eggenschwiler J, Efstratiadis A, Tilghman SM. Disruption of imprinting caused by deletion of the H19 gene region in mice. Nature. 1995;375(6526):34–9.
151. Gicquel C, Rossignol S, Cabrol S, Houang M, Steunou V, Barbu V, et al. Epimutation of the telomeric imprinting center region on chromosome 11p15 in Silver-Russell syndrome. Nat Genet. 2005;37(9):1003–7.
152. Ludwig T, Eggenschwiler J, Fisher P, D'Ercole AJ, Davenport ML, Efstratiadis A. Mouse mutants lacking the type 2 IGF receptor (IGF2R) are rescued from perinatal lethality in Igf2 and Igf1r null backgrounds. Dev Biol. 1996;177(2):517–35.
153. Frank D, Fortino W, Clark L, Musalo R, Wang W, Saxena A, et al. Placental overgrowth in mice lacking the imprinted gene Ipl. Proc Natl Acad Sci USA. 2002;99(11):7490–5.
154. Apostolidou S, Abu-Amero S, O'Donoghue K, Frost J, Olafsdottir O, Chavele KM, et al. Elevated placental expression of the imprinted PHLDA2 gene is associated with low birth weight. J Mol Med. 2007;85(4):379–87.
155. Castrillon DH, Sun D, Weremowicz S, Fisher RA, Crum CP, Genest DR. Discrimination of complete hydatidiform mole from its mimics by immunohistochemistry of the paternally imprinted gene product p57KIP2. Am J Surg Pathol. 2001;25(10):1225–30.
156. Fukunaga M. Immunohistochemical characterization of p57(KIP2) expression in early hydatidiform moles. Hum Pathol. 2002;33(12):1188–92.
157. Monk D, Arnaud P, Frost J, Hills FA, Stanier P, Feil R, et al. Reciprocal imprinting of human GRB10 in placental trophoblast and brain: evolutionary conservation of reversed allelic expression. Hum Mol Genet. 2009;18(16):3066–74.
158. Charalambous M, Smith FM, Bennett WR, Crew TE, Mackenzie F, Ward A. Disruption of the imprinted Grb10 gene leads to disproportionate overgrowth by an Igf2-independent mechanism. Proc Natl Acad Sci USA. 2003;100(14):8292–7.
159. Charalambous M, Cowley M, Geoghegan F, Smith FM, Radford EJ, Marlow BP, et al. Maternally-inherited Grb10 reduces placental size and efficiency. Dev Biol. 2010;337(1):1–8.
160. Ou-Yang RJ, Hui P, Yang XJ, Zynger DL. Expression of glypican 3 in placental site trophoblastic tumor. Diagn Pathol. 2010;5:64.
161. Han VK, Bassett N, Walton J, Challis JR. The expression of insulin-like growth factor (IGF) and IGF-binding protein (IGFBP) genes in the human placenta and membranes: evidence for IGF-IGFBP interactions at the feto-maternal interface. J Clin Endocrinol Metab. 1996;81(7):2680–93.

Genetic Basis of Gestational Trophoblastic Disease

3

Pei Hui

Keywords
Genetic basis of GTD • Genomic imprinting of GTD

Introduction

Related to various trophoblastic cells within the placenta, gestational trophoblastic disease (GTD) consists of a distinct group of proliferative disorders that have unique clinical settings, genetic compositions, and varying biological behaviors. Recent laboratory investigations of biomarker expression have delineated the cellular pathways of differentiation related to each of the entities of GTDs (Fig. 3.1) [1]. The most common hydatidiform moles are proliferative lesions of cells recapitulating chorionic villous trophoblasts. Gestational choriocarcinoma is a fully malignant tumor with proliferating cells recapitulating previllous trophoblasts of the developing placenta. The lesional cells of placental site trophoblastic tumor (PSTT) and exaggerated placental site reaction have cytological features resembling intermediate trophoblasts at the implantation site, whereas epithelioid trophoblastic tumor (ETT) and placental site nodule have proliferating cells resembling intermediate trophoblasts at the chorionic laeve. Biologically, the androgenetic nature of hydatidiform moles clearly indicates that an excessive paternal genome plays an important role in the development of these conditions, likely through an altered genomic imprinting. Recent linkage studies identified mutations of NALP7 on 19q13.4 as causal events in the development of familial biparental complete hydatidiform mole. Future investigations into the biological aspects of NALP7 gene alterations may hold the key to unlock the mystery as how altered genomic imprinting and related gene expression result in the phenotype of diandric hydatidiform mole in general. Recent findings of the preferential requirement of paternal X chromosome by several trophoblastic tumors suggest a unique genetic factor that may render a growth advantage to the neoplastic trophoblasts.

Androgenetic Nature of Hydatidiform Moles

Molecular and genetic investigations in the 1970s were pivotal to understanding the etiology of hydatidiform moles [2–4]. Using direct chromosomal preparations of fresh chorionic villi from

P. Hui, MD, PhD (✉)
Department of Pathology, Yale University School of Medicine, 310 Cedar Street, 254B New Haven, CT 06520-8023, USA
e-mail: pei.hui@yale.edu

P. Hui (ed.), *Gestational Trophoblastic Disease: Diagnostic and Molecular Genetic Pathology*, Current Clinical Pathology, DOI 10.1007/978-1-61779-394-3_3,

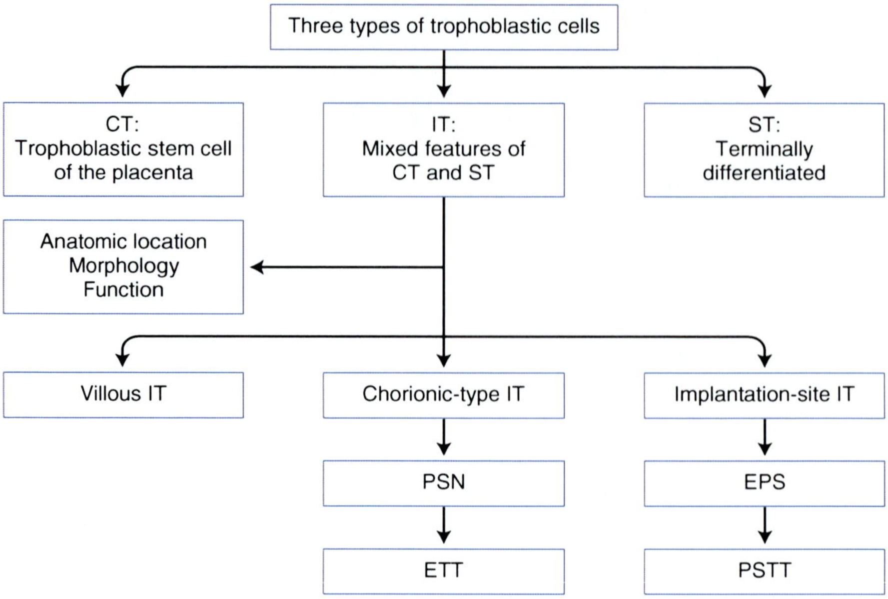

Fig. 3.1 Lineage differentiation of gestational trophoblastic disease (Courtesy of Dr. Katja Gwin, MD, University of Chicago). *CT* cytotrophoblast; *IT* intermediate trophoblast; *ST* syncytiotrophoblast; *PSN* placental site nodule; *ETT* epithelioid trophoblastic tumor; *EPS* exaggerated implantation site; *PSTT* placental site trophoblastic tumor

molar samples and Q- or R-banding analyses, Kajii observed repeatedly paternal homozygosity of the homologous chromosomes in complete moles [2, 5]. The androgenetic nature of complete moles was quickly confirmed by other studies using various approaches including HLA polymorphism typing, isoenzyme, and restriction fragment length polymorphisms (RFLP) [6–9]. In all complete moles except a rare subset of biparental ones, the cellular components inherit an androgenic-only nuclear genome and a maternal-only mitochondrial DNA [10–12], with either 46, XX diploid karyotypes arising from fertilization of an enucleated egg by one spermatozoon followed by duplication (homozygous, 80–90%), or 46 XX or XY karyotypes arising from simultaneous fertilization of an enucleated egg by two spermatozoa (heterozygous, 10–20%) [3, 5, 7, 13, 14]. The mechanism of how the ovum loses its maternal haploid genome is largely unclear. Initially, it was thought that complete moles are the result of fertilization of an ovum where the maternal nucleus is either eliminated or inactivated as a polar body [2, 15]. The current prevailing hypothesis indicates that the pathogenesis of complete mole involves fertilization of an empty ovum (null genome) by a haploid sperm with duplications of the sperm DNA to reconstitute a diploid genome in the majority of the cases [7]. The remaining complete moles arise from fertilization of an empty ovum (null genome) either by a diploid sperm resulting from failure of the second meiotic division [7] or, a more favored mechanism, by two independent haploid sperms [16]. The existence of a small subset of biparental complete mole points to a different pathogenesis, however (see the following). A complete hydatidiform mole does not support embryonic development but sustains a hyperplastic proliferation of the placental trophoblasts.

The genetic profile of partial hydatidiform moles is triploid with a diandric, monogynic genome arising from fertilization of a haploid egg by either two heterozygous spermatozoa (heterozygous, 90%) or one spermatozoon with duplication (homozygous, 10%) [17, 18]. Rare tetraploid partial moles have also been reported, with three haploid paternal chromosome sets and a 92XXXX, 92XXYY, or 92XXXY karyotype [19, 20]. Studies of rare tetraploid partial moles with a 92,XXXY karyotype by chromosomal heteromorphisms, isoenzymes, and RFLPs

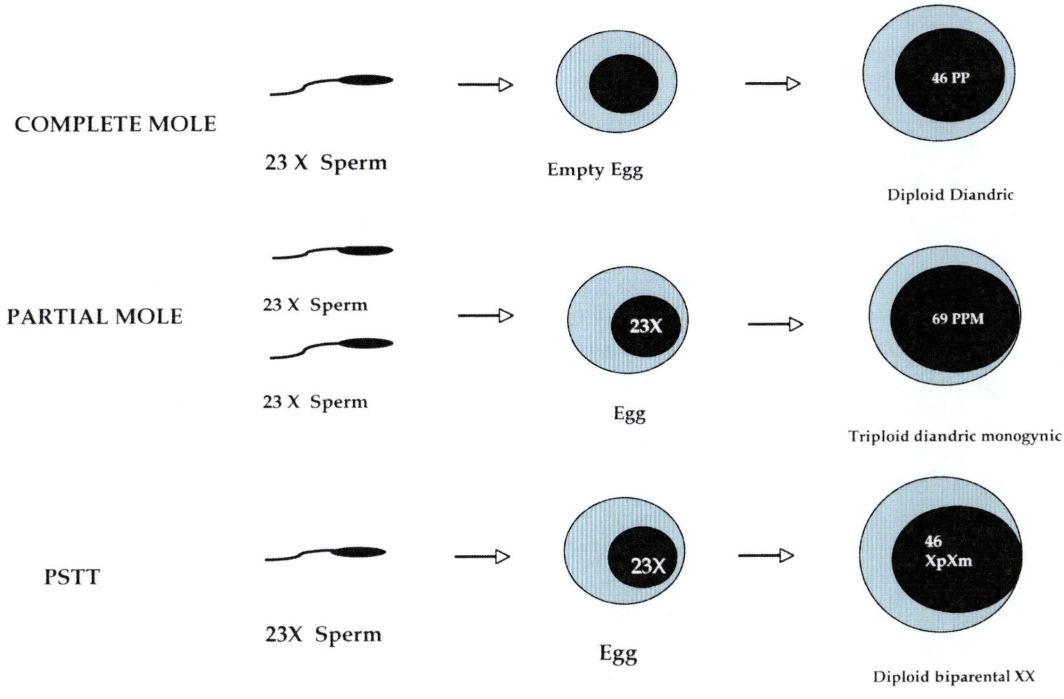

Fig. 3.2 Genetic composition of hydatidiform moles and proposed genetic requirement by PSTT

revealed a combination of a haploid ovum with three haploid sets of paternal chromosomes either by the mechanism of trispermy (involving three separate haploid spermatozoa) or through dispermy (involving one haploid and one diploid sperm) [19]. It is important to realize that non-molar triploids have an extra set of chromosomes derived from the mother [18], and they do not have the biological, histological, and clinical characteristics of diandric monogynic partial mole. Diploid partial moles probably do not exist, although some early reports raised the possibility because of the presence of fetal red blood cells and/or fetal tissues [21–23]. A study of a larger series of putative diploid partial moles revealed that the majority of the cases were misclassified by morphological examination, while the rest of cases proved to be triploid up on repeat ploidy analysis [21]. Additional discussion of the genetic aspects of partial mole can be found in chapter 5.

It is important to emphasize that the presence of an excess paternal genome is the key genetic element in the pathogenesis of both complete and partial hydatidiform moles (Fig. 3.2).

Genomic Imprinting and Hydatidiform Moles

Pronuclear transfer experiments in early 1980s implied that the hyperplastic nature of complete mole is a result of excess paternal genome representation in the ovum [24–26]. Mouse embryos with two female pronuclei had abnormally underdeveloped extraembryonic placental issue, whereas, those with only two male pronuclei (reminiscent to the genome of a homozygous complete mole), although the embryo failed to develop, produced hyperplastic placental tissue morphologically similar to that of complete mole [25]. These findings suggested that the maternal genome is important for the embryonic development, while the paternal genome is essential for the development of extraembryonic tissue, that is, the placenta, supporting the theory of "parental conflict of interest" of genomic imprinting (see Chap. 2). A disruption of the normal, balanced genomic imprinting in gestation may result in abnormal trophoblastic proliferation leading to molar pregnancy.

With their obvious lack (complete mole) or relatively deficiency (partial mole) of maternal genome, abnormal genomic imprinting has long been implicated in the development of hydatidiform moles. The genetic composition of hydatidiform moles suggests that the excessive trophoblastic proliferation is due to the expression of two doses of paternally imprinted genes. The absence of an embryo in complete moles may be related to the absence of imprinted, maternal gene expression. Consistent with the "parental conflict interest" theory, a lack of the maternal genome together with a global genome demethylation and abnormal paternal imprinting gene expression are key molecular features of complete hydatidiform mole. IGF2 and H19 tightly linked on human chromosome 11 are of special interest because of their reciprocal imprinting and association with GTD. Normally, IGF2 gene is expressed from the paternal allele [27, 28], whereas H19 gene is expressed from the maternal allele [29–31]. Although double representation of the paternal genome may be a prerequisite for the pathogenesis of complete moles, the trophoblast expresses abnormally both IGF2 (normally expressed only from paternal alleles) and H19 (normally expressed only from maternal alleles) [32–34], suggesting a failure of allele-specific gene expression in CHM. It has been suggested that a mutated promoter is responsible for overcoming transcriptional suppression by imprinting control of H19 gene [35]. However, such imprinting alteration is selective because retention of other paternal imprinted genes, that is, p57, exists [36, 37]. It has also been suggested that abnormal expression of imprinted genes in trophoblasts may be connected to the global genome demethylation [38] that occurs only in trophoblastic cells of complete moles. Therefore, the pathogenesis of androgenic complete hydatidiform moles is likely to involve, in addition to a loss of maternal genome, the combination of gain of paternal expression of imprinted genes and additional alterations of epigenetic gene silencing through global genome demethylation.

Alterations of genomic imprinting are not unique to molar gestations and have been implicated in the development of other GTDs including gestational choriocarcinoma, a bona fide malignant tumor [39]. Choriocarcinoma, which may develop from complete hydatidiform mole, showed similar expression of IGF2 and enhanced expression of H19, although a biallelic expression of IGF2 or H19 was not consistently found [33–35]. Limited data have suggested that there is a lack of correlation between IGF2 and H19 imprinting status, and in fact, the imprinting status of H19 and IGF2 was found differentially modulated, indicating that allele-specific expression of IGF2 operates in the absence of a parental imprint in choriocarcinoma [40].

The implication of altered genomic imprinting in the pathogenesis of mole has been extensively investigated recently in a small subset of familial biparental complete mole (FBCM) at genetic and molecular levels [41]. Familial recurrent complete moles occur with a frequency of 0.6–2.57% of all hydatidiform moles [42, 43], among which FBCM is an exceptional condition. Initially reported 30 years ago, Ambani described recurrent moles in multiple pregnancies of sisters in three unrelated families [44]. Additional cases were reported thereafter [45, 46]. Helwani successfully performed a genetic study on eight independent moles occurring in two sisters from a large consanguineous Lebanese family. Karyotyping and genotyping results revealed a diploid and biparental constitution in seven of the eight analyzed moles, suggesting a common mechanism underlying the etiology of these molar pregnancies in the family [47]. Fisher reported three recurrent complete moles in a patient, and all had biparental genomic contributions. Two of the three had even different male partners' genomes with two moles being XX and one XY [48]. At present, up to 21 families of FBCM have been reported in the literature [49].

A thorough review in 2004 by Fisher indicated that the clinical sequelae of biparental complete moles are similar to conventional diandric complete mole [50]. Although the genome of familial biparental moles is contributed by both parents, gene expression patterns are also found similar to those seen in androgenetic complete moles [51]. These findings together with the imprinting theory have supported the hypothesis that the causative alteration in FBCM would involve imprinted genes and/or their expression. Methylation studies of imprinted genes in biparental mole found that there is acquisition of paternal methylation patterns by the maternal alleles [52]. Additional study by the same group suggested that the abnormal methylation in familial biparental molar tissues was acquired de novo in the patients' germline as a result of a false reprogramming during the postzygotic development of the conceptuses [53]. Patients with FBCM showed a pattern of failure to acquire or maintain DNA methylation at DMRs (PEG3, SNRPN, KCNQ1OT1, GNAS exon 1A) that normally acquire CpG methylation during oogenesis, but not at H19, which acquires CpG methylation during spermatogenesis [54], suggesting the presence of a complex pattern of imprinting abnormalities in FBCM tissues [55] [41]. It has been proposed that genetic alterations in biparental complete mole result in abnormal genomic imprinting to shut down maternal gene expression during oogenesis, leading to the expression of alleles only [41, 56].

Genetic linkage studies of patients with familial biparental mole by Moglabey initially identified an abnormal locus on 19q13.3–14.4 [57], which was soon confirmed by Sensi's studies of FBCMs in two sisters of an Italian family [58]. Further genetic refinement and physical mapping of a biparental complete mole by Hodges narrowed the locus to chromosome 19q13.4 region [59]. The candidate region of 19q13.4 contains several Kruppel-type zinc finger genes with functions of transcription regulation of downstream genes [60]. Since these zinc finger genes involve silencing the imprinted H19–Igf2 axis, it was suggested that alterations of the Kruppel-type zinc finger gene locus on 19q13.4 deregulate the normal imprinting control, leading to a global imprinting alteration, responsible for the pathogenesis of FBCMs [61]. Instead of finding a zinc finger gene, however, subsequent analysis of candidate genes on 19q13.4 led to Murdoch's discovery of NALP7/NLRP7 (nucleotide-binding, leucine-rich repeat, pyrin domains) gene in 2006 [62], of which homozygous or compound heterozygous mutations have been found in the majority of FBCM as causative events of the disease (FRHM) [49, 54, 62, 63].

NALP7 is one of 14 NALP proteins, a large subfamily of the CATERPILLER protein family involved in intracellular regulation of bacterial-induced inflammation [62]. NALP7 contains an amino-terminal PYRIN domain involved in protein–protein interaction, a NACHT domain, found in neuronal apoptosis inhibitor proteins and in those involved in major histocompatibility complex (MHC) class II transactivation and caspase-recruitment proteins, a nuclear localization signal (NLS) present within the NACHT domain and a leucine-rich repeat (LRR) domain essential for nuclear transport, cell cycle regulation, mitotic spindle formation, and postmitotic nuclear envelope reorganization. The normal expression of the NALP7 gene is autosomal recessive and is transcribed in unfertilized oocyte at or before meiosis I. NALP7 gene is also transcribed in the endometrium. NALP7 is the first maternal effect gene (genes that are expressed in the oocyte to support embryonic development until activation of the embryonic genome occurs) identified in human and is also responsible for recurrent spontaneous abortions [62]. Recent epigenetic and mutational analyses of FBCM patients from 11 families revealed methylation defect(s) at some imprinted loci, and biallelic NLRP7 mutations were found in almost all families of FBCM [56]. Different mutations were identified, and missense mutations were found to be clustered in the leucine-rich region (LRR) [64]. It is interesting that NLRP7 mutations preferentially affect female reproduction but not male reproduction [64]. Contrary to what was hoped to find a causal genetic defect related to DNA imprinting, as a member of the CATERPILLER protein family, the principle function of NALP7 is to mediate inflammatory response through activation of proinflammatory caspases (CASP1) and apoptotic pathways [62]. Women heterozygous for NALP7 mutations are at risk for reproductive wastage without manifestation of a molar phenotype [63]. One hypothesis is that defects of NALP7 regulation of cytokine secretion (e.g., interleukin-1beta) may cause alterations in folliculogenesis, ovulation, blastocyst implantation, and trophoblast biology [49]. Another recent suggestion is that NALP7 plays a role in controlling the timing of oocyte growth or in transducing signals for the initiation of imprint establishment [56]. However, exactly how NALP7/NLRP7 mutations result in familial biparental moles is largely unclear. Conventional androgenic complete moles are unlikely caused by NALP7 mutations. Further investigations of NALP7 alterations in FBCM may eventually elucidate the key converging molecular event that underscores the pathogenesis of complete hydatidiform mole of both androgenetic and biparental nature.

Genetic Basis of Gestational Trophoblastic Tumors

Gestational Trophoblastic Tumors

Tumors arising from extraembryonic tissues are rare and include gestational choriocarcinoma and intermediate trophoblastic tumors, that is, PSTT and ETT. In oncology, these tumors are extraordinary with respect to their fetal origin (semi-allograft) and the maternal tissue matrix (endomyometrium) that supports their growth. These tumors have variably clinical behaviors with choriocarcinoma as one of the most malignant tumors in human if untreated [65]. PSTT and ETT are very rare neoplastic proliferations of extravillous intermediate trophoblasts at the implantation site or at chorionic laeve, respectively (Fig. 3.1) [1, 66, 67]. The clinical presentation of PSTT and ETT generally involves a young woman who has a history of full-term pregnancy, abortion or uncommonly, complete mole. As a whole, however, our understanding of the pathogenesis of these tumors is lacking, largely due to their rarity.

Preferential Requirement of Paternal X Chromosome in Placental Site Trophoblast Tumor

During conception, tissue having paternally derived genetic material is implanted in the female uterus. Rarely, this event leads to the development of a disease in the mother in the form of GTD. PSTT has been proposed as a neoplastic proliferation of trophoblasts with morphological and biological features of extravillous (intermediate) trophoblasts at the implantation site. It is a true neoplastic proliferation with invasion into the maternal endomyometrium, of which the normal immunologic barriers to the overgrowth of allogeneic tissues are overcome. In this respect, PSTT is similar to two other forms of proliferative gestational diseases, that is, partial and complete hydatidiform moles, in which distinctive chromosomal abnormalities have long been recognized [2, 3] as discussed earlier. The question can be asked whether the pathogenesis of the trophoblastic tumor may also require a certain genetic prerequisite. At the cytogenetic level, most trophoblastic tumors (PSTT and choriocarcinoma) analyzed were diploid [68–70]. Most of PSTTs showed only rare genetic imbalances analyzed by comparative genomic hybridization (Fig. 3.3) [71]. Interestingly, a recurrent gain of chromosome 22q12 was found in two of four cases of PSTT, but not in three cases of ETTs [72, 73]. Comparative genomic hybridization investigation of 12 cases of gestational choriocarcinoma found consistently deletions at 8p (five cases) and amplifications at 7q (four cases) [74].

One would expect, a priori, gestational trophoblastic tumors to occur with equal frequency after male and female conceptuses. A decade ago, a review of 72 cases of PSTT in the literature [75] identified 21 cases with detailed clinical and pathology information regarding the sex of the antecedent gestations, among which 18 had a female antecedent gestation by history [75] and was confirmed by DNA analysis in four cases [76, 77]. In one case, in which the preceding gestational event was a complete mole, the DNA analyses confirmed that the tumor indeed arose from the mole and harbored two androgenic X chromosomes [76]. Only two patients who developed PSTT had an antecedent delivery of male infant by history [78, 79]. A single case was reported to suggest the presence of a Y chromosome upon genetic analysis, although the antecedent gestation was female and Southern blots using five

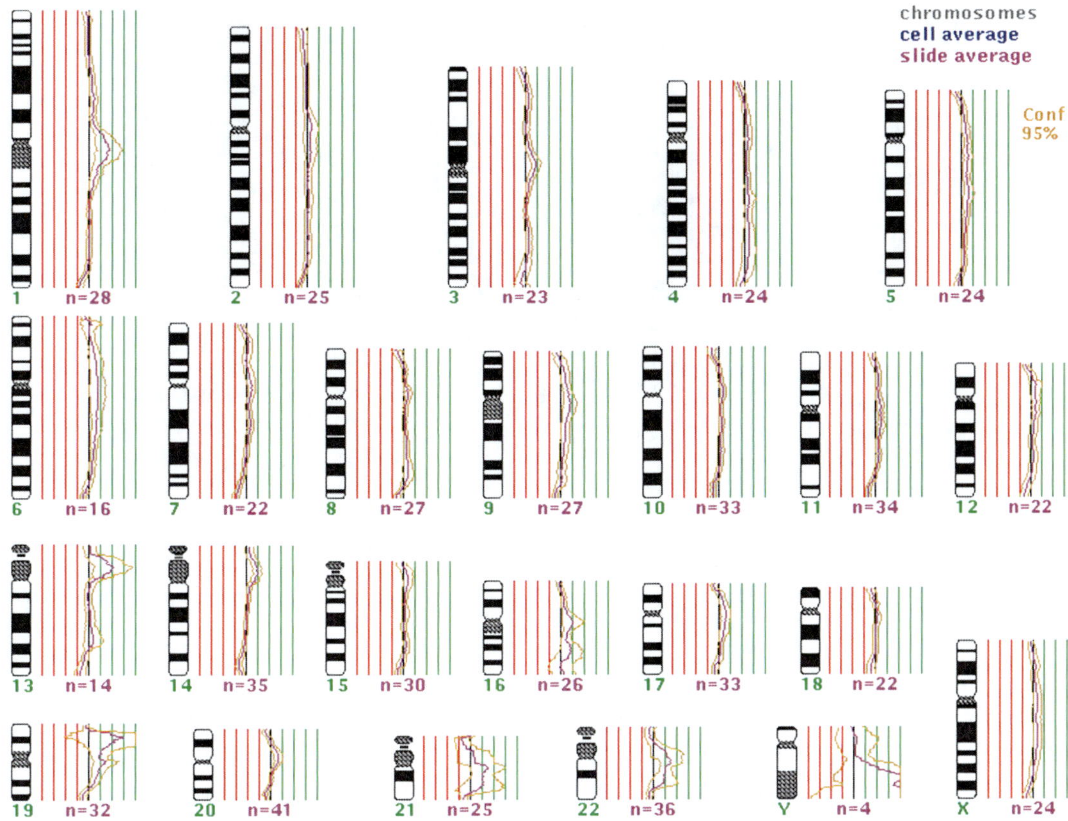

Fig. 3.3 Comparative genomic hybridization profile of PSTT. Note the presence of general balanced chromosomal profiles except regional gains at 21q21 and 22q1 in this particular case. (Modern Pathology 17:248, 2004)

autosomal RFLP markers showed that the tumor DNA had identical hybridization patterns to DNA from the patient's second daughter [80].

One early investigation into the sex chromosomal component of PSTT by analyzing the human androgen receptor gene identified the presence of a paternal X chromosome in four of five cases. An absence of a Y chromosomal element was consistently observed in all five PSTTs by the semi-nested PCR amplification of SRY (human sex-determining region on the Y chromosome) (Fig. 3.4) [75]. Four other cases of PSTT in the literature had, by molecular analysis, an XX female chromosomal composition [76, 77, 81]. Overall, 89% of the cases (23 of 26) showed a XX genome either by history or by genetic analysis [75]. Since then, additional case reports of PSTT have been published and, again, a female antecedent pregnancy was documented in 12 out of 14 cases [82, 83]. One cell line from a PSTT was established and confirmed by karyotyping to have XX genome. [84]. However, the results of our investigations were in contrast to that of a genetic analysis of 23 PSTTs, in which 50% of PSTTs were found to contain a Y chromosome [85]. In this paper, the detection of the Y chromosome was performed by amplifying the SRY locus using DNA material extracted from paraffin-embedded formalin-fixed tissues, a single 50 cycle-PCR amplification followed by gel electrophoresis. However, such a technical approach likely carried the risk of PCR artifacts due to the high cycle number and potential amplification of contaminating template [85, 86].

To definitively resolve the issue, a multi-institutional study was taken to investigate\ 20 new cases of PSTT by the highly accurate

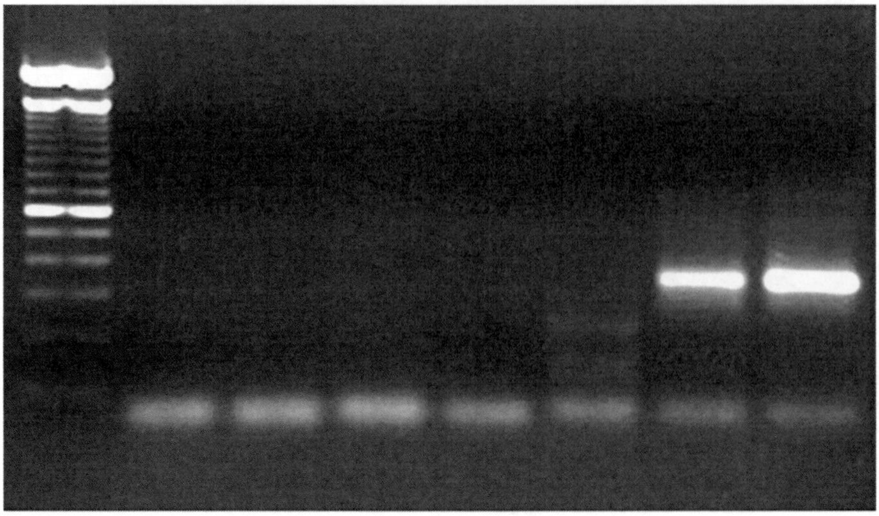

Fig. 3.4 Absence of Y chromosomal element in five cases of PSTT analyzed by semi-nested PCR analysis of SRY gene (Laboratory Investigation 80:965, 2000)

microsatellite genotyping method using the AmpFlSTR® Identifiler™ PCR Amplification Assay. The assay consists of one multiplex PCR that amplifies 15 tetranucleotide microsatellite loci plus the amelogenin locus shared by the X and Y chromosomes. The small products generated from the X and Y amelogenin alleles permit efficient analysis of DNA template extracted from formalin-fixed paraffin-embedded tissue. In conjunction with capillary electrophoresis, which precisely sizes the two X and Y PCR products, this approach ensures a highly consistent and reliable assessment of sex chromosome status. Using this STR genotype platform, the presence of XX genome was consistently observed in all 20 cases of PSTT in this largest series (Fig. 3.5) [87]. Combined results from other two studies confirmed the presence of a haploid paternal set of chromosomes in all PSTTs and an absence of Y chromosomal element. A more recent paper approached the issue using polymorphism analysis at amelogenin, PRKX/PRKY and ZFX/ZFY loci. Of 15 cases of PSTT, an absence of Y chromosome element was observed in 14 cases [86]. The remaining one case was reported to have a detectable Y chromosomal allele. It is of interest that the detectable amplification of the Y chromosomal allele in this case was minimal in comparison with that of the X allele, again raising concerns for tissue or PCR amplicon cross-contamination [86]. It is of great interest, however, that this recent study revealed also a shortfall of Y chromosome in gestational choriocarcinoma and ETT [86], suggesting a general genetic prerequisite for all gestational trophoblastic tumors.

Overall, the results of these molecular investigations imply that the presence of a paternal X chromosome is associated with the neoplastic proliferation of PSTTs. One simple explanation is that PSTT may arise from a persistent lesional tissue of an antecedent complete hydatidiform mole, a much more common GTD with uniparental disomy of the paternal genome and an exclusive paternal X chromosome. Such a view was based on the assumption that 5% of complete moles (dispermic with 46XY chromosomal compliment) will progress to gestational choriocarcinoma, leading to the small percentage of choriocarcinoma with a Y chromosome [86]. In one previous study [75], indeed, a PSTT was proven to have developed from an antecedent homozygous a complete mole [76]. However, only a small percentage (7–10%) of PSTTs have been reported to follow a complete mole [75, 76, 88]. An assumption that many complete moles

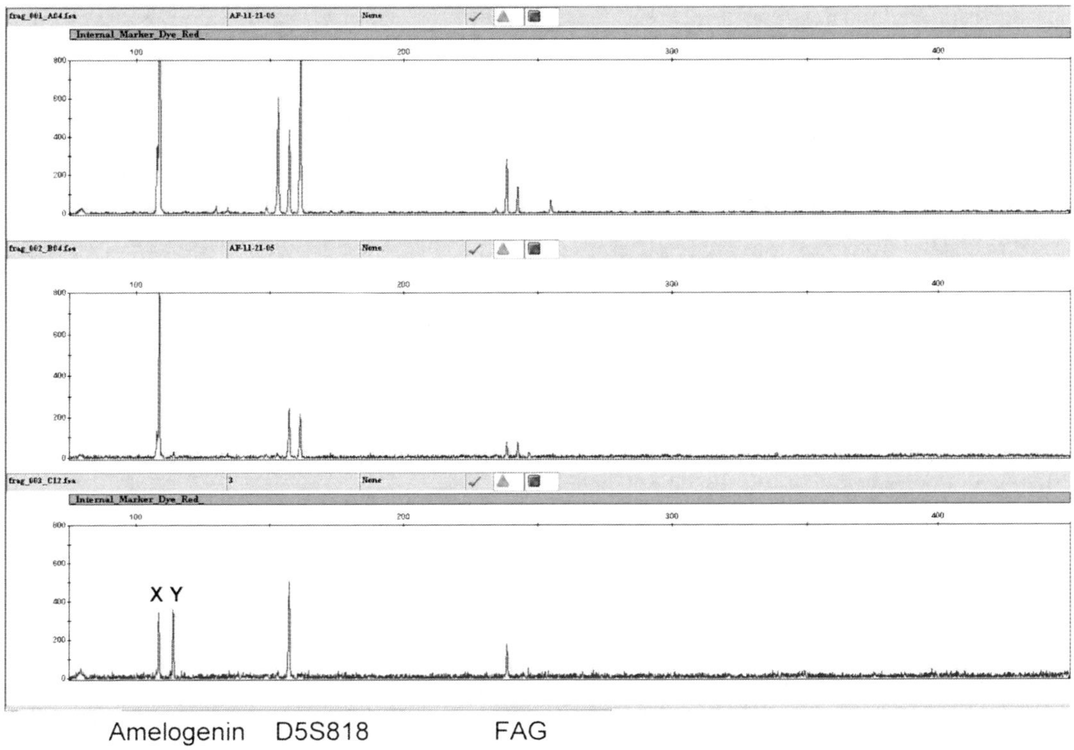

Fig. 3.5 Absence of Y chromosomal allele at the amelogenin locus in PSTT. AmpFlSTR® Identifiler™ PCR amplifies the amelogenin, D5S818 and FGA (alpha fibrinogen) tetranucleotide polymorphic loci in PSTT (upper panel), paired normal myometrium (middle panel), and unrelated, normal male control tissue (lower panel). The PCR products were analyzed by capillary electrophoresis (*Y*-axis – fluorescence intensity of labeled product and *X*-axis – PCR product size in base pairs). The tumor demonstrates paternal alleles at D5S818 and FAG loci together with the maternal alleles detected in the paired myometrium. Normal male control sample shows both X and Y products (107 and 113 base pairs, respectively) at the amelogenin locus, while only the X product is seen in the tumor and paired myometrium

are under-recognized, and most of PSTT primarily arise from a prior complete mole [86] can not be justified [89–91]. Alternatively, the paternal X chromosome may play an important, active role in the pathogenesis of PSTT (Fig. 3.2) [87].

Genomic Imprinting and Paternal X Chromosome Requirement in Trophoblastic Tumors

Epigenetic imprinting, the selective suppression of various genes derived from one parent or the other, has been proposed to be an important regulatory mechanism in the development of the placenta in eutherian mammals (for details see Chap. 2). The "parental conflict hypothesis" views that parents of opposite sex have conflicting interests in allocating resources to their offspring by the mother [92–95]. The intent of the paternal genome would be to maximize resources for the father's own progeny. In contrast, the interest of the maternal genome would be to distribute resources equally among the offspring. This implies that growth-promoting genes are mainly expressed from the paternally inherited genome and are silent in the maternally inherited counterpart. Analyses of many imprinted genes in mammals support this theory [96, 97]. X chromosome inactivation plays a central role in compensation for the double dose of X-linked genes in cells of a female relative to cells of a male. The paternal X chromosome is preferentially imprinted and silent in mouse trophectoderm [98–104], a tissue type corresponding to that from which PSTT and hydatidiform moles arise in humans. In marsupial mammals, the paternal X chromosome is preferentially inactivated in all lineages [105, 106]. The paternal X chromosome is preferentially imprinted and silent in mouse trophectoderm, and genes on the X chromosome are expressed only from the maternal alleles (see Chap. 2). Therefore, in mouse placenta, X chromosome inactivation represents a special form of genomic imprinting, that is, imprinted X chromosome inactivation.

In theory, imprinted X inactivation may have co-evolved with genomic imprinting when placental mammals emerged as discussed in Chap. 2 [107]. Existing study results indicate there are X chromosome-linked, genetically imprinted genes that specifically regulate the development of extraembryonic tissues [100, 108], and that the X chromosome inactivation in an XX embryo is crucial to the development of normal extraembryonic tissue [25]. In mice, the paternally derived X chromosome is preferentially inactivated in the primitive trophectoderm cell lineages [109]. Epigenetic regulation of gene expression through imprinting and its implication in placental development and trophoblastic tumorigenesis have drawn great attention recently. Somatic chromosomal imprinting studies suggest that uniparental gene expression can function as cancer predisposing and/or initiating events [110].

Considering all the information available it has been hypothesized that PSTT is a neoplastic condition of the extraembryonic trophoblast of an antecedent female conceptus, and a paternal X chromosome is necessary for the neoplastic transformation. The paternal X chromosome may be involved in this tumor in two possible ways. One is that in PSTT, paternal X chromosome harbors a dominant oncogene, although another is that the tumorigenesis results from an abnormal dosage of functional X chromosomes. Although no definitive candidate oncogenes exist, possibilities include Esx1[100], Pem [101], MYCL2 [111], and IAP [112]. Further studies are needed to substantiate the involvement of any of these genes in PSTT. However, because PSTT is an extremely rare neoplasm while female conceptuses harboring a paternal X chromosome are extremely common, the hypothesis of a dominant oncogene on the paternal X chromosome would require either mutational activation of such a gene, or one or more cooperating oncogenic events. In addition, there exists no published data to support a familial susceptibility to PSTT. The contention that the paternal X chromosome of PSTT harbors a dominant oncogene would require that this X chromosome be active. The presence of an active (hypomethylated) AR locus of paternal X chromosome in one prior study is of interest and requires further investigations (Fig. 3.6) [75].

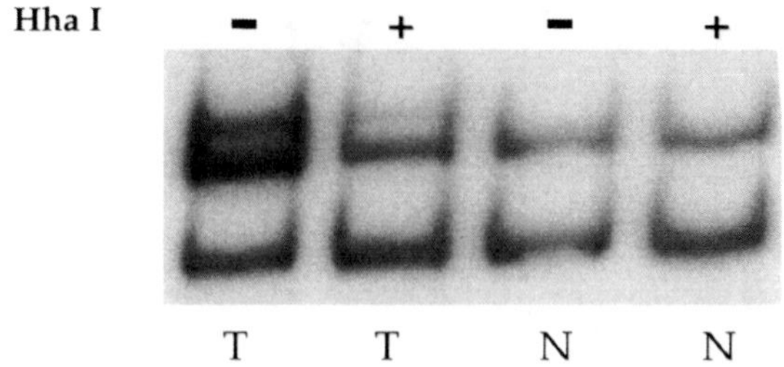

Fig. 3.6 Presence of an active paternal X chromosome in PSTT (methylation sensitive analysis at the HUMARA locus). The unique paternal X allele present in PSTT (top band in first 2 lanes) is preferentially digested by DNA methylation-sensitive enzyme Hha I (lane 2). *T*, tumor sample; *N*, maternal myometrial sample (Laboratory Investigation 80:965, 2000)

PSTT is perhaps another GTD whose pathogenesis requires unique genetic composition (Fig. 3.2) that may be related to placental imprinting. The unique chromosome composition of PSTT may reflect a role for abnormal gene dosage resulting in a proliferative advantage to the trophoblast. It has been demonstrated that the paternal genome is essential for the invasive and proliferative capacity of the placenta during early implantation [92, 113]. During the past decade, oncogenic genes have been discovered to transit from functional haploidy to diploidy through loss of imprinting [114]. Among autosomal genes, examples include H19 and IGF2 [115], which are paternally imprinted in extraembryonic tissue. This imprinting seems to be relaxed in trophoblast-derived choriocarcinoma and hydatidiform mole [116–118]. Considering the fact that X chromosomal imprinting is absolutely required for the development of mouse placental trophoblasts, relaxation of an imprinted paternal X in trophoblast would explain the requirement by PSTT as it will bring growth advantage according to the theory of parental conflict of interest. It has been intriguing that the mode of X inactivation appears random in human extraembryonic tissue by the most recent data [119, 120]. However, it remains possible that a relaxation of the X inactivation (random or imprinted) or inappropriate expression of paternal X-linked genes will result in double dosing of X chromosomal genes in trophectoderm leading to trophoblast hyperplasia and eventually PSTTs.

Perspectives

The introduction of imprinting genes and imprinted X chromosome inactivation during the evolution coincided with the appearance of eutherian mammals, leading to the first time that the fetal tissue came in to direct contact with maternal endomyometrium. Genomic imprinting and preferential X inactivation in placental trophoblasts likely regulate many of the complex biological interactions, and play important roles in the pathogenesis of some reproductive disorders, such as GTDs. Imprinting alterations leading to over-representation of the paternal genes in trophoblasts underline the development of hydatidiform moles. The propensity to malignancy of complete hydatidiform mole is likely associated with its genetic compositions, and the growth advantage conferred by the selective inheritance of the diandric-only genome. Paternal homozygosity would lead to an inactivation of tumor suppressor gene by a signal event occurring at the DNA level. Alternatively, paternal transmission of imprinted alleles would result in the silencing of particular tumor suppressor genes in a complete hydatidiform mole. The genetic requirement of an excess paternal genome is intriguing this and little is known about the mechanism of malignant transformation of trophoblasts. In-depth investigations of these aspects are important to understand the pathogenesis of hydatidiform moles, a rather common disease of human reproduction. As epigenetic regulation of X chromosome inactivation in trophectoderm has significant biological implications, PSTTs may provide an important tumor model with which the sex chromosome biology and the proliferative advantage conferred by paternal X chromosome in trophoblastic tumors may be further explored.

References

1. Shih IM, Kurman RJ. The pathology of intermediate trophoblastic tumors and tumor-like lesions. Int J Gynecol Pathol. 2001;20(1):31–47.
2. Kajii T, Ohama K. Androgenetic origin of hydatidiform mole. Nature. 1977;268(5621):633–4.
3. Szulman AE. Syndromes of hydatidiform moles. Partial vs. complete. J Reprod Med. 1984;29(11):788–91.
4. Vassilakos P, Riotton G, Kajii T. Hydatidiform mole: two entities. A morphologic and cytogenetic study with some clinical consideration. Am J Obstet Gynecol. 1977;127(2):167–70.
5. Kajii T. The road to diploid androgenesis (the Japan Society of Human Genetics award lecture). Jinrui Idengaku Zasshi. 1986;31(2):61–71.
6. Yamashita K, Wake N, Araki T, Ichinoe K, Makoto K. Human lymphocyte antigen expression in hydatidiform mole: androgenesis following fertilization by a haploid sperm. Am J Obstet Gynecol. 1979;135(5):597–600.
7. Jacobs PA, Wilson CM, Sprenkle JA, Rosenshein NB, Migeon BR. Mechanism of origin of complete hydatidiform moles. Nature. 1980;286(5774):714–6.
8. Lawler SD, Povey S, Fisher RA, Pickthall VJ. Genetic studies on hydatidiform moles. II. The origin of complete moles. Ann Hum Genet. 1982;46(Pt 3):209–22.
9. Hoshina M, Boothby MR, Hussa RD, Pattillo RA, Camel HM, Boime I. Segregation patterns of polymorphic restriction sites of the gene encoding the alpha subunit of human chorionic gonadotropin in trophoblastic disease. Proc Natl Acad Sci USA. 1984;81(8):2504–7.
10. Wallace DC, Surti U, Adams CW, Szulman AE. Complete moles have paternal chromosomes but maternal mitochondrial DNA. Hum Genet. 1982;61(2):145–7.
11. Edwards YH, Jeremiah SJ, McMillan SL, Povey S, Fisher RA, Lawler SD. Complete hydatidiform moles combine maternal mitochondria with a paternal nuclear genome. Ann Hum Genet. 1984;48(Pt 2):119–27.
12. Azuma C, Saji F, Tokugawa Y, Kimura T, Nobunaga T, Takemura M, et al. Application of gene amplification by polymerase chain reaction to genetic analysis

of molar mitochondrial DNA: the detection of anuclear empty ovum as the cause of complete mole. Gynecol Oncol. 1991;40(1):29–33.
13. Ohama K, Okamoto E, Nomura K, Fujiwara A, Fukuda Y. Genetic studies of hydatidiform mole with 46, XY karyotype (author's transl). Nippon Sanka Fujinka Gakkai Zasshi. 1981;33(10):1664–8.
14. Lipata F, Parkash V, Talmor M, Bell S, Chen S, Maric V, et al. Precise DNA genotyping diagnosis of hydatidiform mole. Obstet Gynecol. 2010;115(4):784–94.
15. Wake N, Takagi N, Sasaki M. Androgenesis as a cause of hydatidiform mole. J Natl Cancer Inst. 1978;60(1):51–7.
16. Sebire NJ, Fisher RA, Rees HC. Histopathological diagnosis of partial and complete hydatidiform mole in the first trimester of pregnancy. Pediatr Dev Pathol. 2003;6(1):69–77.
17. Lawler SD, Fisher RA, Pickthall VJ, Povey S, Evans MW. Genetic studies on hydatidiform moles. I. The origin of partial moles. Cancer Genet Cytogenet. 1982;5(4):309–20.
18. Jacobs PA, Szulman AE, Funkhouser J, Matsuura JS, Wilson CC. Human triploidy: relationship between parental origin of the additional haploid complement and development of partial hydatidiform mole. Ann Hum Genet. 1982;46(Pt 3):223–31.
19. Surti U, Szulman AE, Wagner K, Leppert M, O'Brien SJ. Tetraploid partial hydatidiform moles: two cases with a triple paternal contribution and a 92, XXXY karyotype. Hum Genet. 1986;72(1):15–21.
20. Sheppard DM, Fisher RA, Lawler SD, Povey S. Tetraploid conceptus with three paternal contributions. Hum Genet. 1982;62(4):371–4.
21. Genest DR, Ruiz RE, Weremowicz S, Berkowitz RS, Goldstein DP, Dorfman DM. Do nontriploid partial hydatidiform moles exist? A histologic and flow cytometric reevaluation of nontriploid specimens. J Reprod Med. 2002;47(5):363–8.
22. Paradinas FJ, Fisher RA, Browne P, Newlands ES. Diploid hydatidiform moles with fetal red blood cells in molar villi. 1–Pathology, incidence, and prognosis. J Pathol. 1997;181(2):183–8.
23. Fisher RA, Paradinas FJ, Soteriou BA, Foskett M, Newlands ES. Diploid hydatidiform moles with fetal red blood cells in molar villi. 2–Genetics. J Pathol. 1997;181(2):189–95.
24. Surani MA, Barton SC. Development of gynogenetic eggs in the mouse: implications for parthenogenetic embryos. Science. 1983;222(4627):1034–6.
25. McGrath J, Solter D. Completion of mouse embryogenesis requires both the maternal and paternal genomes. Cell. 1984;37(1):179–83.
26. Barton SC, Surani MA, Norris ML. Role of paternal and maternal genomes in mouse development. Nature. 1984;311(5984):374–6.
27. Ohlsson R, Nystrom A, Pfeifer-Ohlsson S, Tohonen V, Hedborg F, Schofield P, et al. IGF2 is parentally imprinted during human embryogenesis and in the Beckwith-Wiedemann syndrome. Nat Genet. 1993;4(1):94–7.
28. Giannoukakis N, Deal C, Paquette J, Goodyer CG, Polychronakos C. Parental genomic imprinting of the human IGF2 gene. Nat Genet. 1993;4(1):98–101.
29. Rachmilewitz J, Gileadi O, Eldar-Geva T, Schneider T, de Groot N, Hochberg A. Transcription of the H19 gene in differentiating cytotrophoblasts from human placenta. Mol Reprod Dev. 1992;32(3):196–202.
30. Zhang Y, Shields T, Crenshaw T, Hao Y, Moulton T, Tycko B. Imprinting of human H19: allele-specific CpG methylation, loss of the active allele in Wilms tumor, and potential for somatic allele switching. Am J Hum Genet. 1993;53(1):113–24.
31. Ferguson-Smith AC, Sasaki H, Cattanach BM, Surani MA. Parental-origin-specific epigenetic modification of the mouse H19 gene. Nature. 1993;362(6422): 751–5.
32. Mutter GL, Stewart CL, Chaponot ML, Pomponio RJ. Oppositely imprinted genes H19 and insulin-like growth factor 2 are coexpressed in human androgenetic trophoblast. Am J Hum Genet. 1993;53(5): 1096–102.
33. Wake N, Arima T, Matsuda T. Involvement of IGF2 and H19 imprinting in choriocarcinoma development. Int J Gynaecol Obstet. 1998;60 Suppl 1:S1–8.
34. Ariel I, de Groot N, Hochberg A. Imprinted H19 gene expression in embryogenesis and human cancer: the oncofetal connection. Am J Med Genet. 2000;91(1):46–50.
35. Arima T, Matsuda T, Takagi N, Wake N. Association of IGF2 and H19 imprinting with choriocarcinoma development. Cancer Genet Cytogenet. 1997;93(1): 39–47.
36. Fukunaga M. Immunohistochemical characterization of p57(KIP2) expression in early hydatidiform moles. Hum Pathol. 2002;33(12):1188–92.
37. Castrillon DH, Sun D, Weremowicz S, Fisher RA, Crum CP, Genest DR. Discrimination of complete hydatidiform mole from its mimics by immunohistochemistry of the paternally imprinted gene product p57KIP2. Am J Surg Pathol. 2001;25(10):1225–30.
38. Mann MR, Lee SS, Doherty AS, Verona RI, Nolen LD, Schultz RM, et al. Selective loss of imprinting in the placenta following preimplantation development in culture. Development. 2004;131(15):3727–35.
39. Hashimoto K, Azuma C, Koyama M, Ohashi K, Kamiura S, Nobunaga T, et al. Loss of imprinting in choriocarcinoma. Nat Genet. 1995;9(2):109–10.
40. He L, Cui H, Walsh C, Mattsson R, Lin W, Anneren G, et al. Hypervariable allelic expression patterns of the imprinted IGF2 gene in tumor cells. Oncogene. 1998;16(1):113–9.
41. Slim R, Mehio A. The genetics of hydatidiform moles: new lights on an ancient disease. Clin Genet. 2007;71(1):25–34.
42. Parazzini F, La Vecchia C, Franceschi S, Mangili G. Familial trophoblastic disease: case report. Am J Obstet Gynecol. 1984;149(4):382–3.
43. Sand PK, Lurain JR, Brewer JI. Repeat gestational trophoblastic disease. Obstet Gynecol. 1984;63(2): 140–4.

44. Ambani LM, Vaidya RA, Rao CS, Daftary SD, Motashaw ND. Familial occurrence of trophoblastic disease - report of recurrent molar pregnancies in sisters in three families. Clin Genet. 1980;18(1):27–9.
45. Sunde L, Vejerslev LO, Jensen MP, Pedersen S, Hertz JM, Bolund L. Genetic analysis of repeated, biparental, diploid, hydatidiform moles. Cancer Genet Cytogenet. 1993;66(1):16–22.
46. Seoud M, Khalil A, Frangieh A, Zahed L, Azar G, Nuwayri-Salti N. Recurrent molar pregnancies in a family with extensive intermarriage: report of a family and review of the literature. Obstet Gynecol. 1995;86(4 Pt 2):692–5.
47. Helwani MN, Seoud M, Zahed L, Zaatari G, Khalil A, Slim R. A familial case of recurrent hydatidiform molar pregnancies with biparental genomic contribution. Hum Genet. 1999;105(1–2):112–5.
48. Fisher RA, Khatoon R, Paradinas FJ, Roberts AP, Newlands ES. Repetitive complete hydatidiform mole can be biparental in origin and either male or female. Hum Reprod. 2000;15(3):594–8.
49. Williams D, Hodgetts V, Gupta J. Recurrent hydatidiform moles. Eur J Obstet Gynecol Reprod Biol. 2010;150(1):3–7.
50. Fisher RA, Hodges MD, Newlands ES. Familial recurrent hydatidiform mole: a review. J Reprod Med. 2004;49(8):595–601.
51. Fisher RA, Hodges MD, Rees HC, Sebire NJ, Seckl MJ, Newlands ES, et al. The maternally transcribed gene p57(KIP2) (CDNK1C) is abnormally expressed in both androgenetic and biparental complete hydatidiform moles. Hum Mol Genet. 2002;11(26): 3267–72.
52. El-Maarri O, Seoud M, Coullin P, Herbiniaux U, Oldenburg J, Rouleau G, et al. Maternal alleles acquiring paternal methylation patterns in biparental complete hydatidiform moles. Hum Mol Genet. 2003;12(12):1405–13.
53. El-Maarri O, Seoud M, Riviere JB, Oldenburg J, Walter J, Rouleau G, et al. Patients with familial biparental hydatidiform moles have normal methylation at imprinted genes. Eur J Hum Genet. 2005; 13(4):486–90.
54. Kou YC, Shao L, Peng HH, Rosetta R, del Gaudio D, Wagner AF, et al. A recurrent intragenic genomic duplication, other novel mutations in NLRP7 and imprinting defects in recurrent biparental hydatidiform moles. Mol Hum Reprod. 2008;14(1):33–40.
55. Slim R, Fallahian M, Riviere JB, Zali MR. Evidence of a genetic heterogeneity of familial hydatidiform moles. Placenta. 2005;26(1):5–9.
56. Hayward BE, De Vos M, Talati N, Abdollahi MR, Taylor GR, Meyer E, et al. Genetic and epigenetic analysis of recurrent hydatidiform mole. Hum Mutat. 2009;30(5):E629–39.
57. Moglabey YB, Kircheisen R, Seoud M, El Mogharbel N, Van den Veyver I, Slim R. Genetic mapping of a maternal locus responsible for familial hydatidiform moles. Hum Mol Genet. 1999;8(4):667–71.
58. Sensi A, Gualandi F, Pittalis MC, Calabrese O, Falciano F, Maestri I, et al. Mole maker phenotype: possible narrowing of the candidate region. Eur J Hum Genet. 2000;8(8):641–4.
59. Hodges MD, Rees HC, Seckl MJ, Newlands ES, Fisher RA. Genetic refinement and physical mapping of a biparental complete hydatidiform mole locus on chromosome 19q13.4. J Med Genet. 2003;40(8):e95.
60. Loukinov DI, Pugacheva E, Vatolin S, Pack SD, Moon H, Chernukhin I, et al. BORIS, a novel male germ-line-specific protein associated with epigenetic reprogramming events, shares the same 11-zinc-finger domain with CTCF, the insulator protein involved in reading imprinting marks in the soma. Proc Natl Acad Sci USA. 2002;99(10):6806–11.
61. Wolffe AP. Transcriptional control: imprinting insulation. Curr Biol. 2000;10(12):R463–5.
62. Murdoch S, Djuric U, Mazhar B, Seoud M, Khan R, Kuick R, et al. Mutations in NALP7 cause recurrent hydatidiform moles and reproductive wastage in humans. Nat Genet. 2006;38(3):300–2.
63. Qian J, Deveault C, Bagga R, Xie X, Slim R. Women heterozygous for NALP7/NLRP7 mutations are at risk for reproductive wastage: report of two novel mutations. Hum Mutat. 2007;28(7):741.
64. Wang CM, Dixon PH, Decordova S, Hodges MD, Sebire NJ, Ozalp S, et al. Identification of 13 novel NLRP7 mutations in 20 families with recurrent hydatidiform mole; missense mutations cluster in the leucine-rich region. J Med Genet. 2009;46(8):569–75.
65. Berkowitz RS, Goldstein DP. Current management of gestational trophoblastic diseases. Gynecol Oncol. 2009;112(3):654–62.
66. Shih IM, Kurman RJ. Placental site trophoblastic tumor–past as prologue. Gynecol Oncol. 2001;82(3): 413–4.
67. Shih IM, Kurman RJ. Epithelioid trophoblastic tumor: a neoplasm distinct from choriocarcinoma and placental site trophoblastic tumor simulating carcinoma. Am J Surg Pathol. 1998;22(11):1393–403.
68. Kotylo PK, Michael H, Davis TE, Sutton GP, Mark PR, Roth LM. Flow cytometric DNA analysis of placental-site trophoblastic tumors. Int J Gynecol Pathol. 1992;11(4):245–52.
69. Fukunaga M, Ushigome S. Metastasizing placental site trophoblastic tumor. An immunohistochemical and flow cytometric study of two cases. Am J Surg Pathol. 1993;17(10):1003–10.
70. Fukunaga M, Ushigome S. Malignant trophoblastic tumors: immunohistochemical and flow cytometric comparison of choriocarcinoma and placental site trophoblastic tumors. Hum Pathol. 1993;24(10): 1098–106.
71. Xue WC, Guan XY, Ngan HY, Shen DH, Khoo US, Cheung AN. Malignant placental site trophoblastic tumor: a cytogenetic study using comparative genomic hybridization and chromosome in situ hybridization. Cancer. 2002;94(8):2288–94.
72. Hui P, Riba A, Pejovic T, Johnson T, Baergen RN, Ward D. Comparative genomic hybridization study

of placental site trophoblastic tumour: a report of four cases. Mod Pathol. 2004;17(2):248–51.
73. Xu ML, Yang B, Carcangiu ML, Hui P. Epithelioid trophoblastic tumor: comparative genomic hybridization and diagnostic DNA genotyping. Mod Pathol. 2009;22(2):232–8.
74. Ahmed MN, Kim K, Haddad B, Berchuck A, Qumsiyeh MB. Comparative genomic hybridization studies in hydatidiform moles and choriocarcinoma: amplification of 7q21-q31 and loss of 8p12-p21 in choriocarcinoma. Cancer Genet Cytogenet. 2000; 116(1):10–5.
75. Hui P, Parkash V, Perkins AS, Carcangiu ML. Pathogenesis of placental site trophoblastic tumor may require the presence of a paternally derived X chromosome. Lab Invest. 2000;80(6):965–72.
76. Fisher RA, Paradinas FJ, Newlands ES, Boxer GM. Genetic evidence that placental site trophoblastic tumours can originate from a hydatidiform mole or a normal conceptus. Br J Cancer. 1992;65(3): 355–8.
77. Kodama S, Kase H, Aoki Y, Yahata T, Tanaka K, Motoyama T, et al. Recurrent placental site trophoblastic tumor of the uterus: clinical, pathologic, ultrastructural, and DNA fingerprint study. Gynecol Oncol. 1996;60(1):89–93.
78. Dessau R, Rustin GJ, Dent J, Paradinas FJ, Bagshawe KD. Surgery and chemotherapy in the management of placental site tumor. Gynecol Oncol. 1990;39(1): 56–9.
79. Hoffman JS, Silverman AD, Gelber J, Cartun R. Placental site trophoblastic tumor: a report of radiologic, surgical, and pathologic methods of evaluating the extent of disease. Gynecol Oncol. 1993;50(1): 110–4.
80. Arima T, Imamura T, Amada S, Tsuneyoshi M, Wake N. Genetic origin of malignant trophoblastic neoplasms. Cancer Genet Cytogenet. 1994;73(2):95–102.
81. Lathrop JC, Lauchlan S, Nayak R, Ambler M. Clinical characteristics of placental site trophoblastic tumor (PSTT). Gynecol Oncol. 1988;31(1):32–42.
82. Hassadia A, Gillespie A, Tidy J, Everard RGNJ, Wells M, Coleman R, et al. Placental site trophoblastic tumour: clinical features and management. Gynecol Oncol. 2005;99(3):603–7.
83. Khan S, Dancey G, Lindsay I, Sebire NJ, Fisher RA, Seckl MJ, et al. Placental site trophoblastic tumour derived from an oocyte donation pregnancy. BJOG. 2006;113(3):344–6.
84. Kobel M, Pohl G, Schmitt WD, Hauptmann S, Wang TL, Shih Ie M. Activation of mitogen-activated protein kinase is required for migration and invasion of placental site trophoblastic tumor. Am J Pathol. 2005;167(3):879–85.
85. Oldt 3rd RJ, Kurman RJ, Shih Ie M. Molecular genetic analysis of placental site trophoblastic tumors and epithelioid trophoblastic tumors confirms their trophoblastic origin. Am J Pathol. 2002;161(3): 1033–7.
86. Yap KL, Hafez MJ, Mao TL, Kurman RJ, Murphy KM, Shih Ie M. Lack of a y-chromosomal complement in the majority of gestational trophoblastic neoplasms. J Oncol. 2010;2010:364508.
87. Hui P, Wang HL, Chu P, Yang B, Huang J, Baergen RN, et al. Absence of Y chromosome in human placental site trophoblastic tumor. Mod Pathol. 2007;20(10): 1055–60.
88. Baergen RN, Rutgers JL, Young RH, Osann K, Scully RE. Placental site trophoblastic tumor: a study of 55 cases and review of the literature emphasizing factors of prognostic significance. Gynecol Oncol. 2006;100(3):511–20.
89. Keep D, Zaragoza MV, Hassold T, Redline RW. Very early complete hydatidiform mole. Hum Pathol. 1996;27(7):708–13.
90. Buza N, Hui P. Gestational trophoblastic disease: histopathological diagnosis in the molecular era. Diagn Histopathol. 2010;16(11):526–37.
91. Sebire NJ. Histopathological diagnosis of hydatidiform mole: contemporary features and clinical implications. Fetal Pediatr Pathol. 2010;29(1):1–16.
92. Barlow DP. Gametic imprinting in mammals. Science. 1995;270(5242):1610–3.
93. Haig D, Westoby M. An earlier formulation of the genetic conflict hypothesis of genomic imprinting. Nat Genet. 2006;38(3):271.
94. Abu-Amero S, Monk D, Apostolidou S, Stanier P, Moore G. Imprinted genes and their role in human fetal growth. Cytogenet Genome Res. 2006;113(1–4): 262–70.
95. Solter D. Imprinting. Int J Dev Biol. 1998;42(7): 951–4.
96. Tilghman SM. The sins of the fathers and mothers: genomic imprinting in mammalian development. Cell. 1999;96(2):185–93.
97. Constancia M, Kelsey G, Reik W. Resourceful imprinting. Nature. 2004;432(7013):53–7.
98. Wagschal A, Feil R. Genomic imprinting in the placenta. Cytogenet Genome Res. 2006;113(1–4):90–8.
99. Hemberger M. Epigenetic landscape required for placental development. Cell Mol Life Sci. 2007; 64(18):2422–36.
100. Li Y, Lemaire P, Behringer RR. Esx1, a novel X chromosome-linked homeobox gene expressed in mouse extraembryonic tissues and male germ cells. Dev Biol. 1997;188(1):85–95.
101. Lin TP, Labosky PA, Grabel LB, Kozak CA, Pitman JL, Kleeman J, et al. The Pem homeobox gene is X-linked and exclusively expressed in extraembryonic tissues during early murine development. Dev Biol. 1994;166(1):170–9.
102. Salido EC, Yen PH, Mohandas TK, Shapiro LJ. Expression of the X-inactivation-associated gene XIST during spermatogenesis. Nat Genet. 1992;2(3): 196–9.
103. Sado T, Ferguson-Smith AC. Imprinted X inactivation and reprogramming in the preimplantation mouse embryo. Hum Mol Genet. 2005;14(Spec No 1): R59–64.
104. Huynh KD, Lee JT. Inheritance of a pre-inactivated paternal X chromosome in early mouse embryos. Nature. 2003;426(6968):857–62.

105. Cooper DW, VandeBerg JL, Sharman GB, Poole WE. Phosphoglycerate kinase polymorphism in kangaroos provides further evidence for paternal X inactivation. Nat New Biol. 1971;230(13):155–7.
106. Graves JA. Mammals that break the rules: genetics of marsupials and monotremes. Annu Rev Genet. 1996;30:233–60.
107. Reik W, Lewis A. Co-evolution of X-chromosome inactivation and imprinting in mammals. Nat Rev Genet. 2005;6(5):403–10.
108. Li E, Beard C, Jaenisch R. Role for DNA methylation in genomic imprinting. Nature. 1993;366(6453): 362–5.
109. Takagi N, Sasaki M. Preferential inactivation of the paternally derived X chromosome in the extraembryonic membranes of the mouse. Nature. 1975; 256(5519):640–2.
110. Pulford DJ, Falls JG, Killian JK, Jirtle RL. Polymorphisms, genomic imprinting and cancer susceptibility. Mutat Res. 1999;436(1):59–67.
111. Redolfi E, Pizzuti A, Di Bacco A, Susani L, Labella T, Affer M, et al. Mapping of the MYCL2 processed gene to Xq22-23 and identification of an additional L MYC-related sequence in Xq27.2. FEBS Lett. 1999;446(2–3):273–7.
112. Deveraux QL, Takahashi R, Salvesen GS, Reed JC. X-linked IAP is a direct inhibitor of cell-death proteases. Nature. 1997;388(6639):300–4.
113. Barlow DP. Imprinting: a gamete's point of view. Trends Genet. 1994;10(6):194–9.
114. Glassman ML, de Groot N, Hochberg A. Relaxation of imprinting in carcinogenesis. Cancer Genet Cytogenet. 1996;89(1):69–73.
115. Jinno Y, Ikeda Y, Yun K, Maw M, Masuzaki H, Fukuda H, et al. Establishment of functional imprinting of the H19 gene in human developing placentae. Nat Genet. 1995;10(3):318–24.
116. Ariel I, Lustig O, Oyer CE, Elkin M, Gonik B, Rachmilewitz J, et al. Relaxation of imprinting in trophoblastic disease. Gynecol Oncol. 1994;53(2):212–9.
117. Rachmilewitz J, Elkin M, Rosensaft J, Gelman-Kohan Z, Ariel I, Lustig O, et al. H19 expression and tumorigenicity of choriocarcinoma derived cell lines. Oncogene. 1995;11(5):863–70.
118. Walsh C, Miller SJ, Flam F, Fisher RA, Ohlsson R. Paternally derived H19 is differentially expressed in malignant and nonmalignant trophoblast. Cancer Res. 1995;55(5):1111–6.
119. Looijenga LH, Gillis AJ, Verkerk AJ, van Putten WL, Oosterhuis JW. Heterogeneous X inactivation in trophoblastic cells of human full-term female placentas. Am J Hum Genet. 1999;64(5):1445–52.
120. Migeon BR, Lee CH, Chowdhury AK, Carpenter H. Species differences in TSIX/Tsix reveal the roles of these genes in X-chromosome inactivation. Am J Hum Genet. 2002;71(2):286–93.

4 Complete Hydatidiform Mole

Pei Hui

Keywords
Complete mole • Early complete mole • Diagnostic features

Introduction

Complete mole, also known as "classic" hydatidiform mole, is the prototype of molar gestation bearing the traditional description of "hydatid," for example, grape-like structures at the time of evacuation, a term that was used throughout the last century. The historical tale of "365 babies" of the Dutch's Countess Margaret of Henneberg (Chap. 1) clearly documented a case of well-developed complete mole some 700 years ago. It is important to note that essentially all meaningful epidemiology data of hydatidiform mole in the literature have been based on studies of complete mole rather than partial mole. Epidemiological data on partial hydatidiform mole have been at best unreliable, largely because of a significant diagnostic inaccuracy in practice, even at the present time (see Chap. 1).

P. Hui, MD, PhD (✉)
Department of Pathology, Yale University School of Medicine, 310 Cedar Street,
254B New Haven, CT 06520-8023, USA
e-mail: pei.hui@yale.edu

Pathogenesis

Recapitulating the chorionic villous trophoblast, complete mole is a proliferative disorder of cytotrophoblast and syncytiotrophoblast without embryonic development. Some investigators consider all hydatidiform moles are simply degenerative or immature placenta with excessive edema [1]. Complete hydatidiform mole appears to develop exclusively in human with only a few exceptions documented in chimpanzees [2] and other animals. The true androgenetic nature of a complete mole was confirmed in a reported case of cattle [3].

On the genetic level, complete moles are diploid in most cases, and their genetic material is entirely paternally derived (see Chap. 3). The androgenetic nature of complete moles disrupts the normal embryogenesis and placental development because of unbalanced gene expression likely through altered genomic imprinting. While the majority of compete moles are diploid diandric in their chromosomal composition, tetraploid and even triploid complete moles are possible as long as theoretically all the extra copies of the chromosomal sets are paternally derived [4, 5]. Homozygous and heterozygous complete moles

P. Hui (ed.), *Gestational Trophoblastic Disease: Diagnostic and Molecular Genetic Pathology*, Current Clinical Pathology, DOI 10.1007/978-1-61779-394-3_4,

may have different biological and clinical implications [6].

Recurrent complete moles have been well described in the literatures. Among 150 or so reported cases [7, 8], the subset of familial biparental complete moles (FBCMs) is of greater interest and has invited numerous investigations in recent years as to their seemingly paternal-only expression of imprinted genes despite of the presence of the maternal haploid genome. FBCM is defined as the occurrence of multiple complete moles arising in different conceptions and affecting more than one woman from the same pedigree [9]. Only 21 families of FBCM have been documented in the literature [8]. They have histological features indistinguishable from those of conventional diandric, uniparental complete moles. Various mutations of NALP7/NLRP7 of the maternal allele located on 19q13.4 have been found to be the causal genetic alterations. It is believed that various NALP7 mutations result in an abnormal imprinting pattern similar to that of diandric complete mole, despite of the presence of haploid maternal genome in FBCM [8, 10–15]. Detailed discussion of the genetic aspects of FBCM can be found in Chap. 3. One clinical aspect of FBCM is, in contrast to the conventional diandric complete mole, that the patients have an exceedingly rare chance of a subsequent normal pregnancy [8], although exception has been reported [7]. Further investigations into the molecular aspects of biparental complete mole are important to understand how altered genomic imprinting relates to the development of hydatidiform mole in general [8].

Clinical Presentation

In the past, the first manifestation of complete mole in more than 85% of the patients was vaginal bleeding during the second trimester (average at 16th weeks) of pregnancy [16]. Frequently, vaginal bleeding was accompanied by passing tissues resembling grape-like structures. Upon physical examination, 50% of the patients had an excessive uterine size [17]. Other manifestations included hyperemesis, toxemia, and hyperthyroidism and pulmonary embolism [18]. Markedly elevated serum human chorionic gonadotropin (hCG) was a typical laboratory finding in over 50% of the patients and frequently reaching over 100,000 mIU/mL [19]. Ultrasound showed no evidence of fetal development or fetal heart beat; instead, the classic "snowstorm" or mixed echogenic appearance due to well-developed molar vesicles admixed with blood was characteristically seen. In fact, the combination of characteristic ultrasound findings along with an inappropriate elevation of hCG for the gestational age are highly suspicious for the presence of well-developed complete mole. Preeclampsia (pregnancy-induced hypertension, edema, and proteinuria) occurred in about 25% of the patients with well-developed complete mole. Near a third of the patients also developed ovarian theca lutein cysts leading to marked enlargement of the ovary that were also detectable by ultrasound [20, 21].

In the past 20 years or so, increasing usage of highly sensitive methods of serum hCG detection and early ultrasound exams have drastically changed the clinical landscape of diagnosis and management of hydatidiform moles. The aforementioned classic features of complete hydatidiform mole have become rare in modern clinical practice and are seldom encountered during gross specimen examination in a pathology lab [18, 22, 23]. An absence of fetal heart beat by ultrasound as early as 6 weeks of gestation can lead to therapeutic abortion by dilatation and curettage [24]. Therefore, most patients of complete mole present now as missed abortions in the first trimester (6.5 to 12 weeks of gestational age) before the classic symptoms and ultrasound appearance develop [24, 25]. Vaginal bleeding is still the most common presenting symptom seen in 84% of the cases, comparing with 97% in the past [22]. A comparative study in late 1990s by the New England Trophoblastic Center showed a mean gestational age of 8.5 weeks among cases of complete mole diagnosed between 1994 and 1997, compared to 17 weeks of those classic, well-developed complete moles diagnosed between 1969 and 1975 [26]. Among complete mole patients managed in the late 1980s through early 1990s, uterine size larger than gestational age was seen only in 28%, theca lutein cysts in 9%, hyperemesis gravidarum in 6%, preeclampsia in 1.3%, and none developed hyperthyroidism or respiratory distress [22].

Pathology

Gross Pathology

Morphological presentation (size and extent of villous edema) of complete mole depends on the gestational age at time of evacuation. The specimen of a well-developed complete mole consists of bulky volume of bloody tissue with grossly identifiable, enlarged, and edematous villi. The hydropic changes are diffuse and uniformly transform chorionic villi into transparent vesicles of variable sizes ranging from a few millimeters to 3.0 cm with an average of 1.5 cm, thereby resembling clusters of grapes (Fig. 4.1a, b). When collapsing molar villi admix with the maternal gestational endometrial tissue in a curettage specimen, floating the tissue sample in a water or saline bath may help to identify the hydropic chorionic villi. Normal placental structures are grossly absent and identifiable fetal development is lacking. Evacuated at a much earlier stage, the gross appearance of an early complete mole becomes subtle or there may be no gross evidence of abnormal edematous villi, particularly when the patient presents with a missed abortion. Occasionally, an early complete mole may be evacuated in an elective abortion procedure without any clinical suspicion for abnormal pregnancy.

Histological Pathology

Well-developed complete hydatidiform mole (Table 4.1a): Microscopically, a well-developed complete mole presents two salient morphological features: diffuse villous edema and marked trophoblastic hyperplasia. The hydropic changes involve all chorionic villi that show markedly edematous villous stroma with cistern formation involving frequently many villi as central cystic spaces that are completely devoid of cellular components (Fig. 4.2). The villous outlines are generally smooth, round to ovoid. Stromal

Table 4.1 Histological features of well-developed complete hydatidiform mole

Diffusely enlarged chorionic villi with marked stromal hydropic changes
Villous cistern formation
Multifocal to circumferential trophoblastic hyperplasia with cytological atypia
Absence of nucleated RBC and fetal parts
Negative nuclear staining of p57 in cytotrophoblasts and villous stromal cells

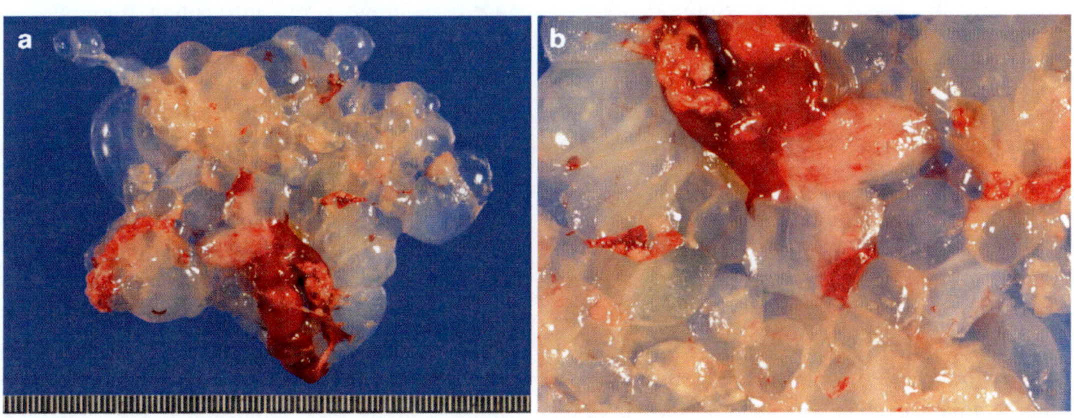

Fig. 4.1 Gross appearance of well-developed complete hydatidiform mole (**a**, **b**) (courtesy of Dr. Bart Kenney, Yale University). Note markedly enlarged chorionic villi and diffuse hydropic changes

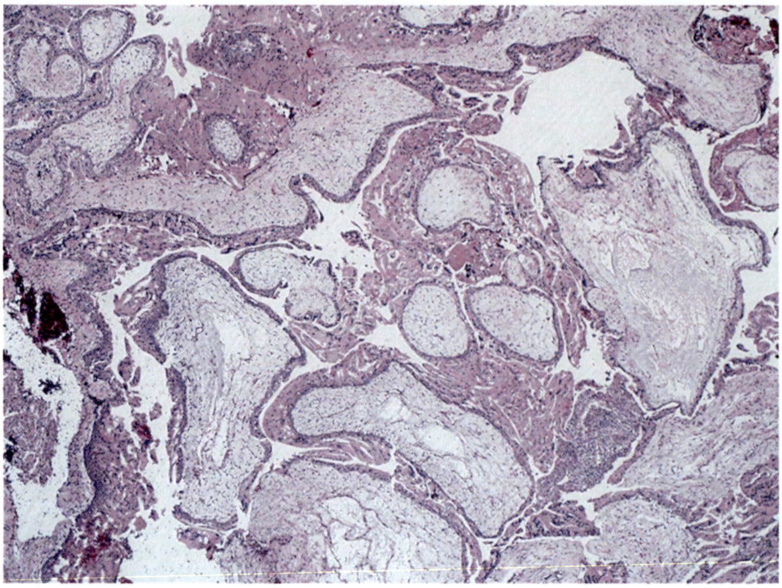

Fig. 4.2 Histological appearance of well-developed complete hydatidiform mole. Note the markedly diffuse hydropic changes involving all chorionic villi with cistern formation at this low magnification

trophoblastic inclusions are generally present. Trophoblastic hyperplasia is characterized by irregular yet diffuse trophoblastic proliferation involving a significant portion of chorionic villi. This hyperplasia is non-polar, multifocal to frequently circumferential around the involved villi (Fig. 4.3a, b). Occasional interconnections or bridges are formed by the proliferating trophoblast between the villi (Fig. 4.3c). Sheets or confluent aggregates of intermediate trophoblast are admixed with cytotrophoblast and syncytiotrophoblast (Fig. 4.4a). Significant cytological atypia is almost always present in syncytiotrophoblast and intermediate trophoblast (Fig. 4.4b). Mitosis is frequently present among cytotrophoblast and intermediate trophoblast. Although the villous stroma is generally hypocellular, cellular stroma can be found, particularly near the tips of some chorionic villi, where stellate spindle cells are embedded in a myxoid matrix along with numerous apoptotic bodies (karyorrhexis) (Fig. 4.5). There are no fetal parts or nonvillous placental structures, including amnion, yolk sac, and chorionic membrane. Fetal nucleated red blood cells are lacking. Fetal capillaries, however, may be identifiable by histology and/or immunohistochemistry, particularly in a very early complete mole (see the following).

Very early complete hydatidiform mole (VECM): Very early complete mole is defined as a complete mole evacuated before 12 weeks of gestation. The first documentation of early complete mole was made by Keep who described four cases of the condition [24]. The gestational ages of these four patients were 6.5–11 weeks and all were initially misdiagnosed as missed abortion based on clinical and ultrasound findings, and only retrospectively confirmed as complete mole by DNA analysis [24]. These early complete mole may not be suspected in most of the cases by clinicians as well as pathologists due to their subtle clinical and pathological presentation. No gross pathological characteristics distinguish very early complete mole from conventional missed abortion in a curettage specimen. Although ultrasonography may still detect abnormalities (absence of fetal heart beat), a significant proportion of the cases (1/3–2/3) demonstrate minimal hydropic change and are therefore unidentifiable clinically, even with improved sonographic expertise [27, 28]. In the absence of

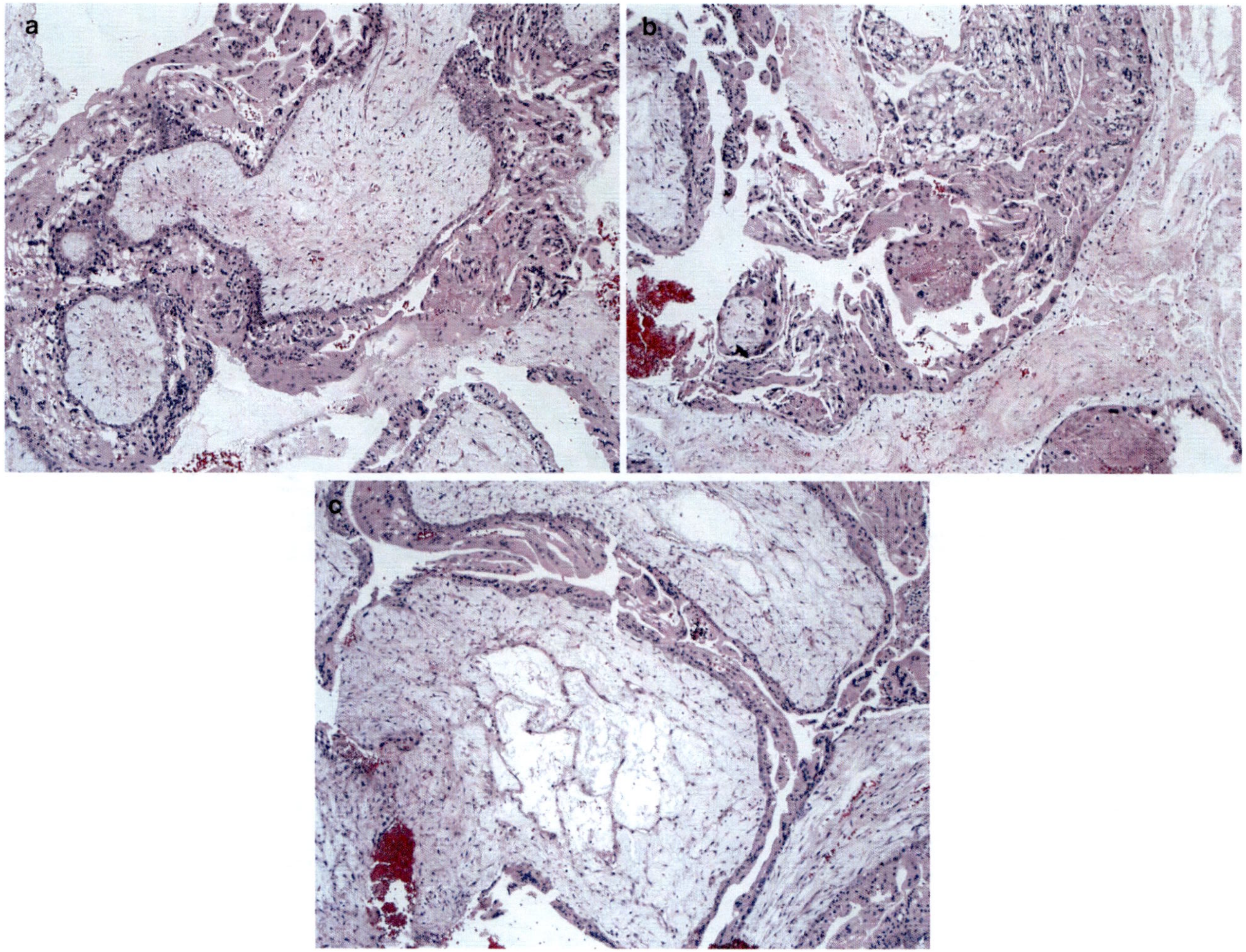

Fig. 4.3 Well-developed complete hydatidiform mole with marked trophoblastic hyperplasia. Note the circumferential hyperplasia of the villous trophoblast (**a**, **c**) and the trophoblastic bridging between villi (**b**) at intermediate magnification

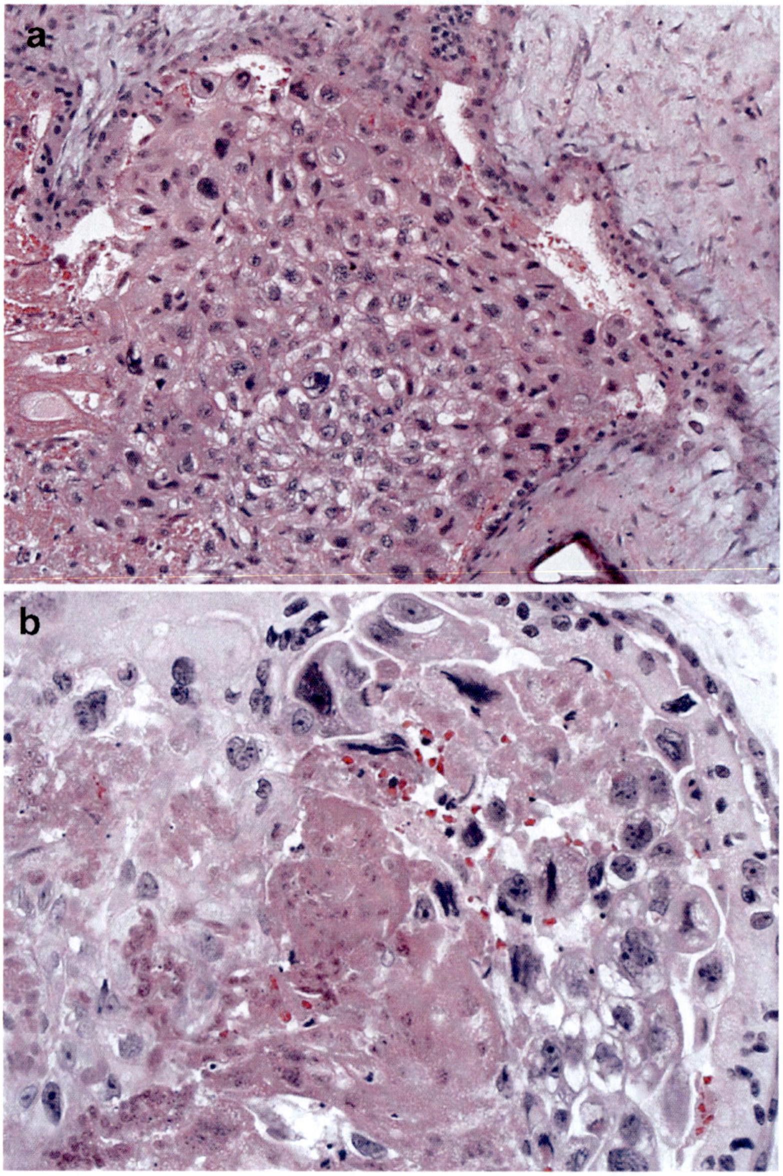

Fig. 4.4 High-power view of the trophoblast of well-developed complete mole. Sheets or confluent aggregates of villous intermediate trophoblast admixed with cytotrophoblast and syncytiotrophoblast (**a**). Significant cytological atypia is present (**b**)

the typical clinical and imaging characteristics, the role of pathologist has become more critical in the diagnosis of very early complete mole.

Histologically, the two diagnostic hallmarks of a well-developed complete mole, enlarged villi with cistern formation and exuberant or circumferential trophoblastic proliferation, are not present in a very early complete mole. However, the histological changes of the villous stroma in VECM are highly characteristic (Table 4.2). In VECM, the chorionic villi usually display abnormal bulbous, polypoid to phyllodes-like configurations without significant edema (Fig. 4.6a–d). The villi are small or slightly enlarged, relatively uniform and usually do not have irregular contour or trophoblastic inclusions (Fig. 4.7). The villous

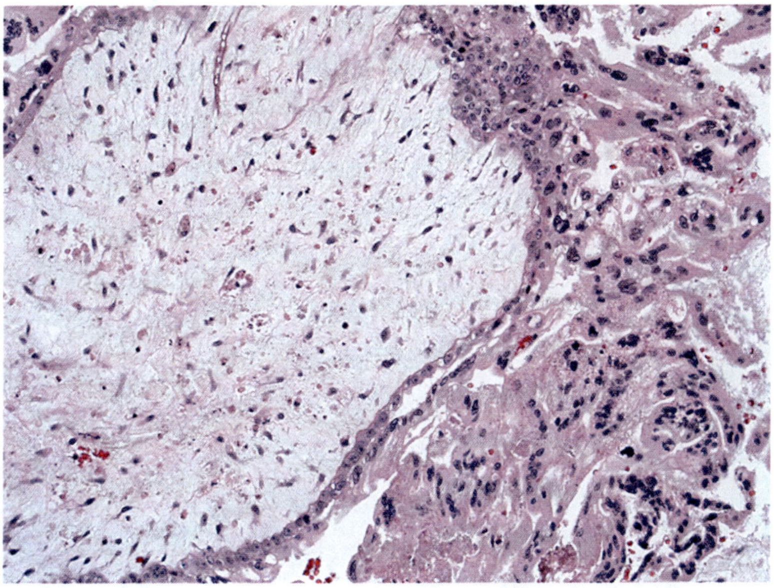

Fig. 4.5 Cellular and myxoid villous stroma with prominent karyorrhexis involving some smaller villi in well-developed complete mole

Table 4.2 Histological features of very early complete hydatidiform mole (VECM)

Polypoid or cauliflower-like chorionic villi of normal sizes
Cellular and myxoid villous stroma with prominent karyorrhexis
Mild to moderate trophoblastic hyperplasia in random or circumferential fashion
Negative nuclear staining of p57 in cytotrophoblasts and villous stromal cells

stroma frequently has a primitive appearance resembling the mesenchymal villi during the early placental formation (Fig. 4.8a). They are characteristically hypercellular and composed of stellate to plump fibroblasts embedded in a bluish myxoid matrix with prominent karyorrhexis or apoptotic bodies (Fig. 4.8b). These stromal fibroblasts are relatively large with slightly hyperchromatic nuclei. Stromal hydropic changes are rare or not prominent. Linear rudimentarily developed capillaries may be found, particularly by immunohistochemical staining of endothelial markers, see the following. Trophoblastic proliferation – a hallmark of CHM – is only focally present or may be completely absent in VECM. In an early complete mole, the pattern of trophoblastic proliferation recapitulates that observed in early placental formation after implantation. When present, it randomly involves some villi with circumferential distribution of both cytotrophoblastic and syncytiotrophoblastic cells (Fig. 4.9).

Vasculature in complete mole: Well-formed villous vessels, as discussed earlier, should not be found in a fully developed complete mole, although immunohistochemistry with endothelial cell markers (CD34 and QBEND10) may highlight the presence of endothelial cells in a linear fashion [29, 30]. This is, however, not true for an early complete mole, which may present with histologically identifiable vessels. They are in the form of capillaries (Fig. 4.10) and occasionally may contain identifiable fetal nucleated red blood cells [29, 31, 32], some of which may appear megaloblastic. CD34 immunostain may highlight numerous capillaries within the stroma [29]. These villous vessels generally disappear before the mid-second trimester. In addition to the presence of nucleated red blood cells, so-called

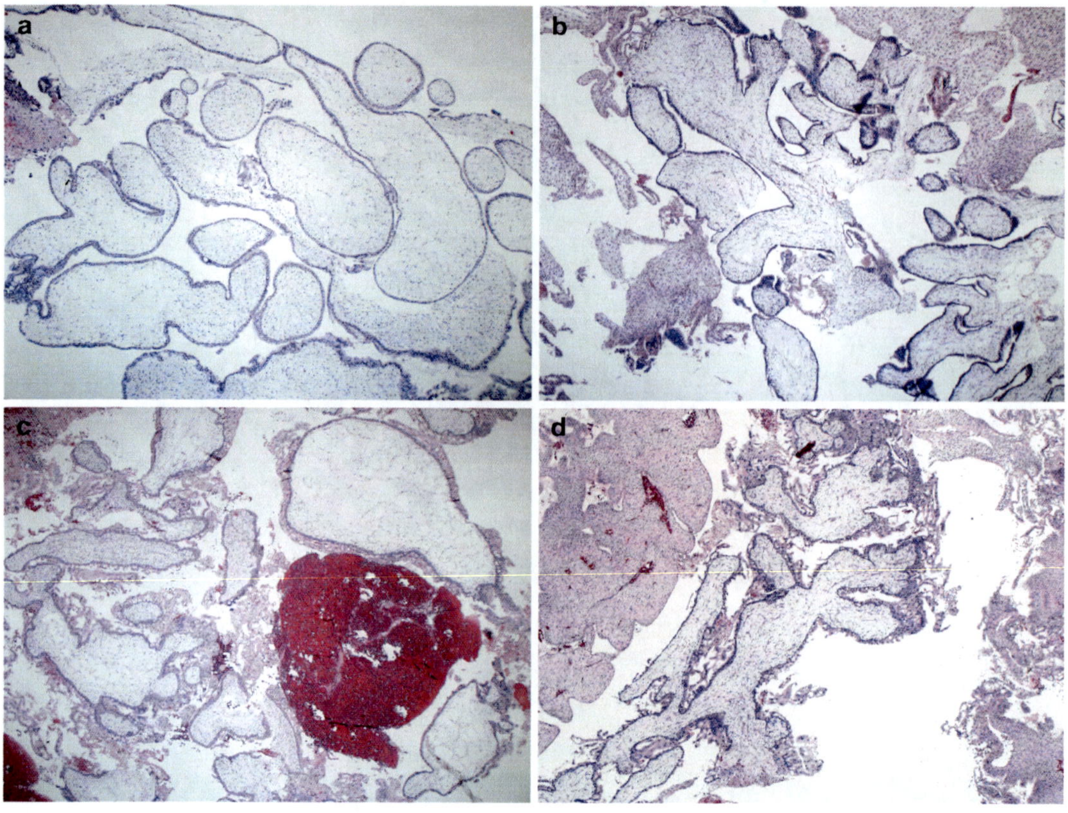

Fig. 4.6 Microscopic presentations of 4 examples early complete moles at low magnification (**a**,**b**,**c** and **d**)

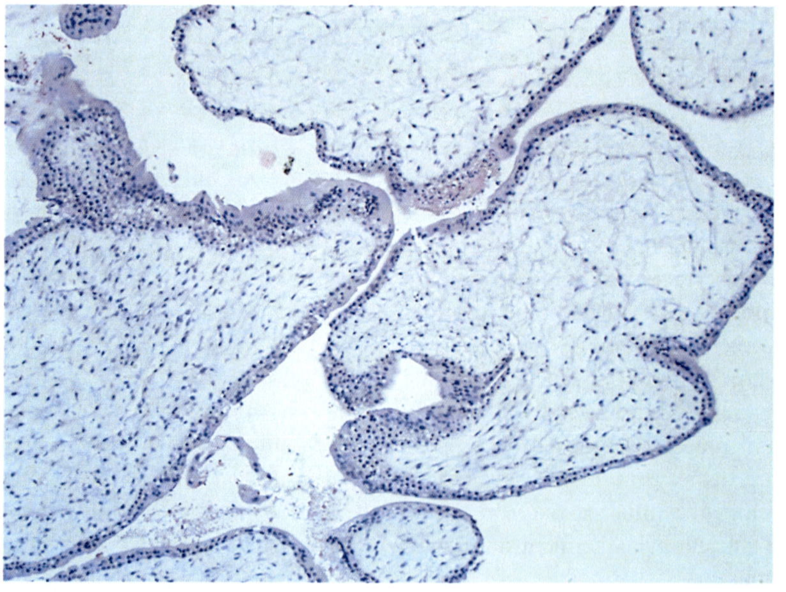

Fig. 4.7 Medium power view of an early complete mole. Note small to mildly enlarged villi that have no significant edema or trophoblastic hyperplasia

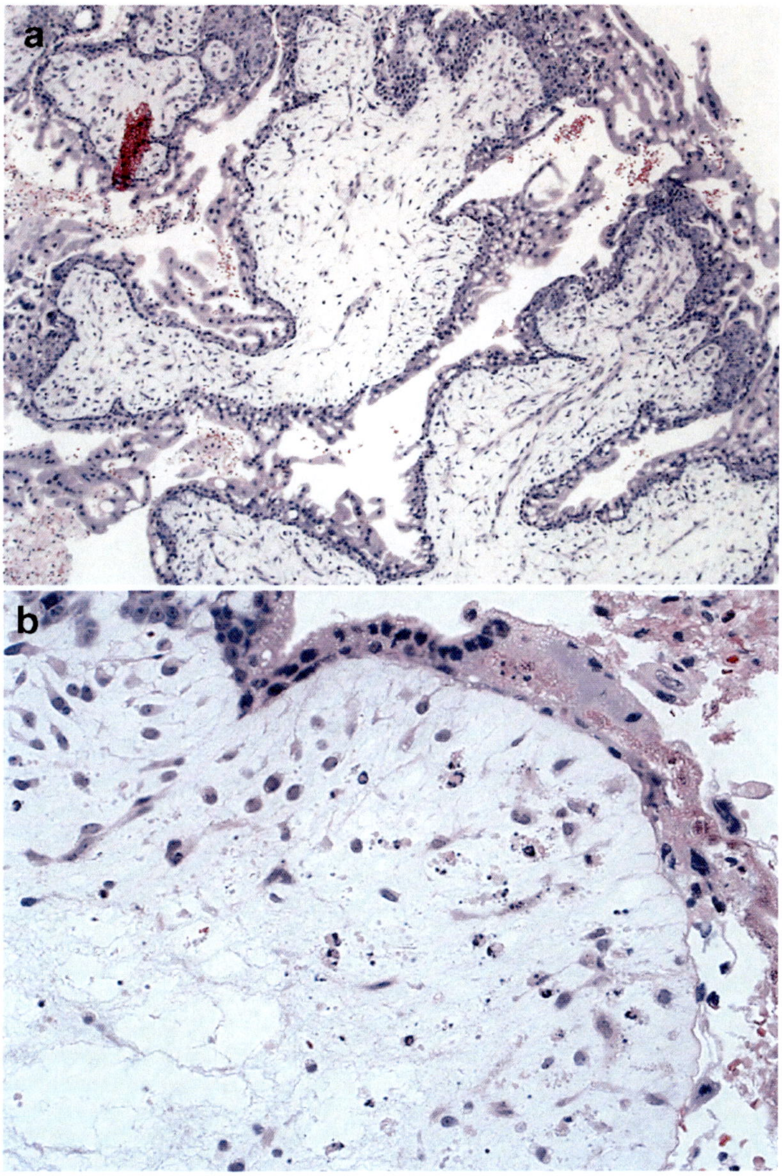

Fig. 4.8 Very early complete mole showing primitive chorionic villi with cellular and myxoid matrix (**a**), stellate to plump stromal cells, and prominent karyorrhexis or apoptotic bodies (**b**)

stunted embryos have been described in the literature as severely abnormal embryonic structures present in a very early complete mole [33]. However, a dead twin embryo with coexisting complete mole is possible [34], and molecular genotyping may be helpful in resolving this issue in the future.

Implantation site reaction in association with complete mole: Frequently associated with complete mole, the implantation site often characteristically shows changes histologically similar to exaggerated placental site reaction (see Chap. 10). The trophoblastic infiltration consists of so-called implantation site intermediate trophoblast. Suction

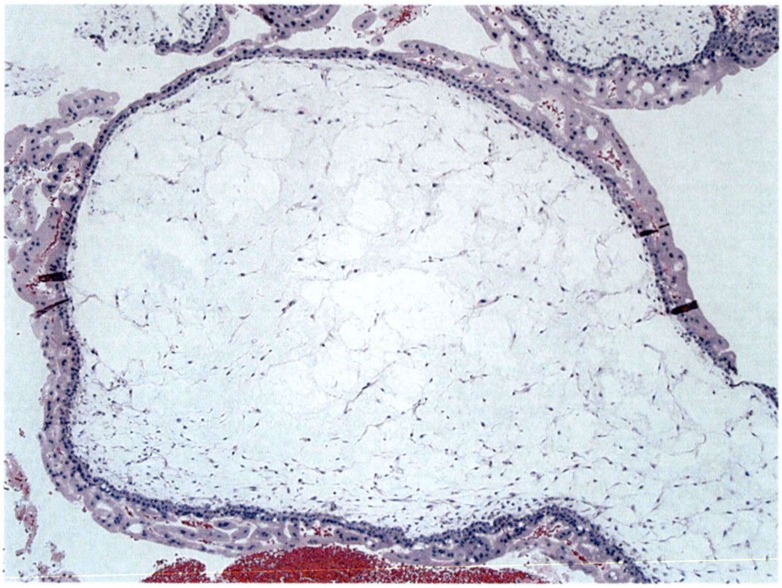

Fig. 4.9 Mild trophoblastic hyperplasia in a random to circumferential distribution in an early complete mole

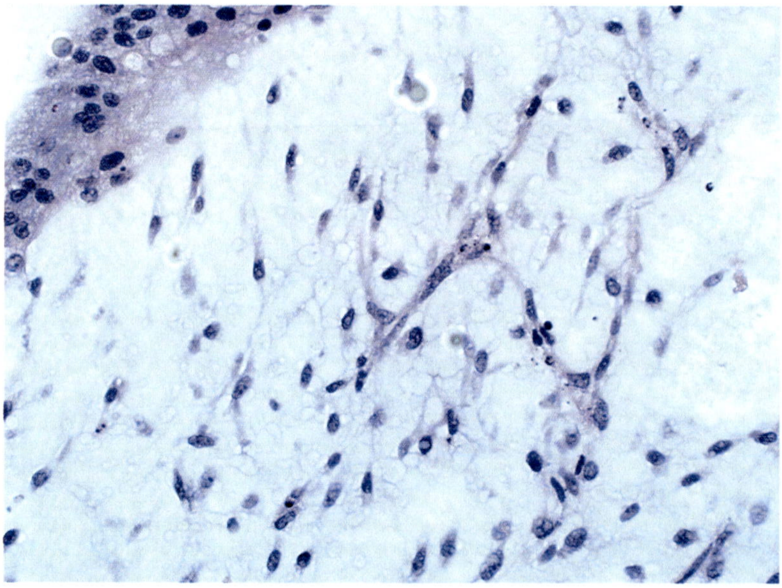

Fig. 4.10 Rudimental capillary vasculatures in an early complete mole

curettage often yields fragments of endometrium and/or superficial myometrium with infiltrating intermediate trophoblasts, frequently showing cytological atypia, and even simulating placental site trophoblastic tumor (Fig. 4.11). However, an absence of mass lesion clinically or by imaging and the presence of concurrent molar gestation should easily confirm a non-neoplastic process. Similar to a well-developed complete mole, an exaggerated placental site reaction with striking trophoblast atypicality may be associated with VECM.

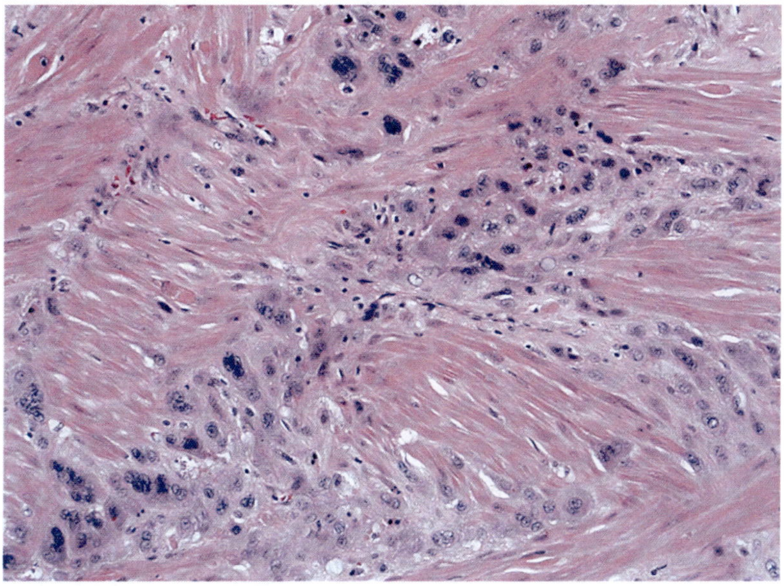

Fig. 4.11 Exaggerated placental site – like reaction associated with complete mole

Ancillary Studies

Most complete moles are diploid by flow cytometry DNA ploidy analysis [35, 36]. It should be noted that ploidy analysis using paraffin-embedded tissue is frequently plagued with technical difficulties and interpretation errors resulting in a significant misclassification of ploidy, and misdiagnosis of hydatidiform mole. This is because the ploidy histograms produced from paraffin-embedded tissue samples tend to have increased cellular debris and broader peaks with a high coefficient of variation [37]. Effects of various fixatives and fixation conditions may significantly affect DNA ploidy analysis as well [37].

The unique androgenic nature of complete hydatidiform mole has been explored to identify imprinting markers for diagnostic purposes. P57 is a cyclin-dependent kinase inhibitor protein, encoded by a paternally imprinted gene. This gene is silent in subsets of cells of complete moles as their genetic material is entirely paternally derived [9, 38]. Hydropic abortuses and partial moles show strong nuclear p57 expression in cytotrophoblast, intermediate trophoblast, villous stromal cell, and decidual stromal cell (see Chap. 5), whereas p57 staining is absent or very weak in cytotrophoblasts and villous stromal cells of complete mole (Fig. 4.12). It should be noted that in complete mole, P57 can be expressed in syncytiotrophoblast, intermediate trophoblast, and stromal endothelial cell. Occasionally scattered weak nuclear staining of p57 in cytotrophoblast may also be seen in complete mole, therefore posing diagnostic difficulties.

Molecular genotyping is the most recently developed technique that has been found practical and highly accurate in the differential diagnosis of hydatidiform moles. Polymerase chain reaction (PCR) amplification of multiple short tandem repeat (STR) loci of maternal decidua and villous tissue provides information about the parental genetic contribution, and therefore, it can reliably distinguish diandric complete mole from diandric monogynic partial mole and biparental diploid hydropic gestation (additional details of STR genotyping diagnosis are discussed in Chap. 11).

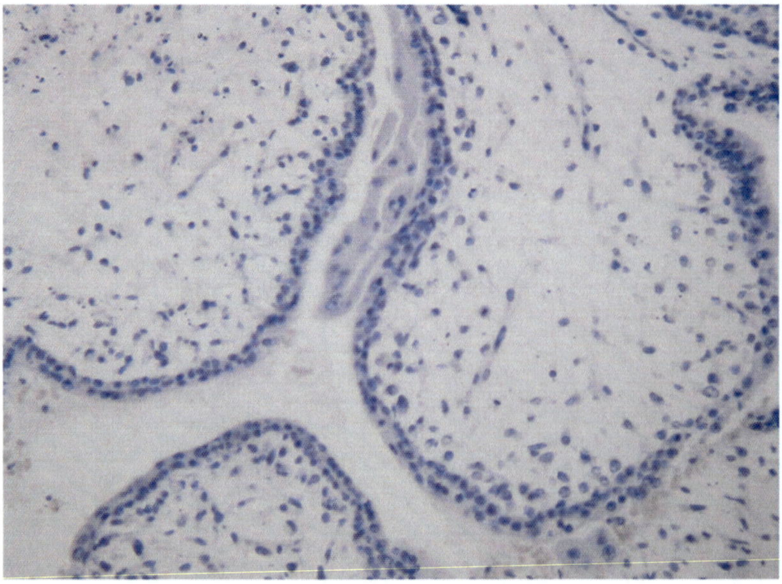

Fig. 4.12 Absence of p57 immunostaining in cytotrophoblastic cells and villous stromal cells in complete mole

Differential Diagnosis

Well-developed complete hydatidiform moles are generally diagnosed without difficulties by routine histological examination with additional help of p57 immunohistochemistry (Figs. 4.12 and 5.5). Although the morphological features of very early complete moles are quite characteristic, the pathologist needs to have a high index of suspicion and be aware of its histological and cytological features. Normal early pregnancy, hydropic non-molar gestation, ectopic pregnancy (particularly tubal pregnancy), and partial mole are common differential diagnoses. Molecular genotyping offers an ultimate diagnosis/confirmation of a complete mole by demonstration of androgenic-only genome in the villous tissue. A recently published diagnostic algorithm suggested that cases morphologically suspicious for complete mole should first be stained for p57, and a negative result would be confirmatory without further analysis. Cases that lack well-developed morphologic features of CHM and have equivocal p57 results should be evaluated by molecular genotyping [39]. However, it has long been suggested [40, 41], and recently confirmed [6] that heterozygous (dispermic) complete moles are more aggressive than homozygous (monospermic) ones in the development of postmolar gestational trophoblastic neoplasia. Therefore, a precise genotyping subclassification of complete moles may be clinically desirable.

Complete mole vs. spontaneous abortion: Early spontaneous abortions usually show obvious hydropic degeneration with large, round villi enriched with edematous fluid. Microscopically, the edema of the chorionic villi may be remarkable, even with cistern formation. However, significant enlargement of chorionic villi is not present in a non-molar missed abortion. There may be reactive trophoblastic proliferation as well, but generally in a polarized distribution (located at one pole of chorionic villi) as opposed to circumferential or multifocal distribution seen in early complete mole. Nevertheless, rare cases of spontaneous non-molar abortus may have circumferential proliferation of trophoblasts, similar to that seen in complete mole.

Complete mole vs. partial mole: Well-developed complete moles are distinguished from partial moles by the extent of hydropic changes, the degree of trophoblastic hyperplasia, and the

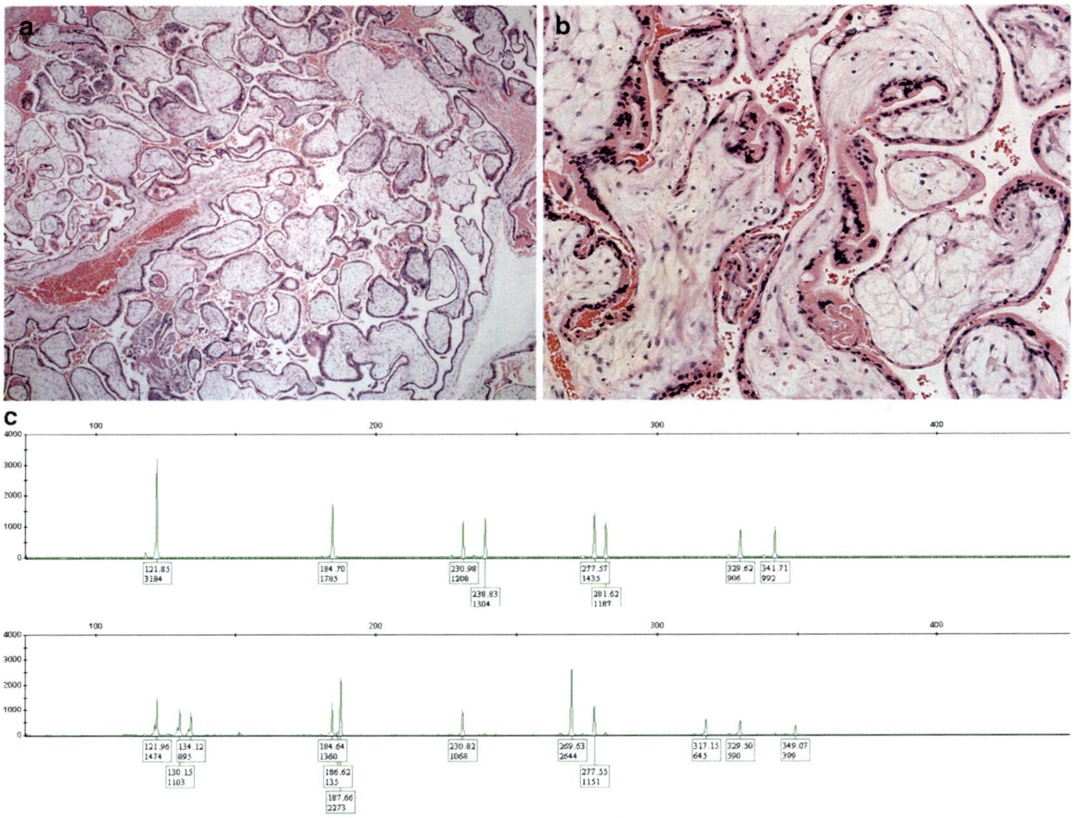

Fig. 4.13 Early partial mole simulating early complete mole by its diffuse villous edema and mild trophoblastic hyperplasia (**a**, **b**). Genotyping confirms the diandric monogynic genome in this partial mole (**c**). Note the presence of dispermic heterozygous paternal and monogynic alleles in the chorionic villi (c, *lower panel*) comparing with the normal biparental allelic pattern in the maternal endometrium (c, *upper panel*)

absence of fetal tissue. In contrast to the diffuse edema involving all villi in a complete mole, a partial hydatidiform mole shows two populations of villi: small fibrotic ones and hydropically dilated ones with marked border irregularities, trophoblastic inclusions, cistern formation, and low levels of trophoblastic hyperplasia in the form of syncytiotrophoblastic knuckles. A diagnostic separation of a very complete mole from a partial mole may be very difficult on mere morphological ground, primarily because of the absence of cistern formation and less trophoblastic hyperplasia in early complete mole (Fig. 4.13 a,b,c). Flow cytometry DNA ploidy analysis is one of the earliest and – until recently – the most frequently used method to distinguish a complete mole from a partial mole. An absence of nuclear p57 staining of cytotrophoblastic cells and villous stromal cells should confirm a diagnosis of complete mole. In a difficult case where ploidy and p57 are inconclusive, DNA genotyping (see Chap. 11) offers an ultimate confirmation (Fig. 4.13c).

Early complete mole vs. early gestation: Early gestation may show overlapping histology with VECM. Generally, normal early gestation demonstrates elongated narrow chorionic villi, a paucicellular stroma with nonbranching capillaries and prominent nucleated red blood cells. Polarized trophoblast proliferation is generally found in an early gestation (Figs. 2.5 and 4.14), in contrast to a random or circumferential pattern seen in complete mole (Figs. 4.3 and 4.9). Ectopic pregnancy, particularly of tubal location, may remarkably simulates an early complete

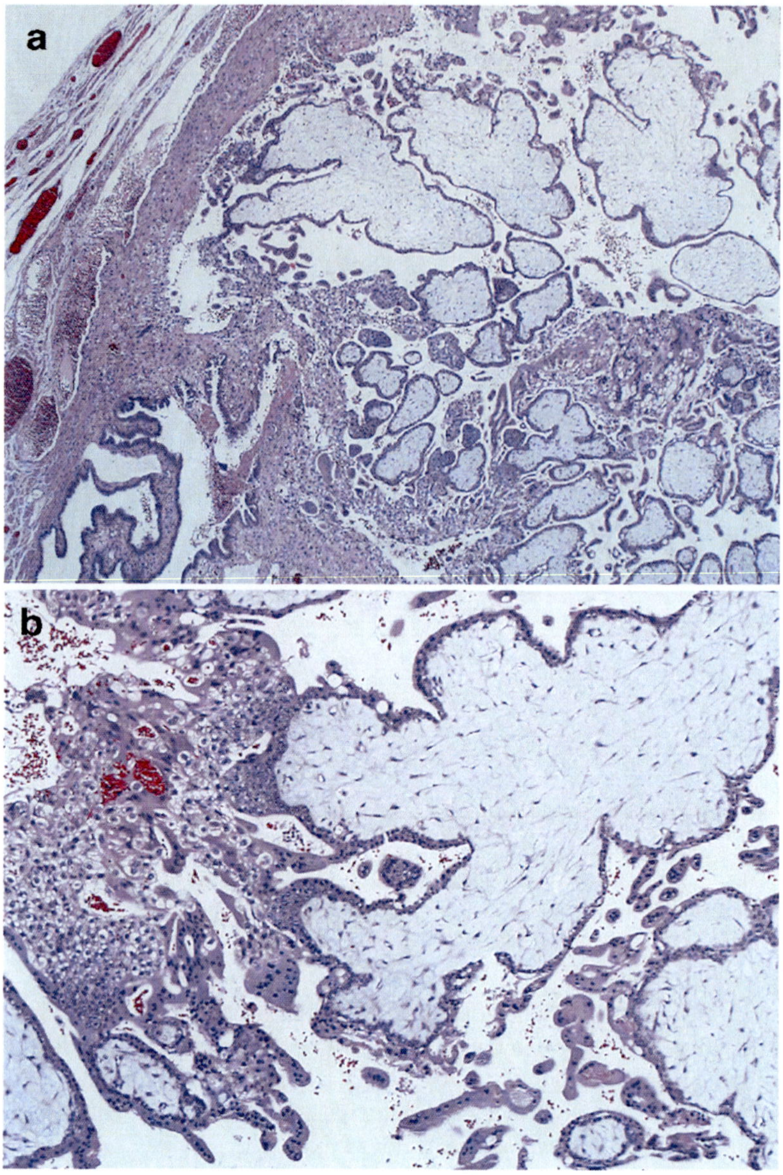

Fig. 4.14 An early tubal pregnancy with histological features simulating an early complete mole at low (**a**) and intermediate magnifications (**b**)

mole (Fig. 4.14a). Since most of the tubal pregnancies terminate with gestational sac ruptured and bleeding at an early stage, the chorionic villi may show primitive appearance with stromal hypercellularity and myxoid changes, greatly overlapping with very early complete mole. However, again, the trophoblastic proliferation is focal and polarized at one end of the chorionic villi (Fig. 4.14b). It is important, however, to note that an early complete mole can arise from tubal gestation (Fig. 4.15a, b). Immunohistochemistry of p57 or genotyping may resolve the issue if in doubt.

Complete mole in twin gestation: Complete mole arising from twin gestation may present, in a curettage specimen, admixed edematous molar and normal chorionic villi, simulating a

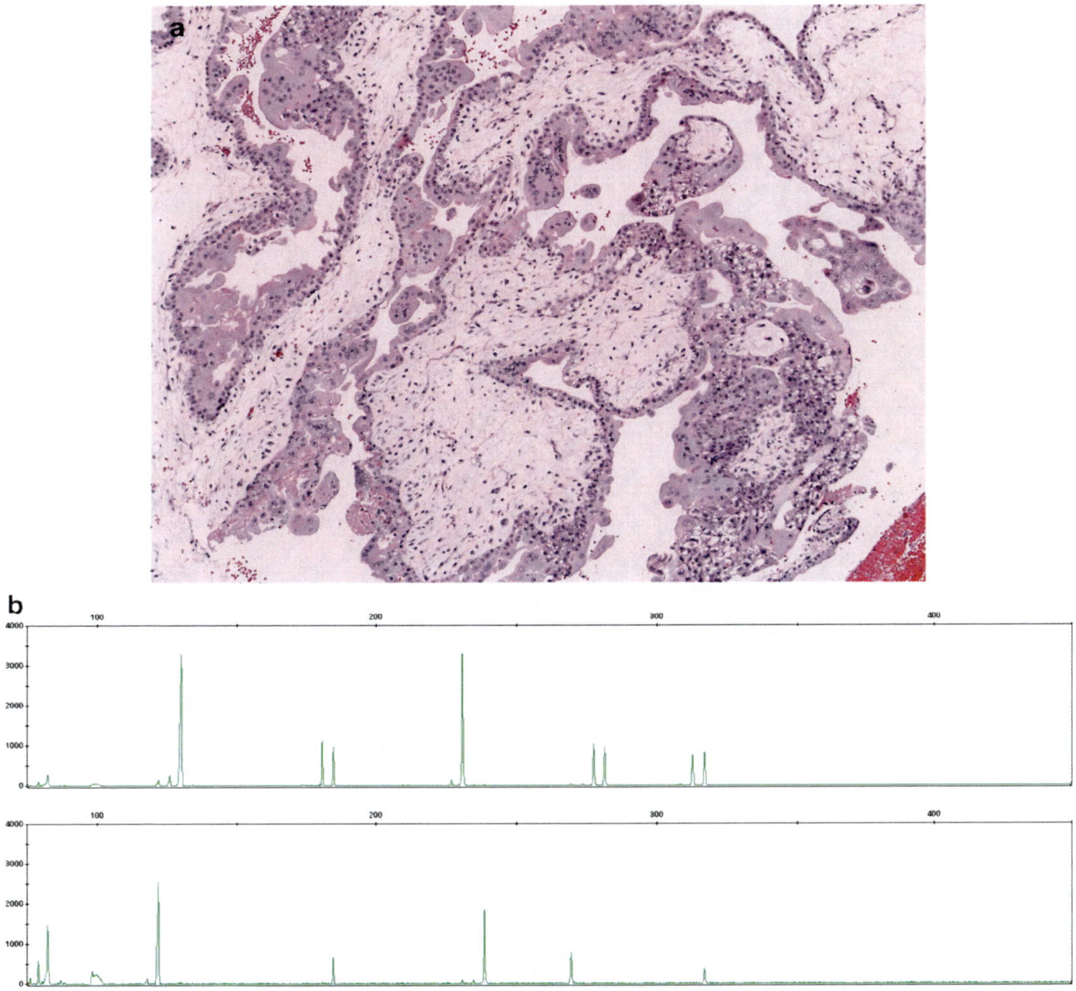

Fig. 4.15 An early complete mole arising from a tubal pregnancy (**a**) with confirmation by DNA genotyping (**b**). Note the presence of homozygous paternal-only alleles in chorionic villi (b, *lower panel*) compared with the normal biparental alleles in maternal endometrium (b, *upper panel*)

partial mole. Careful morphological assessment is crucial to ascertain the true molar hydropic villi, which may be confirmed by p57 immunohistochemistry.

Complete mole vs. choriocarcinoma: Complete mole may present with significant trophoblastic hyperplasia and marked cytological atypia in some cases. In isolation, such exuberant trophoblastic changes may mimic choriocarcinoma histologically when the villi are not represented in the tissue section (Fig. 4.16a, b). In current practice, a diagnosis of choriocarcinoma should not be made in the presence of identifiable chorionic villi, and a diagnosis of choriocarcinoma also requires the presence of tissue necrosis, destructive growth, and extensive hemorrhage (see Chap. 8). Submission of additional tissue or deeper sections of tissue blocks may reveal villous structures. It is possible, however, that an emerging or in-situ choriocarcinoma coexists with normal or molar chorionic villi (see Chap. 9). Since up to 30% of gestational choriocarcinomas follow a term

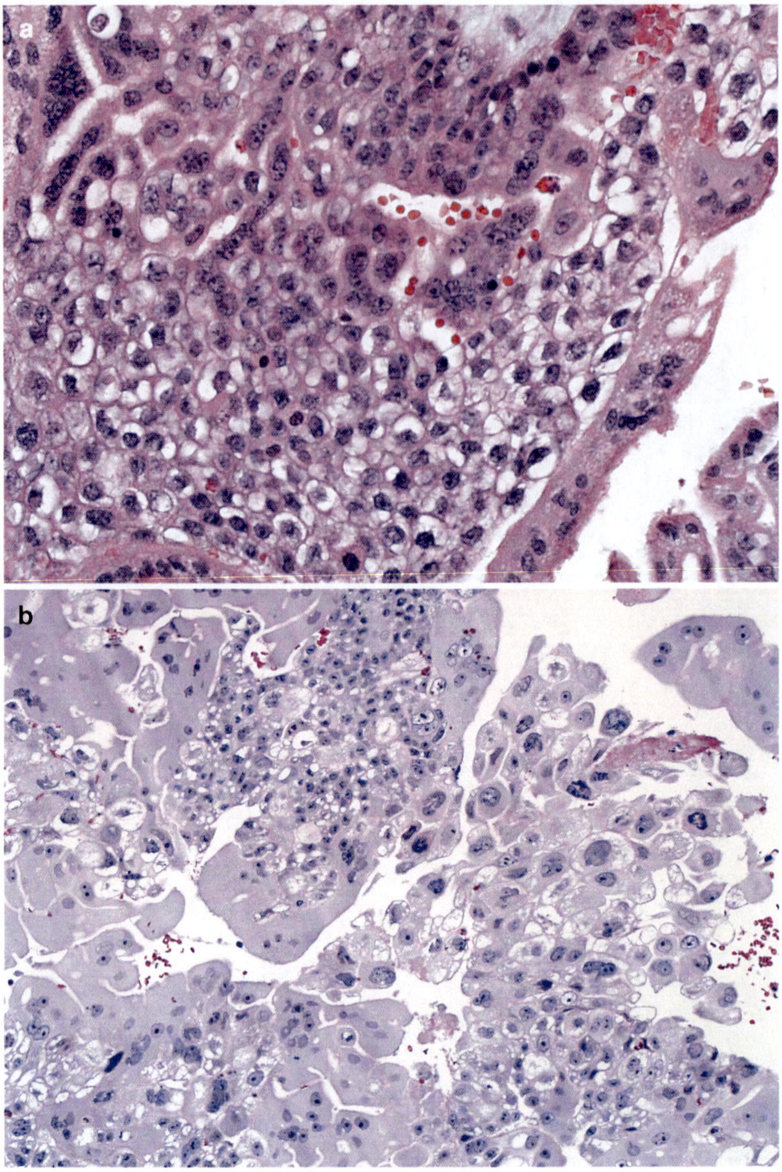

Fig. 4.16 Curettage specimen of an early complete mole shows markedly atypical trophoblasts along with the presence of chorionic villi (**a**). In isolation, such atypical trophoblasts may be misinterpreted as choriocarcinoma (**b**)

pregnancy, recent finding of in-situ choriocarcinoma in an otherwise normal placenta has drawn greater interest. Moreover, in very rare cases, choriocarcinoma may be identified in a missed abortion specimen within degenerative or ghost villi. The presence of sheets of highly atypical trophoblast with bilamellar arrangements should prompt a consideration of in-situ or early choriocarcinoma.

Clinicopathological Correlations

There is a finite increase of subsequent molar gestations after the diagnosis of complete mole. The absolute risk is about 1% after one prior mole and up to 15–18% after two consecutive moles [42, 43]. It is important to note that patients with familial biparental moles have a minimal likelihood to have a subsequent normal pregnancy, and egg donation may be the only option [8, 44, 45]. However, heterozygous NLRP7 mutation carriers appear without increased risk of adverse reproductive events [8, 14].

In 2002, FIGO introduced the term "persistent trophoblastic neoplasia – GTN" to include persistent mole, invasive mole, metastatic mole, choriocarcinoma, and trophoblastic tumors under one clinical term for management purpose [46], because all patients with such a diagnosis require chemotherapy [18]. This is a rather important development resulting in clinical treatment decision based on clinical and serum hCG marker evaluation without a need of tissue diagnosis. Therefore, precise histological diagnoses of the persistent disease after molar pregnancy have become blurred. Clinical parameters including plateaued hCG level for 2–4 weeks, rising hCG levels, continued uterine bleeding or signs of metastatic disease signify the presence of persistent GTN. The incidence of persistent gestational trophoblastic neoplasia after the evacuation of complete hydatidiform moles ranges from 18 to 29% [16, 47–50]. Traditionally, among GTN, choriocarcinoma occurs in about 2–3% of patients after complete moles. In the United States and Western European countries, 50% of gestational choriocarcinomas follow a complete hydatidiform mole (Chap. 12, Fig. 12.2). Chapter 9 provides a thorough discuss of GTN. Histological and immunohistochemical markers have not been well established in predicting the risk of prognosis of complete mole. The amount of trophoblastic hyperplasia and the degree of cytological atypia in complete mole have no apparent prognostic significance. Therefore, grading of complete mole is no longer in practice [51, 52]. Recent investigations have found that an overexpression of Nanog, a stem cell marker, may be correlated with a worse prognosis of complete mole [53, 54]. It is important to realize that evacuation of an early complete mole has not significantly changed the rate of developing persistent gestational neoplasia [18, 22, 55]. Chapter 9 provides an in-depth discussion of persistent trophoblastic neoplasia.

It has been suspected that the risk of GTN is higher for heterozygous complete moles than for homozygous ones [41]. Several groups had worked on the issue using different molecular approaches [41, 56–60]. Using more accurate and comprehensive STR polymorphisms analysis, it has been recently confirmed that heterozygous complete moles indeed have a greater risk of developing GTN [6]. Moreover, the risk of GTN in patients with FBCM was found similar to those with androgenic complete mole [8].

Complete mole with coexisting fetus has a higher incidence of postmolar complications (post-gestational trophoblastic neoplasia). Among 72 patients with coexistent twin pregnancies reported in Japan, 45.2% of 31 patients who required uterine evacuation during the second trimester for medical indications developed GTN, compared to 20.8 and 17.6% who delivered in the first and third trimester, respectively [61]. When comparing with singleton molar pregnancy, complete mole with coexisting twin fetus developed a higher incidence of metastatic or persistent mole that required chemotherapy [61, 62].

References

1. Benirschke K, Kaufmann P, Baergen RN. Pathology of the human placenta. 5th ed. New York: Springer; 2006.
2. Bebyser IWJ, Soma H, Zwart P. Partial hydatidiform mole in a pregnant chimpanzee (Pan troglodytes). Zoo Biol. 1993;12:6.
3. Gopal T, Leipold HW, Dennis SM. Hydatidiform moles in Holstein cattle. Vet Rec. 1980;107(17):395–7.
4. Lage JM, Weinberg DS, Yavner DL, Bieber FR. The biology of tetraploid hydatidiform moles: histopathology, cytogenetics, and flow cytometry. Hum Pathol. 1989;20(5):419–25.
5. Vejerslev LO, Dissing J, Hansen HE, Poulsen H. Hydatidiform mole: genetic origin in polyploid conceptuses. Hum Genet. 1987;76(1):11–9.
6. Baasanjav B, Usui H, Kihara M, Kaku H, Nakada E, Tate S, et al. The risk of post-molar gestational trophoblastic neoplasia is higher in heterozygous than in homozygous complete hydatidiform moles. Hum Reprod. 2010;25(5):1183–91.
7. Fisher RA, Hodges MD, Newlands ES. Familial recurrent hydatidiform mole: a review. J Reprod Med. 2004;49(8):595–601.
8. Williams D, Hodgetts V, Gupta J. Recurrent hydatidiform moles. Eur J Obstet Gynecol Reprod Biol. 2010; 150(1):3–7.

9. Fisher RA, Hodges MD, Rees HC, Sebire NJ, Seckl MJ, Newlands ES, et al. The maternally transcribed gene p57(KIP2) (CDNK1C) is abnormally expressed in both androgenetic and biparental complete hydatidiform moles. Hum Mol Genet. 2002;11(26):3267–72.
10. Panichkul PC, Al-Hussaini TK, Sierra R, Kashork CD, Popek EJ, Stockton DW, et al. Recurrent biparental hydatidiform mole: additional evidence for a 1.1-Mb locus in 19q13.4 and candidate gene analysis. J Soc Gynecol Investig. 2005;12(5):376–83.
11. Murdoch S, Djuric U, Mazhar B, Seoud M, Khan R, Kuick R, et al. Mutations in NALP7 cause recurrent hydatidiform moles and reproductive wastage in humans. Nat Genet. 2006;38(3):300–2.
12. Moglabey YB, Kircheisen R, Seoud M, El Mogharbel N, Van den Veyver I, Slim R. Genetic mapping of a maternal locus responsible for familial hydatidiform moles. Hum Mol Genet. 1999;8(4):667–71.
13. Hodges MD, Rees HC, Seckl MJ, Newlands ES, Fisher RA. Genetic refinement and physical mapping of a biparental complete hydatidiform mole locus on chromosome 19q13.4. J Med Genet. 2003;40(8):e95.
14. Hayward BE, De Vos M, Talati N, Abdollahi MR, Taylor GR, Meyer E, et al. Genetic and epigenetic analysis of recurrent hydatidiform mole. Hum Mutat. 2009;30(5):E629–39.
15. Slim R, Mehio A. The genetics of hydatidiform moles: new lights on an ancient disease. Clin Genet. 2007; 71(1):25–34.
16. Berkowitz RS, Goldstein DP. Chorionic tumors. N Engl J Med. 1996;335(23):1740–8.
17. Goldstein DP, Berkowitz RS. Current management of complete and partial molar pregnancy. J Reprod Med. 1994;39(3):139–46.
18. Berkowitz RS, Goldstein DP. Clinical practice. Molar pregnancy. N Engl J Med. 2009;360(16):1639–45.
19. Berkowitz R, Ozturk M, Goldstein D, Bernstein M, Hill L, Wands JR. Human chorionic gonadotropin and free subunits' serum levels in patients with partial and complete hydatidiform moles. Obstet Gynecol. 1989; 74(2):212–6.
20. Szulman AE, Surti U. The syndromes of hydatidiform mole. I. Cytogenetic and morphologic correlations. Am J Obstet Gynecol. 1978;131(6):665–71.
21. Szulman AE. Syndromes of hydatidiform moles. Partial vs. complete. J Reprod Med. 1984;29(11):788–91.
22. Soto-Wright V, Bernstein M, Goldstein DP, Berkowitz RS. The changing clinical presentation of complete molar pregnancy. Obstet Gynecol. 1995;86(5):775–9.
23. Felemban AA, Bakri YN, Alkharif HA, Altuwaijri SM, Shalhoub J, Berkowitz RS. Complete molar pregnancy. Clinical trends at King Fahad Hospital, Riyadh, Kingdom of Saudi Arabia. J Reprod Med. 1998;43(1):11–3.
24. Keep D, Zaragoza MV, Hassold T, Redline RW. Very early complete hydatidiform mole. Hum Pathol. 1996;27(7):708–13.
25. Sebire NJ, Rees H, Paradinas F, Seckl M, Newlands E. The diagnostic implications of routine ultrasound examination in histologically confirmed early molar pregnancies. Ultrasound Obstet Gynecol. 2001;18(6): 662–5.
26. Mosher R, Goldstein DP, Berkowitz R, Bernstein M, Genest DR. Complete hydatidiform mole. Comparison of clinicopathologic features, current and past. J Reprod Med. 1998;43(1):21–7.
27. Fowler DJ, Lindsay I, Seckl MJ, Sebire NJ. Histomorphometric features of hydatidiform moles in early pregnancy: relationship to detectability by ultrasound examination. Ultrasound Obstet Gynecol. 2007;29(1):76–80.
28. Benson CB, Genest DR, Bernstein MR, Soto-Wright V, Goldstein DP, Berkowitz RS. Sonographic appearance of first trimester complete hydatidiform moles. Ultrasound Obstet Gynecol. 2000;16(2):188–91.
29. Qiao S, Nagasaka T, Nakashima N. Numerous vessels detected by CD34 in the villous stroma of complete hydatidiform moles. Int J Gynecol Pathol. 1997;16(3): 233–8.
30. Yoshida K, Nagasaka T, Nakashima N, Nishida Y, Saito M, Tomomitsu O. Elucidation of vascular structure of molar villi in complete hydatidiform mole by CD-34 antibody. Int J Gynecol Pathol. 2000;19(3):212–8.
31. Fisher RA, Paradinas FJ, Soteriou BA, Foskett M, Newlands ES. Diploid hydatidiform moles with fetal red blood cells in molar villi. 2 – Genetics. J Pathol. 1997;181(2):189–95.
32. Paradinas FJ, Fisher RA, Browne P, Newlands ES. Diploid hydatidiform moles with fetal red blood cells in molar villi. 1 – Pathology, incidence, and prognosis. J Pathol. 1997;181(2):183–8.
33. Zaragoza MV, Keep D, Genest DR, Hassold T, Redline RW. Early complete hydatidiform moles contain inner cell mass derivatives. Am J Med Genet. 1997;70(3):273–7.
34. Baergen RN, Kelly T, McGinniss MJ, Jones OW, Benirschke K. Complete hydatidiform mole with a coexistent embryo. Hum Pathol. 1996;27(7):731–4.
35. Lage JM, Bagg A. Hydatidiform moles: DNA flow cytometry, image analysis and selected topics in molecular biology. Histopathology. 1996;28(4):379–82.
36. Gschwendtner A, Neher A, Kreczy A, Muller-Holzner E, Volgger B, Mairinger T. DNA ploidy determination of early molar pregnancies by image analysis: comparison to histologic classification. Arch Pathol Lab Med. 1998;122(11):1000–4.
37. Esteban JM, Sheibani K, Owens M, Joyce J, Bailey A, Battifora H. Effects of various fixatives and fixation conditions on DNA ploidy analysis. A need for strict internal DNA standards. Am J Clin Pathol. 1991;95(4): 460–6.
38. Chilosi M, Piazzola E, Lestani M, Benedetti A, Guasparri I, Granchelli G, et al. Differential expression of p57kip2, a maternally imprinted cdk inhibitor, in normal human placenta and gestational trophoblastic disease. Lab Invest. 1998;78(3):269–76.
39. McConnell TG, Murphy KM, Hafez M, Vang R, Ronnett BM. Diagnosis and subclassification of hydatidiform moles using p57 immunohistochemistry and molecular genotyping: validation and prospective analysis in routine and consultation practice settings with development of an algorithmic approach. Am J Surg Pathol. 2009;33(6):805–17.

40. Kajii T, Ferrier A, Niikawa N, Takahara H, Ohama K, Avirachan S. Anatomic and chromosomal anomalies in 639 spontaneous abortuses. Hum Genet. 1980;55(1): 87–98.
41. Wake N, Seki T, Fujita H, Okubo H, Sakai K, Okuyama K, et al. Malignant potential of homozygous and heterozygous complete moles. Cancer Res. 1984;44(3):1226–30.
42. Bagshawe KD, Dent J, Webb J. Hydatidiform mole in England and Wales 1973–83. Lancet. 1986;2(8508): 673–7.
43. Garrett LA, Garner EI, Feltmate CM, Goldstein DP, Berkowitz RS. Subsequent pregnancy outcomes in patients with molar pregnancy and persistent gestational trophoblastic neoplasia. J Reprod Med. 2008; 53(7):481–6.
44. Van den Veyver IB, Al-Hussaini TK. Biparental hydatidiform moles: a maternal effect mutation affecting imprinting in the offspring. Hum Reprod Update. 2006; 12(3):233–42.
45. van der Smagt JJ, Scheenjes E, Kremer JA, Hennekam FA, Fisher RA. Heterogeneity in the origin of recurrent complete hydatidiform moles: not all women with multiple molar pregnancies have biparental moles. BJOG. 2006;113(6):725–8.
46. Kohorn EI. The new FIGO 2000 staging and risk factor scoring system for gestational trophoblastic disease: description and critical assessment. Int J Gynecol Cancer. 2001;11(1):73–7.
47. Curry SL, Hammond CB, Tyrey L, Creasman WT, Parker RT. Hydatidiform mole: diagnosis, management, and long-term followup of 347 patients. Obstet Gynecol. 1975;45(1):1–8.
48. Kohorn EI. Hydatidiform mole and gestational trophoblastic disease in Southern Connecticut. Obstet Gynecol. 1982;59(1):78–84.
49. Lurain JR, Brewer JI, Torok EE, Halpern B. Natural history of hydatidiform mole after primary evacuation. Am J Obstet Gynecol. 1983;145(5):591–5.
50. Morrow CP, Kletzky OA, Disaia PJ, Townsend DE, Mishell DR, Nakamura RM. Clinical and laboratory correlates of molar pregnancy and trophoblastic disease. Am J Obstet Gynecol. 1977;128(4):424–30.
51. Genest DR, Laborde O, Berkowitz RS, Goldstein DP, Bernstein MR, Lage J. A clinicopathologic study of 153 cases of complete hydatidiform mole (1980–1990): histologic grade lacks prognostic significance. Obstet Gynecol. 1991;78(3 Pt 1):402–9.
52. Rice LW, Genest DR, Berkowitz RS, Goldstein DP, Bernstein MR, Redline RW. Pathologic features of sharp curettings in complete hydatidiform mole. Predictors of persistent gestational trophoblastic disease. J Reprod Med. 1991;36(1):17–20.
53. Siu MK, Wong ES, Chan HY, Ngan HY, Chan KY, Cheung AN. Overexpression of NANOG in gestational trophoblastic diseases: effect on apoptosis, cell invasion, and clinical outcome. Am J Pathol. 2008; 173(4):1165–72.
54. Shih Ie M, Kuo KT. Power of the eternal youth: Nanog expression in the gestational choriocarcinoma. Am J Pathol. 2008;173(4):911–4.
55. Paradinas FJ, Browne P, Fisher RA, Foskett M, Bagshawe KD, Newlands E. A clinical, histopathological and flow cytometric study of 149 complete moles, 146 partial moles and 107 non-molar hydropic abortions. Histopathology. 1996;28(2):101–10.
56. Wake N, Fujino T, Hoshi S, Shinkai N, Sakai K, Kato H, et al. The propensity to malignancy of dispermic heterozygous moles. Placenta. 1987;8(3):319–26.
57. Cheung AN, Sit AS, Chung LP, Ngan HY, O'Hanlan K, Wong LC, et al. Detection of heterozygous XY complete hydatidiform mole by chromosome in situ hybridization. Gynecol Oncol. 1994;55(3 Pt 1):386–92.
58. Lawler SD, Fisher RA. Genetic studies in hydatidiform mole with clinical correlations. Placenta. 1987; 8(1):77–88.
59. Niemann I, Sunde L, Petersen LK. Evaluation of the risk of persistent trophoblastic disease after twin pregnancy with diploid hydatidiform mole and coexisting normal fetus. Am J Obstet Gynecol. 2007;197(1):45e1–5.
60. Niemann I, Hansen ES, Sunde L. The risk of persistent trophoblastic disease after hydatidiform mole classified by morphology and ploidy. Gynecol Oncol. 2007;104(2):411–5.
61. Matsui H, Sekiya S, Hando T, Wake N, Tomoda Y. Hydatidiform mole coexistent with a twin live fetus: a national collaborative study in Japan. Hum Reprod. 2000;15(3):608–11.
62. Fishman DA, Padilla LA, Keh P, Cohen L, Frederiksen M, Lurain JR. Management of twin pregnancies consisting of a complete hydatidiform mole and normal fetus. Obstet Gynecol. 1998;91(4):546–50.

5 Partial Hydatidiform Mole

Natalia Buza

Keywords
Partial mole • Diagnostic features • Differential diagnosis

Introduction

Hydatidiform moles are nonneoplastic proliferations of the villous trophoblasts, with two distinct subtypes: complete and partial hydatidiform moles (PHMs). While they share some basic features, that is, hydropic placenta/chorionic villi and trophoblastic hyperplasia, partial and complete moles have significant differences in their genetic composition, clinical presentation, histomorphology, and the subsequent risk of developing persistent gestational trophoblastic disease (GTD) or gestational trophoblastic neoplasia (GTN). At the genetic level, PHMs are typically diandric monogynic triploid gestations, most often arising from two sperms fertilizing an egg. Complete moles on the other hand are most commonly diploid or tetraploid and are entirely paternally derived.

Although cytogenetic abnormalities, including triploidy, have been reported in hydatidiform moles since the 1960s, the two subtypes – complete and partial mole – were not defined and separated until the late 1970s [1–7]. Initially, the basis of division had been the absence or the presence of an embryo/fetus, and partial (or "incomplete") moles were defined as "moles with fetuses" (alive or dead) with a triploid karyotype, slowly progressing hydatidiform swelling of the placenta with focal sparing of villi, and focal, inconspicuous trophoblastic hyperplasia [3]. Over the past 3 decades, the evolution of ancillary techniques – cytogenetics, flow cytometry, immunohistochemistry, and most recently molecular genotyping – has significantly contributed to our understanding of the pathogenesis and biology of complete and PHMs and improved our diagnostic accuracy, as it will be discussed in detail in this chapter.

The incidence of molar pregnancies shows wide regional variation: the reported rates range from 0.63 to 1.1/1,000 pregnancies in the United States and Europe, compared to the much higher rates in Mexico, Nigeria, Japan, and Indonesia (up to 13 hydatidiform moles per 1,000 pregnancies) [8–11]. It is unclear to what extent is this variation attributable to racial differences; however, higher incidence has been reported among Asian, Philippine, and Hispanic women, as well as Native Americans and Alaskan natives [9, 12]. In addition to geographic and ethnic factors,

N. Buza, MD (✉)
Department of Pathology, Yale University School of Medicine, 310 Cedar Street, PO Box 208023, New Haven, CT 06520-8023, USA
e-mail: natalia.buza@yale.edu

P. Hui (ed.), *Gestational Trophoblastic Disease: Diagnostic and Molecular Genetic Pathology*, Current Clinical Pathology, DOI 10.1007/978-1-61779-394-3_5,

extremes of maternal age (younger than 20 or older than 40 years of age), nulliparity or low parity, history of infertility, low dietary intake of carotene and animal fat, and family or personal history of GTD have been found to be associated with an increased risk of hydatidiform moles [8, 9, 11, 13]. The above statistics are, however, largely based on data obtained from studies of complete mole. The exact epidemiology of partial mole is at best uncertain due to significant underdiagnosis and misclassification of triploid gestations, see next section. Although complete hydatidiform mole (CHM) and PHM share many of the risk factors, there are data to suggest that higher education, smoking, irregular menstrual cycles, oral contraceptive use for over 4 years, and only male infants among prior live births significantly increase the risk of PHM in contrast to CHM [11, 14]. The risk of partial mole also increases with maternal age [15]; in several studies, the ratio of PHM to CHM was 2:1 in women older than 35 years, while the reverse was true for women under 20 years of age [16–18]. This may be due to abnormal zona pellucida formation with increasing maternal age, which may facilitate sperm penetration and promote formation of a partial mole [17].

Genetic Background

Virtually, all PHMs have a triploid – diandric monogynic – genome, arising from two sperms fertilizing an egg (dispermic, heterozygous PHM) in approximately 90% of cases. The remaining 10% of cases originate from one sperm fertilizing an egg followed by reduplication of the paternal chromosome set, due to failure of meiosis I or II (monospermic, homozygous PHM) [19–21]. As a result, approximately 70% of partial moles have a 69XXY karyotype, 27% are 69XXX, and 3% 69XYY [21, 22].

Not all triploid gestations manifest as PHMs, however. Triploidy is one of the most common chromosomal abnormalities in humans, occurring in up to 3% of all conceptuses [23, 24], and approximately 8–10% of all spontaneous abortions [25, 26]. Nearly two-thirds of these cases are paternally derived and associated with a partial molar phenotype, but approximately one-third of them are digynic, non-molar gestations, arising from meiotic nondisjunction of maternal chromosomes [21, 23, 27]. Interestingly, the ratio of digynic triploids is much higher among cases with well-formed fetuses and late intrauterine fetal demise, resulting in some discrepancies between datasets in the literature [21, 23, 24]. These data imply that the rate of genetic partial moles among spontaneous abortions might be as high as 3%. Many of these cases may possibly be missed on routine pathologic examination without adjunct tests, due to the early gestational age at evacuation and incomplete histological features.

Rare tetraploid partial moles have also been reported, with three haploid paternal chromosome sets and a 92XXXX, 92XXYY, or 92XXXY karyotype [28, 29]. Early reports have also raised the possibility of diploid PHMs mainly on the basis of presence of fetal red blood cells and/or fetal tissues; however, these cases were later either found to be twin gestations with a complete mole and a normal fetus, or very early complete moles with evidence of early embryonic development [20, 30, 31]. A study on a large series of putative diploid PHMs revealed that the majority of the cases were misclassified on pathologic examination, while the rest of them proved to be triploid on repeat ploidy analysis [20]. These more recent data suggest that diploid partial moles probably do not exist, and misclassification of such cases can be avoided by careful microscopic examination coupled with new ancillary techniques (i.e., immunohistochemistry and molecular genotyping).

Clinical Presentation

Majority of patients with PHM present in the late first trimester or early second trimester with vaginal bleeding or with missed or incomplete abortions [11, 15]. The uterine size is usually small or appropriate for gestational age, and the serum human chorionic gonadotropin (hCG) level is normal or moderately elevated [32]. Preeclampsia, uterine enlargement, hyperthyroidism, hyperemesis, and other classic symptoms of CHM are rarely seen in association with partial mole [8, 15, 33]. Ultrasound findings of PHM may include focal cystic changes in the placenta and increase in the transverse diameter of the gestational sac [8, 32, 34, 35]. Unlike in CHM, a fetus may be detectable by ultrasound [11]. However, there is a high false-negative as well as false-positive rate for PHM associated with sonographic study; therefore, pathologic examination of all nonviable pregnancies should be performed irrespective of the ultrasound findings [36, 37].

Gross and Microscopic Features

The volume of the evacuation specimen of PHM is usually less than that of complete mole, but generally more than that of hydropic abortions. Grossly it often appears as normal villous tissue; however, molar vesicles may occasionally be seen (Fig. 5.1). A gestational sac, fetal parts, or a relatively intact fetus may be grossly apparent, depending on the gestational age at the time of evacuation or at the time of intrauterine demise if it occurred weeks before the evacuation. In cases with prolonged postmortem intrauterine retention, the fetus may have undergone marked autolysis preventing the gross or microscopic identification of fetal parts. The fetus, if present, usually shows mild to moderate symmetrical intrauterine growth restriction (IUGR) and characteristic malformations, that is, syndactyly (involving fingers 3–4 and toes 2–3), but spina bifida, cleft palate, cryptophthalmos, simian crease, and renal hypoplasia have also been reported [3, 27, 38–40]. Although PHM is incompatible with fetal survival, there have been rare case reports of liveborn triploid fetuses that died within a few hours of birth, some of which have been confirmed as partial moles [26, 38].

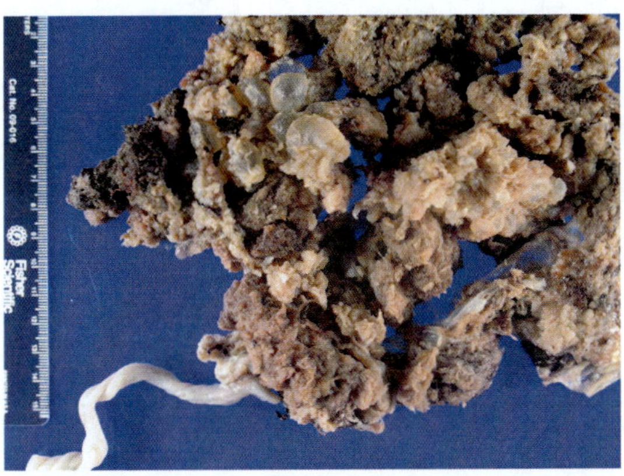

Fig. 5.1 PHM at 20 weeks of gestation with grossly identifiable gestational sac and umbilical cord. Note the semi-transparent hydropic change involving some but not all the chorionic villi. The pregnancy was terminated due to multiple fetal anomalies (ventriculomegaly and omphalocele)

Microscopically partial moles (Table 5.1) are characterized by a dimorphous villous population: large, hydropic, and irregular villi intermixed with smaller, normal appearing or fibrotic chorionic villi (Fig. 5.2a–e). This second villous population with preserved fetal circulation is thought to be responsible for fetal survival in partial moles, in contrast to the typically avascular villi in complete moles [33, 36, 41]. The size of larger hydropic villi is greater than 0.5 mm, generally ranging between 1 and 6 mm [42]. Central cistern formation with a maze-like pattern is seen in advanced cases. The villi are irregularly shaped with scalloped contours. Trophoblastic pseudo-inclusions – resulting from invaginations of the villous surface – are frequently present and are characteristically round or oval in shape. Single cell trophoblastic inclusions ("wandering trophoblasts") are also commonly seen in the villous stroma [42, 43]. There is mild to moderate circumferential – non-polar – trophoblastic hyperplasia without significant atypia [3, 4, 43].

Table 5.1 Histological features of partial hydatidiform mole

1.	Two populations of villi: hydropic enlarged and normal sized
2.	Scalloped villous surface and stromal cistern formation
3.	Round to oval trophoblastic pseudo-inclusions
4.	Mild circumferential trophoblastic hyperplasia and syncytiotrophoblastic sprouts
5.	Presence of nucleated RBC and/or fetal parts
6.	Positive nuclear staining of P57 in cytotrophoblasts and villous stromal cells

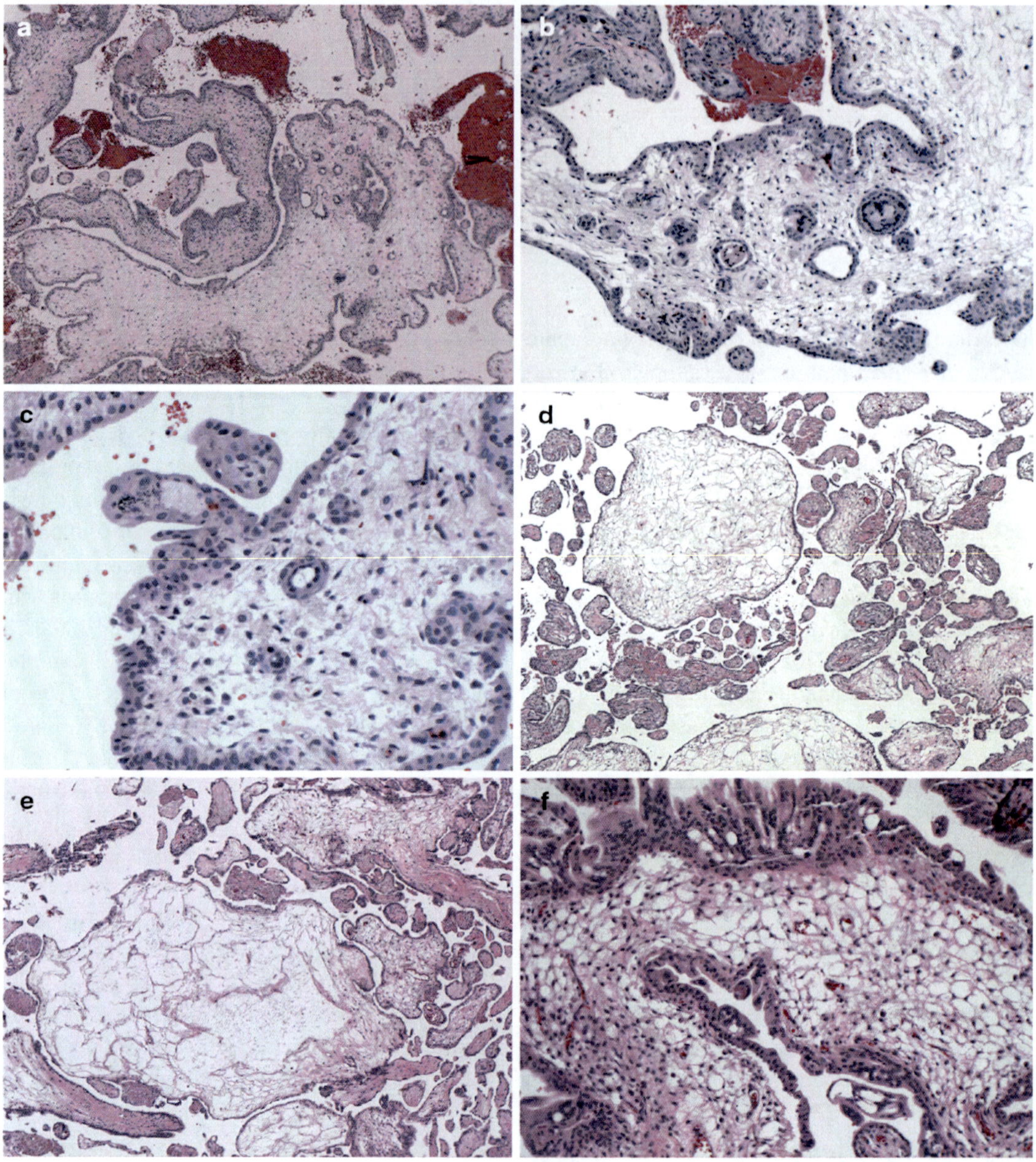

Fig. 5.2 Histomorphologic characteristics of PHM at 12 weeks (**a–c**) and 20 weeks gestational age (**d–f**). There are two populations of chorionic villi, the hydropic, larger villi have markedly irregular contours with several round trophoblastic pseudo-inclusions. Nucleated fetal red blood cells are present (**c**). Central cistern formation can be observed (**e**), and circumferential, non-polar trophoblastic hyperplasia is present

The syncytiotrophoblasts may be focally prominent (syncytiotrophoblast "knuckles" or "sprouts") with intracytoplasmic lacunae. Fetal blood vessels and nucleated red blood cells are often present.

Not all genetically confirmed triploid partial molar gestations show the characteristic histological features, however. At early gestational age (less than 8–9 weeks), the trophoblastic hyperplasia may be only focal, in the form of syncytiotrophoblast sprouts; the villous hydrops is not well developed, and therefore, the dimorphous villous population may not be apparent. Partial moles evacuated at a later developmental stage – involuting or "ancient" PHMs – show two populations of villi with irregular contours, but they may lack villous hydrops, and instead extensive villous fibrosis may be seen [41].

Ancillary Studies

The histological diagnosis of PHM is often challenging, due to the presence of frequent histological mimics and the absence of a single morphologic feature that is entirely specific for partial mole. Consequently, the inter- and intraobserver variability is high even among experts when the diagnosis is based on histology alone [44].

Among ancillary techniques, ploidy analysis – either by cytogenetics or flow cytometry – has been utilized for the longest time [21]. Ploidy analysis is useful in diagnosing triploid gestations and separating them from the diploid, tetraploid, or aneuploid conceptuses (Fig. 5.3). However, it is unable to distinguish between diandric monogynic PHMs and non-molar digynic triploidy, and between diploid CHMs and its non-molar diploid mimics. Furthermore, there are technical limitations associated with these methods. Conventional karyotyping is time- and labor-intensive, and requires fresh tissue, which is often not available, especially if the diagnosis was clinically unsuspected. Flow cytometry analysis, although may be performed on formalin-fixed paraffin-embedded tissues, it is not uncommonly associated with misclassification of ploidy [45]. The role of fluorescent in situ hybridization (FISH) in ploidy analysis for suspected molar gestations has also been advocated; however, it has not become a routine technique due to technical difficulties [46].

The role of immunohistochemistry for various cell cycle proteins (E2F-1, CDK2, cyclin E, p27, p57) and proliferation markers (proliferation cell nuclear antigen [PCNA], Ki-67) has also been explored in various studies [47–49]. Among all these markers, only p57 was found to have practical significance in the differential diagnosis of hydatidiform moles. P57 is a cyclin-dependent kinase inhibitor protein, encoded by a paternally imprinted gene on chromosome 11p15.5 [50]. It is preferentially expressed only from the maternal allele; therefore, CHMs do not express p57 since their genetic material is entirely paternally

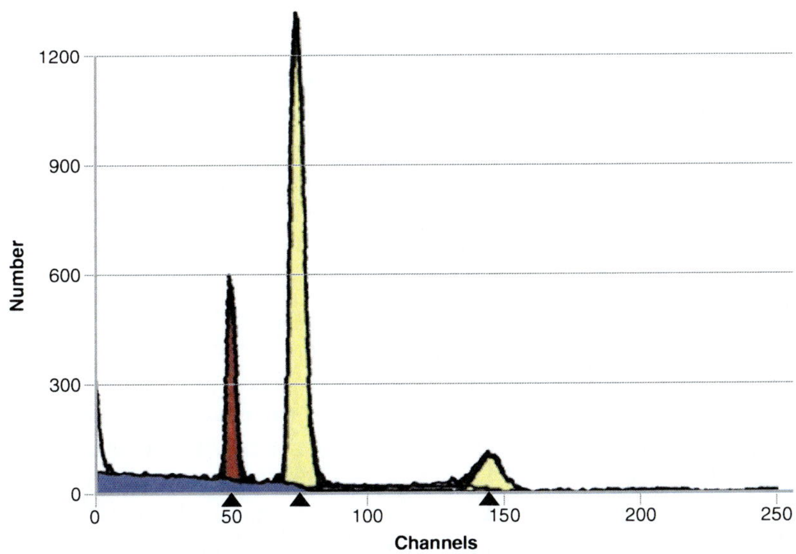

Fig. 5.3 PHM with triploid DNA content by flow cytometric ploidy analysis using isolated nuclei from archived paraffin-embedded tissue. Characteristic triploid DNA content is seen as the *yellow peak* corresponding to a 69 chromosomal composition. The *red peak* corresponds to a 46 chromosomal composition representing the contaminating normal diploid maternal cells

derived. As p57 is a negative regulator of cell cycle, lack of its activity can lead to loss of cell cycle control and hyperproliferation, which may be the explanation for trophoblastic proliferation in CHM. Normal placentas, hydropic abortions, and PHMs show strong nuclear p57 expression in cytotrophoblasts, intermediate trophoblasts, intervillus trophoblast islands, villous stromal cells, and decidual stromal cells, whereas syncytiotrophoblasts are uniformly negative. In complete moles, on the other hand, p57 immunostaining is absent in cytotrophoblasts and villous stromal cells, although its aberrant expression can be seen in intervillous intermediate trophoblasts and villous endothelial cells [50, 51] (Fig. 5.4). The interpretation may be however challenging in rare cases of CHM where an incomplete imprinting of p57 results in weak nuclear staining among the molar cytotrophoblastic cells. Nonetheless, p57 immunostaining is a useful marker in separating CHM from its mimics in the majority of the cases. P57 immunostain cannot, however, differentiate between PHM and other abnormal gestations that contain maternal genetic material (i.e., hydropic abortions, trisomies, digynic triploidy, placental mesenchymal dysplasia).

Most recently, molecular genotyping has been found highly sensitive and specific by multiple groups to aid the diagnosis of hydatidiform moles. Polymerase chain reaction (PCR) amplification of multiple short tandem repeat (STR) loci of maternal decidua and villous tissue provides information about the parental genetic contribution in the villous tissue [19, 52–55]. The alleles in the maternal tissue are compared with the alleles in the chorionic villi: one matching maternal allele and two paternal alleles (heterozygous PHM), or one paternal allele in double quantity (homozygous PHM) in at least two loci is diagnostic of partial mole (Fig. 5.5). Genotyping can reliably distinguish diandric monogynic PHMs from diandric CHMs, biparental diploid hydropic abortions, digynic monoandric triploidy, and the more common chromosomal trisomies [52]. It has been recommended that genotyping should be performed whenever a differential diagnosis of PHM is considered [56].

To best utilize these ancillary techniques, some institutions have developed a diagnostic algorithm: cases morphologically suspicious for CHM are first stained for p57 and a negative result (in the presence of positive internal control) is confirmatory without further analysis, and only those cases that lack well-developed morphologic features of CHM and/or have equivocal p57 results are subjected to genotyping [53]. At our institution, however, all cases with morphologic suspicion of either complete or partial mole are genotyped for final diagnosis and genotypic subclassification [56] for a number of reasons, see discussions in Chap. 11.

Differential Diagnosis

Several conditions may mimic PHM histologically, the separation and precise diagnosis of which are important, as there are marked differences in the prognosis and the clinical management and follow-up of patients with these entities. More commonly, they present in the first trimester of pregnancy, such as typical complete mole, early complete mole, hydropic abortions, and gestations with chromosomal abnormalities. Late gestational mimics include placental mesenchymal dysplasia, chromosomal abnormalities, and twin gestations with complete mole and coexisting normal fetus [27].

In complete moles, the villous hydrops is diffuse and marked, in contrast to the focal and less severe hydropic changes in partial mole (Fig. 5.6a). The villi are round, or may be "cauliflower-shaped" in very early CHM, the trophoblastic hyperplasia is more pronounced, and there is often trophoblastic atypia at the implantation site in the form of exaggerated placental site reaction. Trophoblastic pseudo-inclusions may be present, but in contrast to the round pseudo-inclusions in partial moles, they are more often irregular in shape [43]. Characteristically, the villous stroma is hypercellular and has a slightly basophilic, myxoid matrix with karyorrhectic debris (apoptosis). Unlike in partial moles, fetal parts or fetal tissues are generally absent in complete moles; however, they may be seen in a complete mole arising from

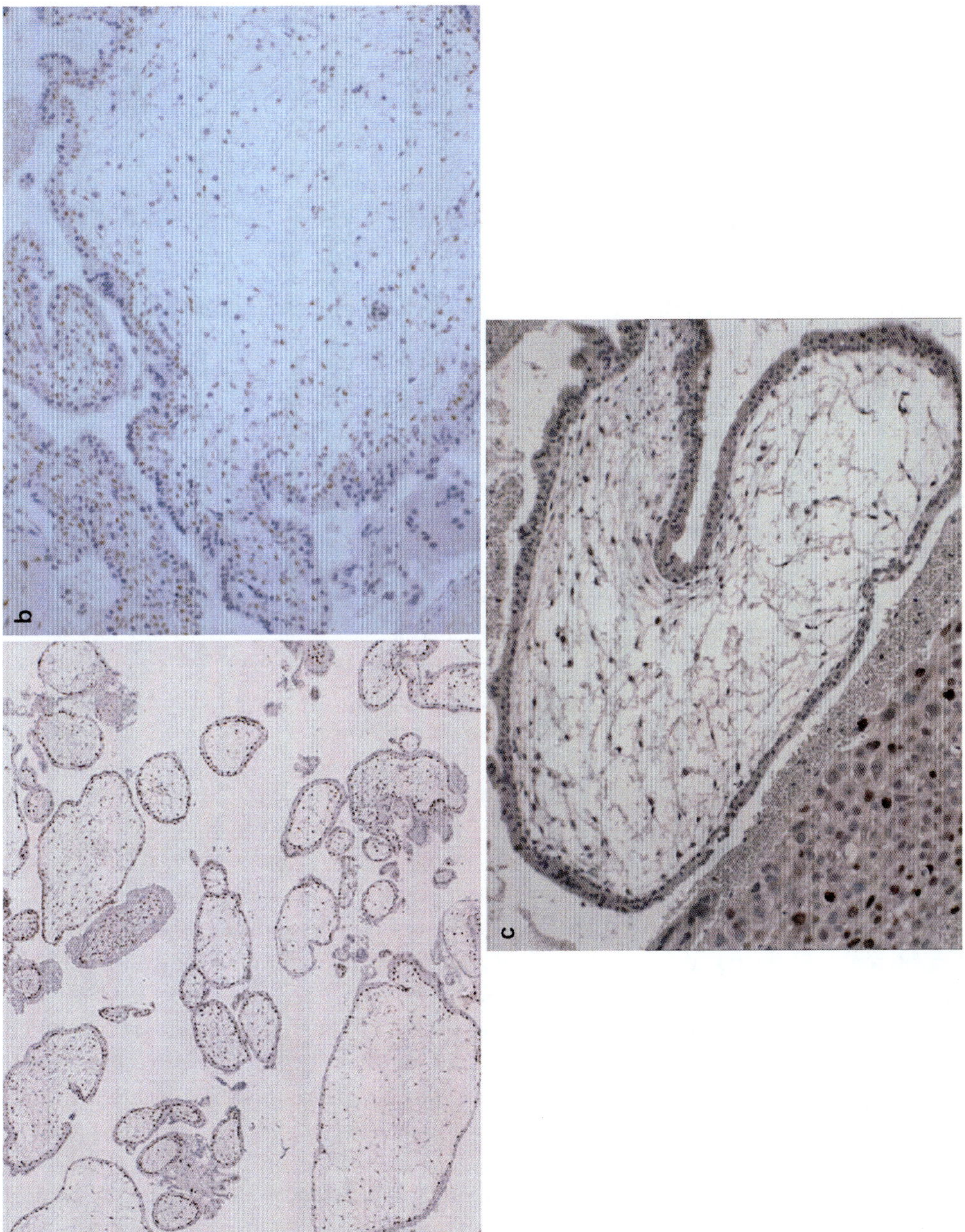

Fig. 5.4 P57 immunohistochemistry: Strong nuclear p57 expression is present in cytotrophoblasts, intermediate trophoblasts, villous stromal cells, and decidual stromal cells in diploid hydropic abortions (**a**) and partial moles (**b**) that contain maternal genetic material. P57 staining is absent in cytotrophoblasts and villous stromal cells in complete mole; positive immunoreaction in the decidual stromal cells serve as positive internal control (**c**)

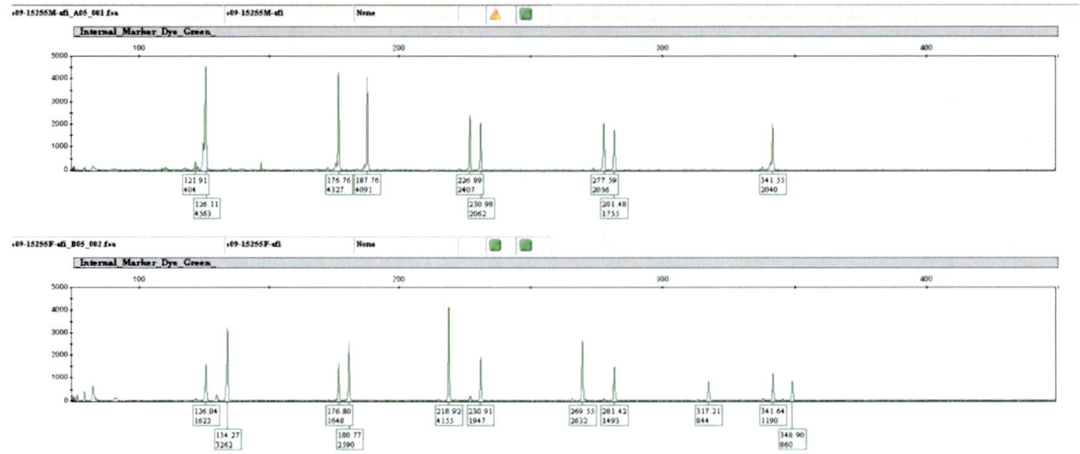

Fig. 5.5 DNA genotyping diagnosis of PHM. Comparing with the biparental alleles in the corresponding gestational endometrium (*upper panel*), the presence of two paternal alleles in addition to one maternal allele at several microsatellite loci (*lower panel*) confirms a dispermic/heterozygous partial mole

a twin gestation [27, 30]. Fetal vessels and nucleated red blood cells, once thought to differentiate between partial and complete moles, can be found in very early complete moles [30, 31, 36].

Hydropic abortions usually have a small volume of tissue on gross examination. The chorionic villi are round with a smooth contour, and demonstrate mild, focal hydropic changes. Trophoblastic hyperplasia – if present – is polar (non-circumferential), limited to the anchoring villi (Fig. 5.6b). There is no atypia or trophoblastic pseudo-inclusions. Hydropic abortion is often used as a general term to include all non-molar – diploid, triploid, and aneuploid – hydropic gestations. In many cases, there is an underlying chromosomal abnormality, discernable by conventional karyotyping or molecular genotyping, which is discussed separately in the following.

It may be very difficult to differentiate between chromosomal abnormalities and partial moles solely on the basis of histology. Closely resembling PHM, gestations with certain chromosomal aberrations (particularly trisomies 6, 7, 13, 15, 16, 18, 21, and 22) often show markedly irregular chorionic villi with trophoblastic pseudo-inclusions and variable degree of hydropic change [52, 57–60] (Fig. 5.7). Similar to partial moles, fetal vessels and fetal red blood cells are commonly seen in the villous stroma. Trophoblastic hyperplasia – equivalent in severity to that seen in partial or complete moles – is also not an unusual feature, especially in trisomies involving chromosomes 7, 15, 21, and 22 [60]. In these cases, it is often not possible to rule out a partial molar gestation without the use of ancillary tests, that is, ploidy analysis, karyotyping, and/or molecular genotyping. The clinical significance of trophoblastic hyperplasia associated with trisomies is not known, however.

Digynic triploid gestations, although are not typically associated with hydropic change or trophoblastic hyperplasia, may also present a diagnostic challenge (Fig. 5.8). Histologically, the chorionic villi are not infrequently irregular in shape, and trophoblastic pseudo-inclusions and syncytiotrophoblast sprouts may also be seen [41]. Fetal vessels and red blood cells are often present. The fetus, if grossly identified, often shows severe asymmetric IUGR [39, 40]. These overlapping morphologic features together with the triploid DNA content on flow cytometry may lead to misclassification as a partial molar gestation. Importantly, unlike partial moles, digynic triploid gestations are not associated with an increased risk of persistent GTD or GTN. Molecular genotyping – as discussed among ancillary techniques – definitively

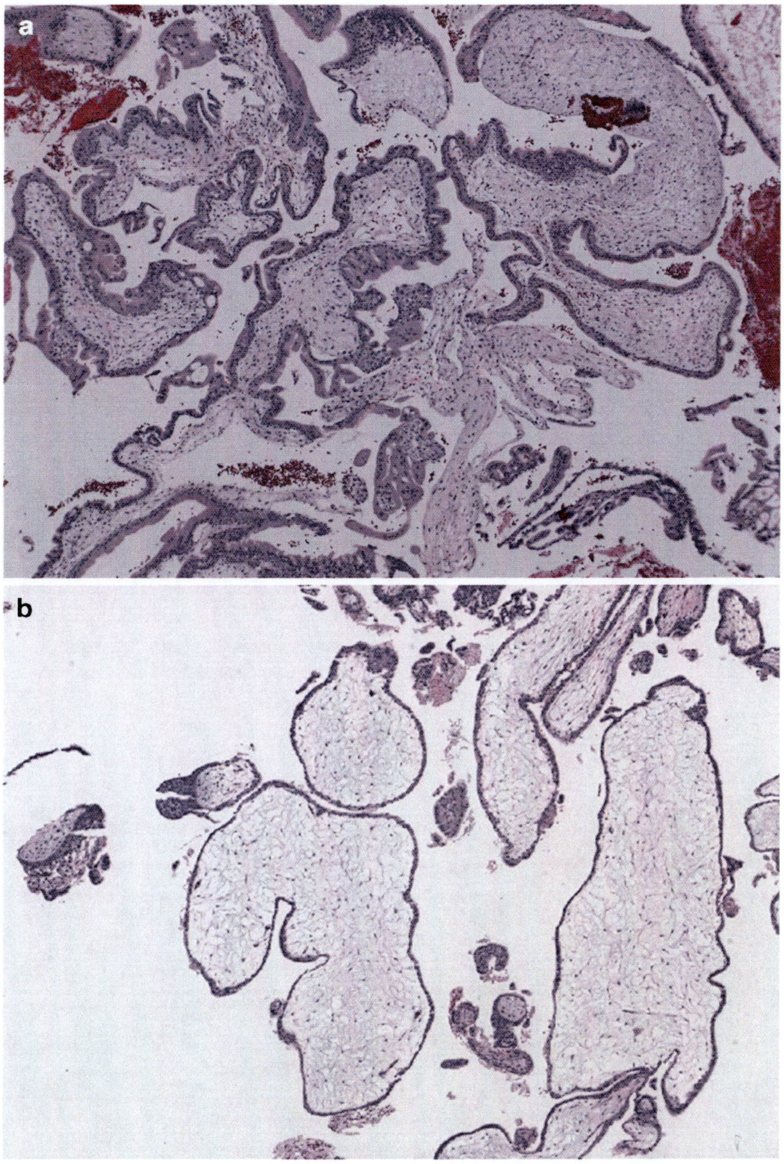

Fig. 5.6 Microscopic mimics of PHM: (**a**) Early complete mole: The villous hydrops and trophoblastic hyperplasia is moderate, not yet fully developed. The villous stroma is characteristically hypercellular and slightly basophilic. (**b**) Hydropic abortion: Villous hydrops is present, but it lacks significant trophoblastic hyperplasia

separates the two entities by identifying the parental origin of haploid chromosomal sets in the triploid genome.

A late gestational age mimic of partial mole, termed placental mesenchymal dysplasia or "pseudo-partial mole," is a rare non-molar disorder characterized by stem villus and terminal villous hydrops, aneurysmal stem villous vessels and peripheral stem villous chorioangiomatoid change [27, 61] (Fig. 5.9). The aneurysmal vessels may suffer from thrombosis, which could potentially explain the high rate of intrauterine fetal demise associated with these cases [62]. In contrast to partial moles, trophoblastic

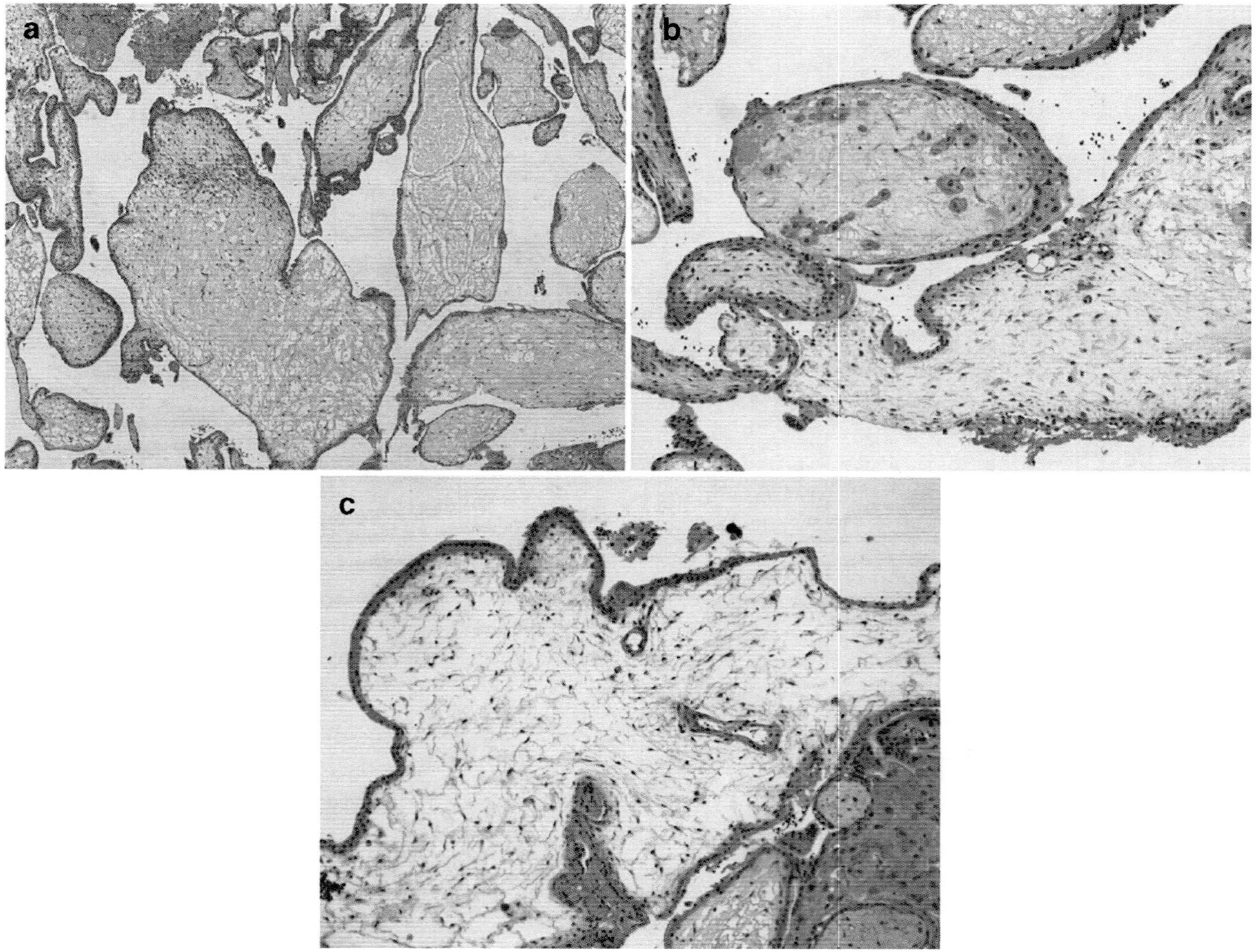

Fig. 5.7 Trisomy 16 syndrome: Irregularly shaped, hydropic villi (**a**) with single cell trophoblastic inclusions (**b**) and irregular to oval trophoblastic pseudo-inclusions (**c**), mimicking a partial mole

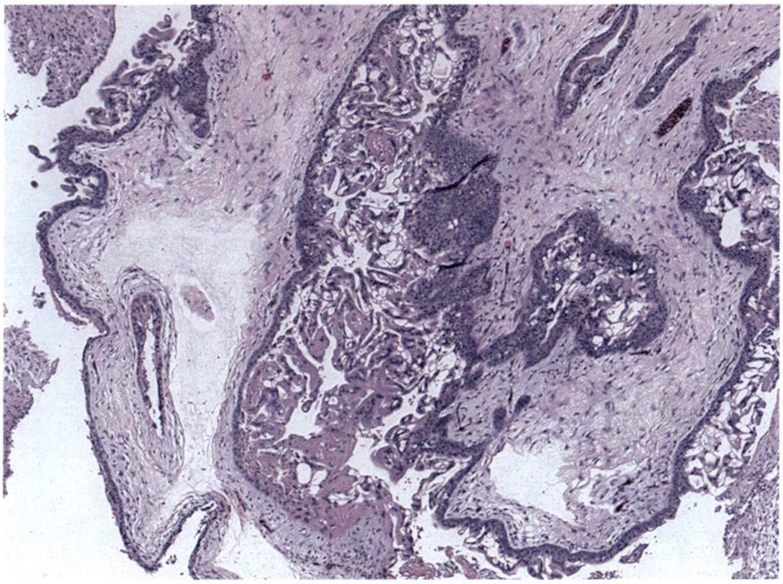

Fig. 5.8 Digynic triploidy. This digynic triploid gestation demonstrates villous hydrops, mild trophoblast hyperplasia, prominent syncytiotrophoblasts with intracytoplasmic lacunae, and irregular to oval trophoblastic pseudo-inclusions, remarkably simulating a diandric partial mole. The diagnosis of digynic triploidy in this case was confirmed by molecular genotyping

hyperplasia and trophoblastic pseudo-inclusions are absent [61]. The stem villi are enlarged, hydropic with rare cistern formation and the villous stroma consists of myxofibroblastic proliferation of spindle and stellate mesenchymal cells without atypia. The fetus has a diploid karyotype and may show evidence of IUGR or Beckwith–Wiedemann syndrome (i.e., macrosomia, visceromegaly, hemihypertrophy, macroglossia, omphalocele, and adrenal cytomegaly) in approximately 50 and 20% of cases, respectively [27, 61, 62].

Clinicopathological Correlations

The preferred method of evacuation in suspected molar pregnancies is suction curettage, which has to be followed by careful hCG monitoring to assure a clinical remission and to help an early detection of persistent GTD [32, 63]. Persistent GTD is a clinical term, encompassing invasive mole, metastatic mole, and choriocarcinoma. Of these, invasive mole, characterized by invasion of molar villi into the myometrium without intervening decidua, is the most common, occurring in approximately 0.5–5% of partial moles and in 15–20% of complete moles [11, 64, 65]. Rarely molar villi also invade intramyometrial vessels and may spread to vagina, vulva, and the broad ligament. Lung metastases can also develop [66]. The risk of developing choriocarcinoma following a partial mole is very minimal – only three cases have been reported recently in the literature –, compared to the 2–3% risk associated with CHMs [67]. Although certain clinical features, as excessive uterine size, theca lutein cysts, maternal age over 40 years and prior molar pregnancy, have been identified as risk factors for persistent GTD in complete moles, no such associations were found in patients with partial moles [68–70].

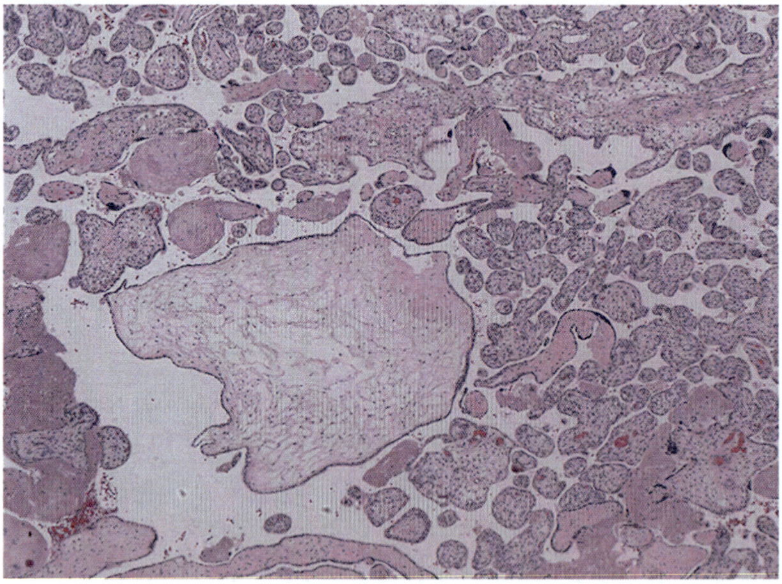

Fig. 5.9 Placental mesenchymal dysplasia: Stem villous hydrops at 23 + 5/7 weeks of gestation. The fetus showed multiple anomalies consistent with Beckwith–Wiedemann syndrome

References

1. Carr DH. Cytogenetics and the pathology of hydatidiform degeneration. Obstet Gynecol. 1969;33(3):333–42.
2. Makino S, Sasaki MS, Fukuschima T. Triploid chromosome constitution in human chorionic lesions. Lancet. 1964;2(7372):1273–5.
3. Szulman AE, Surti U. The syndromes of hydatidiform mole. I. Cytogenetic and morphologic correlations. Am J Obstet Gynecol. 1978;131(6):665–71.
4. Szulman AE, Surti U. The syndromes of hydatidiform mole. II. Morphologic evolution of the complete and partial mole. Am J Obstet Gynecol. 1978;132(1):20–7.
5. Honore LH, Dill FJ, Poland BJ. The association of hydatidiform mole and trisomy 2. Obstet Gynecol. 1974;43(2):232–7.
6. Vassilakos P, Kajii T. Letter: hydatidiform mole: two entities. Lancet. 1976;1(7953):259.
7. Vassilakos P, Riotton G, Kajii T. Hydatidiform mole: two entities. A morphologic and cytogenetic study with some clinical consideration. Am J Obstet Gynecol. 1977;127(2):167–70.
8. Lurain JR. Gestational trophoblastic disease I: epidemiology, pathology, clinical presentation and diagnosis of gestational trophoblastic disease, and management of hydatidiform mole. Am J Obstet Gynecol. 2010; 203(6):531–9.
9. Smith HO. Gestational trophoblastic disease epidemiology and trends. Clin Obstet Gynecol. 2003;46(3): 541–56.
10. Atrash HK, Hogue CJ, Grimes DA. Epidemiology of hydatidiform mole during early gestation. Am J Obstet Gynecol. 1986;154(4):906–9.
11. Hancock BW, Seckl MJ, Berkowitz RS. Gestational trophoblastic disease. London; 2009, Chapter 3, pp. 49–96.
12. Smith HO, Hilgers RD, Bedrick EJ, Qualls CR, Wiggins CL, Rayburn WF, et al. Ethnic differences at risk for gestational trophoblastic disease in New Mexico: a 25-year population-based study. Am J Obstet Gynecol. 2003;188(2):357–66.
13. Berkowitz RS, Cramer DW, Bernstein MR, Cassells S, Driscoll SG, Goldstein DP. Risk factors for complete molar pregnancy from a case-control study. Am J Obstet Gynecol. 1985;152(8):1016–20.
14. Berkowitz RS, Bernstein MR, Harlow BL, Rice LW, Lage JM, Goldstein DP, et al. Case-control study of risk factors for partial molar pregnancy. Am J Obstet Gynecol. 1995;173(3 Pt 1):788–94.
15. Szulman AE, Surti U. The clinicopathologic profile of the partial hydatidiform mole. Obstet Gynecol. 1982;59(5):597–602.
16. Altman AD, Bentley B, Murray S, Bentley JR. Maternal age-related rates of gestational trophoblastic disease. Obstet Gynecol. 2008;112(2 Pt 1):244–50.
17. Tham BW, Everard JE, Tidy JA, Drew D, Hancock BW. Gestational trophoblastic disease in the Asian population of Northern England and North Wales. BJOG. 2003;110(6):555–9.
18. Jeffers MD, O'Dwyer P, Curran B, Leader M, Gillan JE. Partial hydatidiform mole: a common but

underdiagnosed condition. A 3-year retrospective clinicopathological and DNA flow cytometric analysis. Int J Gynecol Pathol. 1993;12(4):315–23.
19. Bifulco C, Johnson C, Hao L, Kermalli H, Bell S, Hui P. Genotypic analysis of hydatidiform mole: an accurate and practical method of diagnosis. Am J Surg Pathol. 2008;32(3):445–51.
20. Genest DR, Ruiz RE, Weremowicz S, Berkowitz RS, Goldstein DP, Dorfman DM. Do nontriploid partial hydatidiform moles exist? A histologic and flow cytometric reevaluation of nontriploid specimens. J Reprod Med. 2002;47(5):363–8.
21. Lawler SD, Fisher RA, Pickthall VJ, Povey S, Evans MW. Genetic studies on hydatidiform moles. I. The origin of partial moles. Cancer Genet Cytogenet. 1982;5(4):309–20.
22. Jacobs PA, Szulman AE, Funkhouser J, Matsuura JS, Wilson CC. Human triploidy: relationship between parental origin of the additional haploid complement and development of partial hydatidiform mole. Ann Hum Genet. 1982;46(Pt 3):223–31.
23. Zaragoza MV, Surti U, Redline RW, Millie E, Chakravarti A, Hassold TJ. Parental origin and phenotype of triploidy in spontaneous abortions: predominance of diandry and association with the partial hydatidiform mole. Am J Hum Genet. 2000;66(6):1807–20.
24. McFadden DE, Robinson WP. Phenotype of triploid embryos. J Med Genet. 2006;43(7):609–12.
25. Hassold T, Chen N, Funkhouser J, Jooss T, Manuel B, Matsuura J, et al. A cytogenetic study of 1000 spontaneous abortions. Ann Hum Genet. 1980;44(Pt 2):151–78.
26. Szulman AE, Philippe E, Boue JG, Boue A. Human triploidy: association with partial hydatidiform moles and nonmolar conceptuses. Hum Pathol. 1981;12(11):1016–21.
27. Genest DR. Partial hydatidiform mole: clinicopathological features, differential diagnosis, ploidy and molecular studies, and gold standards for diagnosis. Int J Gynecol Pathol. 2001;20(4):315–22.
28. Surti U, Szulman AE, Wagner K, Leppert M, O'Brien SJ. Tetraploid partial hydatidiform moles: two cases with a triple paternal contribution and a 92, XXXY karyotype. Hum Genet. 1986;72(1):15–21.
29. Sheppard DM, Fisher RA, Lawler SD, Povey S. Tetraploid conceptus with three paternal contributions. Hum Genet. 1982;62(4):371–4.
30. Paradinas FJ, Fisher RA, Browne P, Newlands ES. Diploid hydatidiform moles with fetal red blood cells in molar villi. 1 – Pathology, incidence, and prognosis. J Pathol. 1997;181(2):183–8.
31. Fisher RA, Paradinas FJ, Soteriou BA, Foskett M, Newlands ES. Diploid hydatidiform moles with fetal red blood cells in molar villi. 2 – Genetics. J Pathol. 1997;181(2):189–95.
32. Berkowitz RS, Goldstein DP. Clinical practice. Molar pregnancy. N Engl J Med. 2009;360(16):1639–45.
33. Czernobilsky B, Barash A, Lancet M. Partial moles: a clinicopathologic study of 25 cases. Obstet Gynecol. 1982;59(1):75–7.
34. Fine C, Bundy AL, Berkowitz RS, Boswell SB, Berezin AF, Doubilet PM. Sonographic diagnosis of partial hydatidiform mole. Obstet Gynecol. 1989;73 (3 Pt 1):414–8.
35. Naumoff P, Szulman AE, Weinstein B, Mazer J, Surti U. Ultrasonography of partial hydatidiform mole. Radiology. 1981;140(2):467–70.
36. Sebire NJ, Fisher RA, Rees HC. Histopathological diagnosis of partial and complete hydatidiform mole in the first trimester of pregnancy. Pediatr Dev Pathol. 2003;6(1):69–77.
37. Fowler DJ, Lindsay I, Seckl MJ, Sebire NJ. Histomorphometric features of hydatidiform moles in early pregnancy: relationship to detectability by ultrasound examination. Ultrasound Obstet Gynecol. 2007;29(1):76–80.
38. Doshi N, Surti U, Szulman AE. Morphologic anomalies in triploid liveborn fetuses. Hum Pathol. 1983; 14(8):716–23.
39. Daniel A, Wu Z, Bennetts B, Slater H, Osborn R, Jackson J, et al. Karyotype, phenotype and parental origin in 19 cases of triploidy. Prenat Diagn. 2001;21(12): 1034–48.
40. McFadden DE, Kalousek DK. Two different phenotypes of fetuses with chromosomal triploidy: correlation with parental origin of the extra haploid set. Am J Med Genet. 1991;38(4):535–8.
41. Redline RW, Hassold T, Zaragoza MV. Prevalence of the partial molar phenotype in triploidy of maternal and paternal origin. Hum Pathol. 1998;29(5):505–11.
42. Fukunaga M. Histopathologic study of partial hydatidiform moles and DNA triploid placentas. Pathol Int. 1994;44(7):528–34.
43. Paradinas FJ, Browne P, Fisher RA, Foskett M, Bagshawe KD, Newlands E. A clinical, histopathological and flow cytometric study of 149 complete moles, 146 partial moles and 107 non-molar hydropic abortions. Histopathology. 1996;28(2):101–10.
44. Fukunaga M, Katabuchi H, Nagasaka T, Mikami Y, Minamiguchi S, Lage JM. Interobserver and intraobserver variability in the diagnosis of hydatidiform mole. Am J Surg Pathol. 2005;29(7):942–7.
45. Frierson Jr HF. Flow cytometric analysis of ploidy in solid neoplasms: comparison of fresh tissues with formalin-fixed paraffin-embedded specimens. Hum Pathol. 1988;19(3):290–4.
46. Yver M, Carles D, Bloch B, Bioulac-Sage P, Martin Negrier ML. Determination of DNA ploidy by fluorescence in situ hybridization (FISH) in hydatidiform moles: evaluation of FISH on isolated nuclei. Hum Pathol. 2004;35(6):752–8.
47. Cheung AN, Ngan HY, Chen WZ, Loke SL, Collins RJ. The significance of proliferating cell nuclear antigen in human trophoblastic disease: an immunohistochemical study. Histopathology. 1993;22(6):565–8.
48. Suresh UR, Hale RJ, Fox H, Buckley CH. Use of proliferation cell nuclear antigen immunoreactivity for distinguishing hydropic abortions from partial hydatidiform moles. J Clin Pathol. 1993;46(1):48–50.

49. Olvera M, Harris S, Amezcua CA, McCourty A, Rezk S, Koo C, et al. Immunohistochemical expression of cell cycle proteins E2F-1, Cdk-2, Cyclin E, p27(kip1), and Ki-67 in normal placenta and gestational trophoblastic disease. Mod Pathol. 2001;14(10):1036–42.
50. Fukunaga M. Immunohistochemical characterization of p57(KIP2) expression in early hydatidiform moles. Hum Pathol. 2002;33(12):1188–92.
51. Castrillon DH, Sun D, Weremowicz S, Fisher RA, Crum CP, Genest DR. Discrimination of complete hydatidiform mole from its mimics by immunohistochemistry of the paternally imprinted gene product p57KIP2. Am J Surg Pathol. 2001;25(10):1225–30.
52. Lipata F, Parkash V, Talmor M, Bell S, Chen S, Maric V, et al. Precise DNA genotyping diagnosis of hydatidiform mole. Obstet Gynecol. 2010;115(4):784–94.
53. McConnell TG, Murphy KM, Hafez M, Vang R, Ronnett BM. Diagnosis and subclassification of hydatidiform moles using p57 immunohistochemistry and molecular genotyping: validation and prospective analysis in routine and consultation practice settings with development of an algorithmic approach. Am J Surg Pathol. 2009;33(6):805–17.
54. Kovacs BW, Shahbahrami B, Tast DE, Curtin JP. Molecular genetic analysis of complete hydatidiform moles. Cancer Genet Cytogenet. 1991;54(2):143–52.
55. Bell KA, Van Deerlin V, Addya K, Clevenger CV, Van Deerlin PG, Leonard DG. Molecular genetic testing from paraffin-embedded tissue distinguishes nonmolar hydropic abortion from hydatidiform mole. Mol Diagn. 1999;4(1):11–9.
56. Hui P. Molecular diagnosis of gestational trophoblastic disease. Expert Rev Mol Diagn. 2010;10(8):1023–34.
57. van Lijnschoten G, Arends JW, Leffers P, De La Fuente AA, Van Der Looij HJ, Geraedts JP. The value of histomorphological features of chorionic villi in early spontaneous abortion for the prediction of karyotype. Histopathology. 1993;22(6):557–63.
58. van Lijnschoten G, Arends JW, Geraedts JP. Comparison of histological features in early spontaneous and induced trisomic abortions. Placenta. 1994;15(7):765–73.
59. Norris-Kirby A, Hagenkord JM, Kshirsagar MP, Ronnett BM, Murphy KM. Abnormal villous morphology associated with triple trisomy of paternal origin. J Mol Diagn. 2010;12(4):525–9.
60. Redline RW, Hassold T, Zaragoza M. Determinants of villous trophoblastic hyperplasia in spontaneous abortions. Mod Pathol. 1998;11(8):762–8.
61. Paradinas FJ, Sebire NJ, Fisher RA, Rees HC, Foskett M, Seckl MJ, et al. Pseudo-partial moles: placental stem vessel hydrops and the association with Beckwith-Wiedemann syndrome and complete moles. Histopathology. 2001;39(5):447–54.
62. Pham T, Steele J, Stayboldt C, Chan L, Benirschke K. Placental mesenchymal dysplasia is associated with high rates of intrauterine growth restriction and fetal demise: a report of 11 new cases and a review of the literature. Am J Clin Pathol. 2006;126(1):67–78.
63. Horowitz NS, Goldstein DP, Berkowitz RS. Management of gestational trophoblastic neoplasia. Semin Oncol. 2009;36(2):181–9.
64. Rice LW, Berkowitz RS, Lage JM, Goldstein DP, Bernstein MR. Persistent gestational trophoblastic tumor after partial hydatidiform mole. Gynecol Oncol. 1990;36(3):358–62.
65. Gaber LW, Redline RW, Mostoufi-Zadeh M, Driscoll SG. Invasive partial mole. Am J Clin Pathol. 1986;85(6):722–4.
66. Honig A, Rieger L, Kristen P, Eck M, Frambach T, Tschammler A, et al. A case of metastasizing invasive hydatidiform mole. Is less–less good? Review of the literature with regard to adequate treatment. Eur J Gynaecol Oncol. 2005;26(2):158–62.
67. Seckl MJ, Fisher RA, Salerno G, Rees H, Paradinas FJ, Foskett M, et al. Choriocarcinoma and partial hydatidiform moles. Lancet. 2000;356(9223):36–9.
68. Feltmate CM, Growdon WB, Wolfberg AJ, Goldstein DP, Genest DR, Chinchilla ME, et al. Clinical characteristics of persistent gestational trophoblastic neoplasia after partial hydatidiform molar pregnancy. J Reprod Med. 2006;51(11):902–6.
69. Curry SL, Hammond CB, Tyrey L, Creasman WT, Parker RT. Hydatidiform mole: diagnosis, management, and long-term followup of 347 patients. Obstet Gynecol. 1975;45(1):1–8.
70. Berkowitz RS, Goldstein DP. Chorionic tumors. N Engl J Med. 1996;335(23):1740–8.

Placental Site Trophoblastic Tumor

6

Pei Hui

Keywords
PSTT • Diagnostic features • Differential diagnosis

Introduction

Placental site trophoblastic tumor or PSTT is a bona fide neoplastic proliferation of cells with cytological features of the intermediate trophoblast present at the implantation site. The recognition of the tumor was made in late 1970s, although similar lesions had been documented in the literature for over a century. The earliest possible description of the lesion was by Marchand in 1895 as "atypical chorioepithelioma" [1]. Other names of the tumor were used including "atypical choriocarcinoma", "syncytioma", a term introduced by Ewing [2–5], and "chorioepitheliosis" [6–8]. Kurman, Scully, and Norris firstly brought the lesion to attention as "trophoblastic pseudotumor" in 1976 based on 12 cases of a trophoblastic lesion involving endomyometrium [9], regardless that some of the cases clearly caused uterine perforation as a result of the lesional infiltrative growth [9, 10]. The term "pseudotumor" was used mainly because of the observed benign clinical course after hysterectomy in this early study [9]. Other case reports in English literature used the term to describe the tumor [10–15], until 1981, when Scully and Young eventually realized that the condition represented in fact a true neoplasm as 2 of their 14 cases had a fatal outcome as a result of metastasis [16]. They then recommended that the term "placental site trophoblastic tumor" to replace "trophoblastic pseudotumor". The term "placental site" was used simply because the proliferating cells had morphological and biological features of implantation site trophoblast. In the following year, Young formally adopted the name in his authoritative review of a total of 42 cases [17] and it was later accepted by WHO [18]. Baergen recently summarized 55 cases of PSTT in her comprehensive review with an intent to identify prognostic factors on the histological ground [19]. To date, around 250 cases of PSTT have been documented in English literature and they represent roughly 3% of gestational trophoblastic disease [20, 21].

P. Hui, MD, PhD (✉)
Department of Pathology,
Yale University School of Medicine, 310 Cedar Street,
254B New Haven, CT 06520-8023, USA
e-mail: pei.hui@yale.edu

P. Hui (ed.), *Gestational Trophoblastic Disease: Diagnostic and Molecular Genetic Pathology*, Current Clinical Pathology, DOI 10.1007/978-1-61779-394-3_6,

Clinical Presentation

Based on the three largest series in English literature, the patient age at presentation ranges from 20 to 63 years with a mean of 30 to 32 years [17, 19, 22]. The oldest patient documented was a 63-year-old who developed a PSTT 12 years after menopause [23]. Gravidity ranged from 1 to 5. The interval between the antecedent pregnancy and the clinical manifestation of the tumor is variable. An estimated 57–70% of the cases had an uneventful full-term pregnancy with tumor development 0.25–204 months (median latency of 12–18 months) after delivery [19, 22, 24]. Antecedent complete hydatidiform mole and abortion (missed or induced) were seen in 11–26% and 10–15% of the cases, respectively. One reported PSTT arose in a background of partial hydatidiform mole [25].

Most of the patients presented with vaginal bleeding (several days to more than a year) and uterine enlargement, clinically thought to be pregnant. Less common symptoms were amenorrhea (months to over a year) and abdominal pain [20, 21, 24]. The most serious complication was uterine perforation, which occurred spontaneously in one reported patient and during curettage in five others. Mild to moderate elevation of serum hCG was seen in nearly 80% of the cases with values ranging from 5 to 26,000 mIU/mL (average 673–691 mIU/mL and median of 74.5 mIU/mL) [19, 22]. Serum hCG was negative at the initial presentation in about 20% of the cases. Metastatic PSTTs had on average higher serum hCG levels with a mean of 1,670 mIU/mL and a median of 116.5 mIU/mL [22]. Nephrotic syndrome was noted in the early studies as an association with PSTT and the symptoms resolved after hysterectomy removal of the tumor [26–28], but was not confirmed by later studies [19, 29, 30]. Erythrocytosis was reported in association with one PSTT [31].

Diagnostic imaging may identify two types of vasculature patterns associated with PSTT: hypervascular and hypovascular [32–34]. Tumors of the hypervascular type show a mass lesion with multiple cystic/vascular spaces by ultrasonography, and a mass lesion with multiple flow voids by MRI. In contrast, PSTTs of the hypovascular type may show no lesion, a solid mass without cystic changes by ultrasonography or a solid mass without prominent vasculature by MRI [32].

The tumor presented at stage I (FIGO) in about 84% of the cases, however tumors at stage III and IV were seen in 5 and 9%, respectively[19]. FIGO Stage II diseases commonly involve adnexa, pelvic lymph nodes, and parametrium. Distant metastasis usually occurs after a second or third local tumor recurrence.

Pathogenesis

PSTT is a true neoplastic proliferation of cells with cytological and histological features recapitulating the implantation site intermediate trophoblast. PSTTs show rare genetic imbalances analyzed by comparative genomic hybridization [35, 36], with recurrent regional chromosomal gains have been identified in a few cases [35]. Recent molecular and genetic investigations have confirmed a preferential requirement of paternal X chromosome, i.e., female gestation, in the tumor genome. This finding suggests that paternal X chromosome may provide a growth advantage likely through altered sex chromosome imprinting inactivation in trophectoderm. A detailed discussion of this aspect can be found in Chap. 3. Related to PSTT at a histological level, exaggerated placental site (EPS) reaction, a benign reactive condition associated with concurrent pregnancy, consists of cells also with features of the implantation site trophoblast. It has been speculated that EPS reaction may be a precursor lesion to PSTT [37]. However, a recent genetic study did not find a genetic linkage between the two conditions [38].

Pathology

Gross Pathology

The majority of the cases of PSTT involve uterine endomyometrium with variable gross appearances. Most tumors are circumscribed, nodular

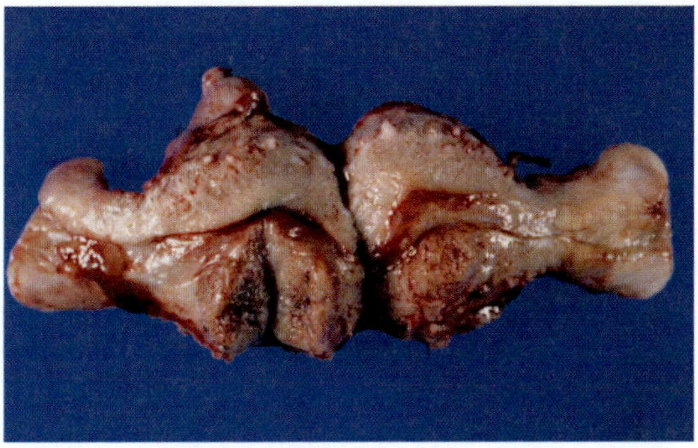

Fig. 6.1 Gross photograph of PSTT. A polypoid intrauterine mass with invasion of the underlying endomyometrium

masses with good demarcation from the surrounding endomyometrium. Some tumors may be polypoid uterine growth with underlying invasion into the myometrium (Fig. 6.1). The tumor size ranges from less than 1.0 to 10.0 cm (average of 5.0 cm). It may enlarge and distort the entire uterine cavity. The cut surfaces of the tumor are usually solid and fleshy with whitish tan to light yellow color (Fig. 6.2). Focal areas of hemorrhage and necrosis are seen in nearly half of the cases (Fig. 6.1). Deep myometrial involvement is common (50%) and transmural invasion is seen in about 10% of the reported cases. Perforation due to deep myometrial invasion may occur with extension into the broad ligament and adnexa in rare cases [39].

Histological Pathology

Table 6.1 summarizes important histological features of PSTT. Microscopic examination usually reveals mass lesions infiltrating endomyometrium (Fig. 6.3a). The tumor consists of single, small aggregates or cords to large sheets of tumor cells (Fig. 6.3b). At the tumor periphery, the proliferating cells characteristically infiltrate and split normal myometrial smooth muscle cells (Fig. 6.4). The tumor cells are large, polyhedral to round, predominantly mononucleated but binucleated and multinucleated forms – resembling syncytiotrophoblasts – are also seen.

Table 6.1 Histological features of PSTT

1. Mass lesion involving endomyometrium
2. Proliferation of implantation site intermediate trophoblasts (large mononuclear cells with occasional multinuclear forms)
3. Infiltrative border with tumor cells splitting myometrial smooth muscle
4. Diffuse positivity for hPL
5. Ki-67 labeling in more than 5–10% of tumor cells

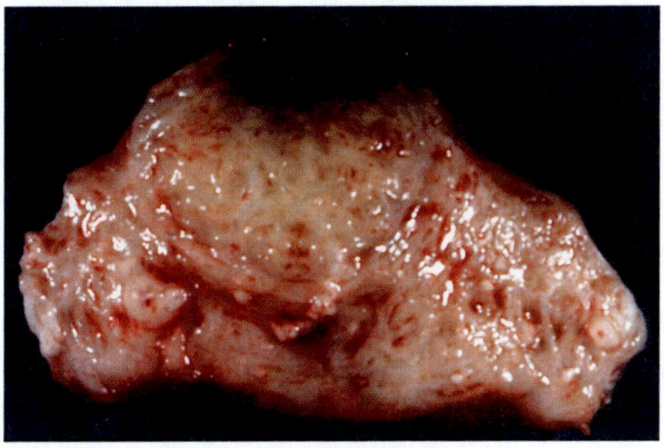

Fig. 6.2 Cross-section of PSTT. Note the solid whitish tan cut surface with areas of hemorrhage [35].

The multinucleated tumor cells are generally irregularly distributed. Occasionally, spindle-shaped tumor cells may also exist particularly at the tumor periphery. The cytoplasm is abundant and amphophilic in nearly half of the cases (Fig. 6.5a). Eosinophilic cytoplasm is present in about 45% (Fig. 6.5b) and a clear cytoplasm is seen in the remaining minority of the cases (5%) (Fig. 6.5c). The nuclei vary considerably in size, shape, and staining patterns. Round small nuclei with pale chromatin pattern are seen in some, but large convoluted nuclei with marked hyperchromasia, nuclear grooves and nuclear pseudoinclusions are seen in most PSTTs. Nucleoli are generally present and may be prominent. There is a variable degree of nuclear atypia (Fig. 6.6a) in some cases at an extreme level (Fig. 6.6b). Mitotic activity ranges from 0 to 22/10 HPF, but most tumors have a mitotic count between 2 and 4/10 HPF. High mitotic activity (over 5 mitoses/10 HPF) has been found to be associated with a worse prognosis. Microscopic to large areas of hemorrhage are quite common

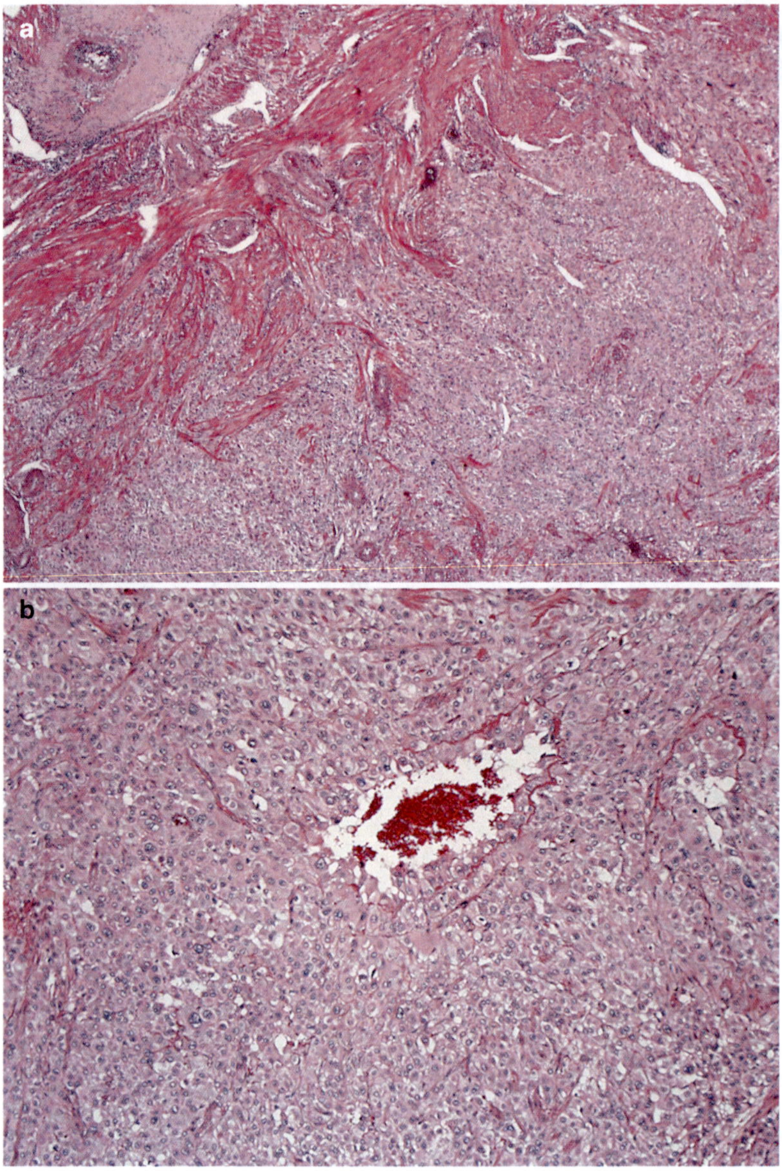

Fig. 6.3 Microscopic findings of PSTT. Note a deep myometrial invasive lesion at low magnification (**a**) and the presence of solid large sheets of trophoblastic cells within the tumor (**b**)

(Fig. 6.7a) and coagulative tumor cell necrosis may be focal or even extensive in about 65% of the cases (Fig. 6.7b).

Other important characteristic features of PSTT include the presence of extracellular fibrin material, similar to that seen at normal implantation site (Fig. 6.7c), and the pattern of vascular invasion of PSTT also recapitulates normal implantation trophoblast with invasion and replacement of the vascular wall (mainly venous structures), while the overall vascular architecture is maintained without collapsing (Fig. 6.8a). Frequently, the replacement is overtly complete by leaving only the original endothelial cells in place (Fig. 6.8b). Concurrent gestation or chorionic villi should be absent by definition, although one case of PSTT was documented arising in a concurrent molar

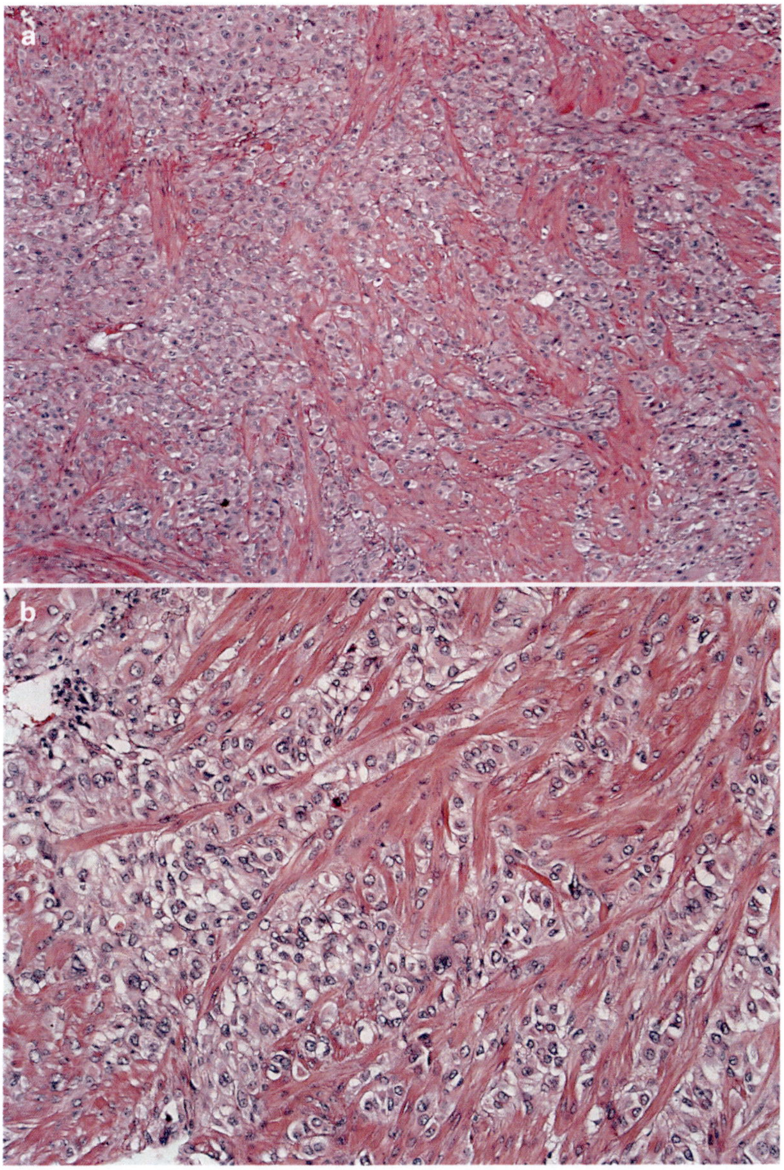

Fig. 6.4 Characteristic growth pattern at the tumor periphery with infiltrating tumor cells splitting the existing myometrial smooth muscle (lower power view, high power view)

gestation [40]. Adjacent endomyometrium may show decidua-like reaction and/or the Arias-Stella changes. In metastatic PSTT, the extra-uterine tumors consist of mainly mononuclear trophoblastic cells.

Some PSTTs may have focal mixed histological and cytological features of other types of trophoblastic tumors, most commonly epithelioid trophoblastic tumor. In such tumors, a diagnosis of mixed PSTT and ETT may be rendered.

Ancillary Studies

Tumor cells of PSTT generally show immunostaining patterns similar to those of implantation site intermediate trophoblast, i.e. hPL, MUC-4, HSD3B1, CD10, HLA-G and Mel-CAM (CD146), and hCG [19, 37, 41, 42]. The staining of hPL is generally strong, and diffuse (Fig. 6.9b) in over 2/3 of the cases. In contrast, protein expression of

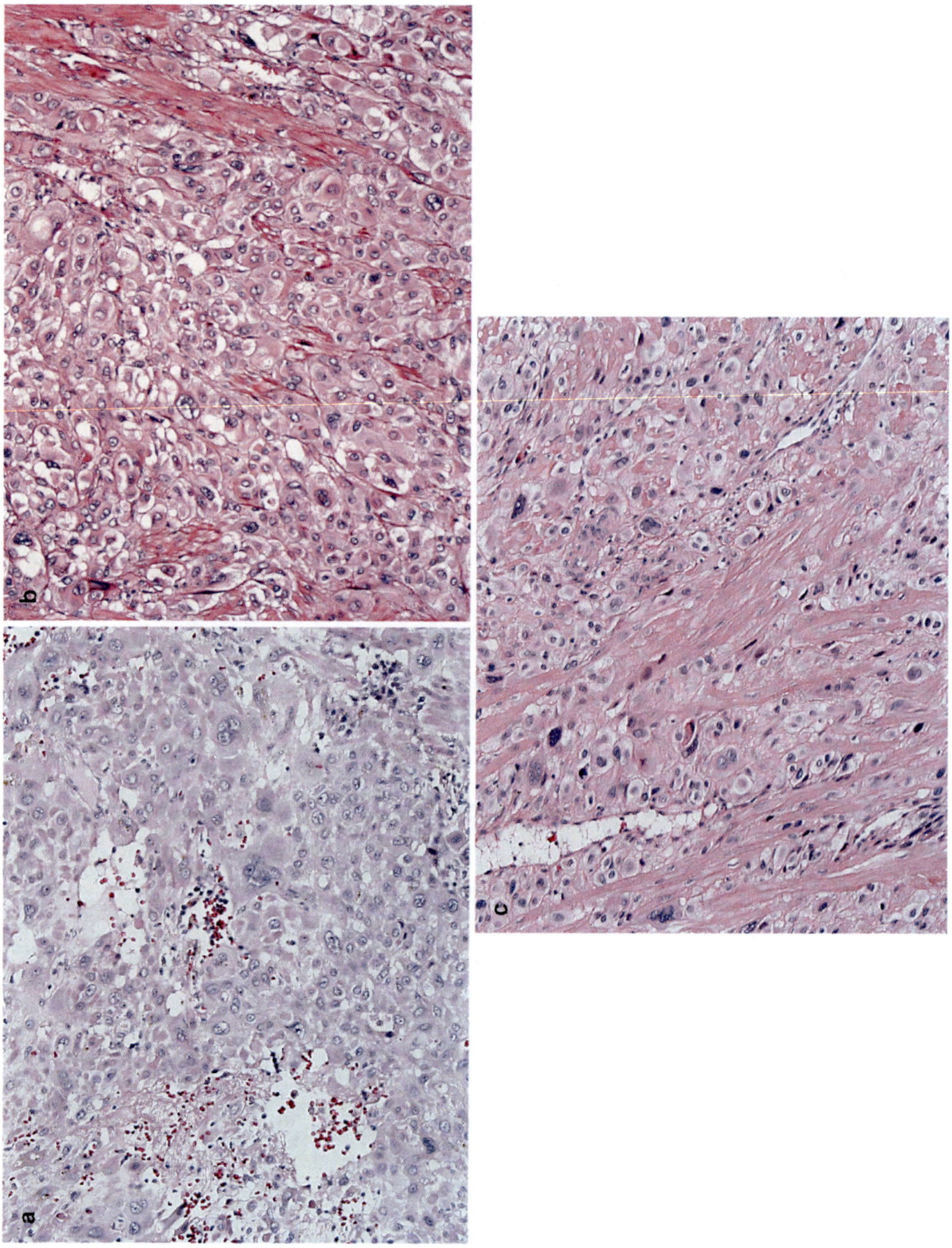

Fig. 6.5 Cytological features of PSTT with variably stained cytoplasm: amphophilic (**a**), eosinophilic (**b**), and clear (**c**)

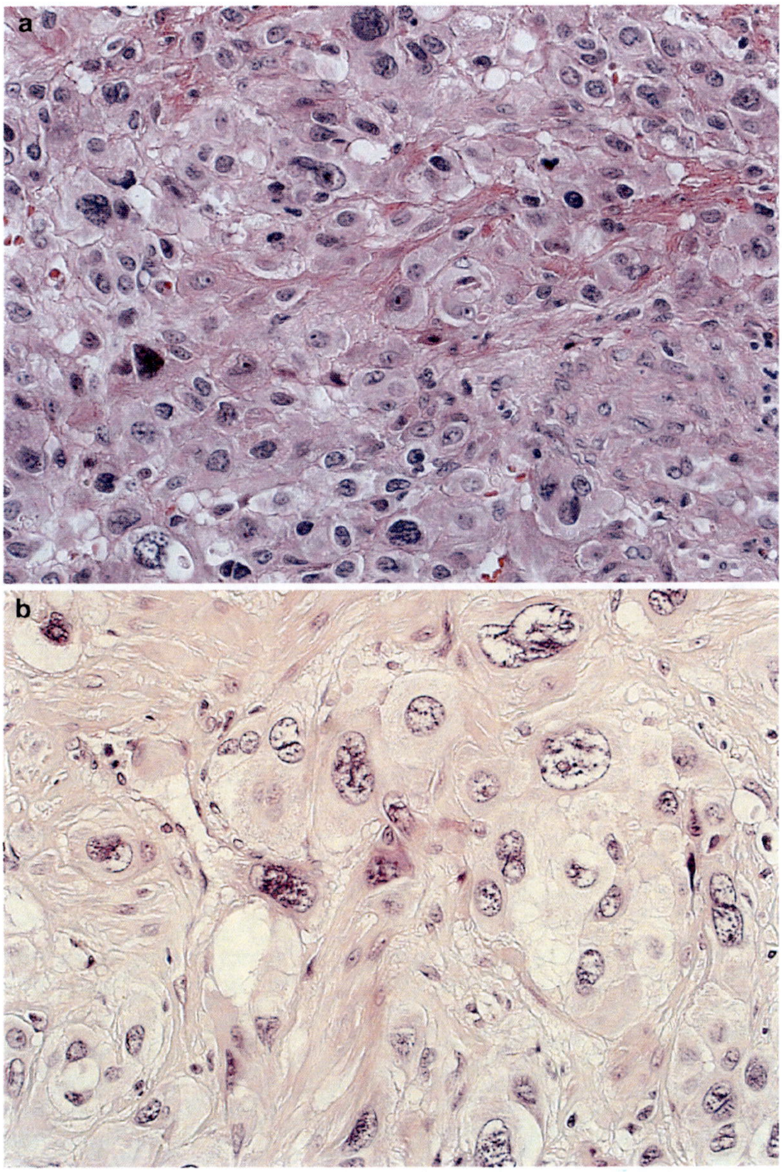

Fig. 6.6 Cytological atypia of PSTT ranging from moderate (**a**) to marked (**b**)

hCG (Fig. 6.9c) and inhibin is only focal, and present in multinucleated tumor cells. Epithelial markers including cytokeratins AE1/3 cocktail and CK18 are strongly expressed in PSTT (Fig. 6.9d). Ki-67 is expressed in the range of 10–30% of the tumor cells and is a highly useful marker in the differential diagnosis of PSTT from its benign mimic, EPS reaction [42]. PSTT has no expression of p63 epithelial marker [37, 42].

Most PSTT tumors analyzed by karyotype or comparative genomic hybridization methods showed generally undisturbed chromosomal profiles, except that a few recurrent regional chromosomal gains have been identified [35].

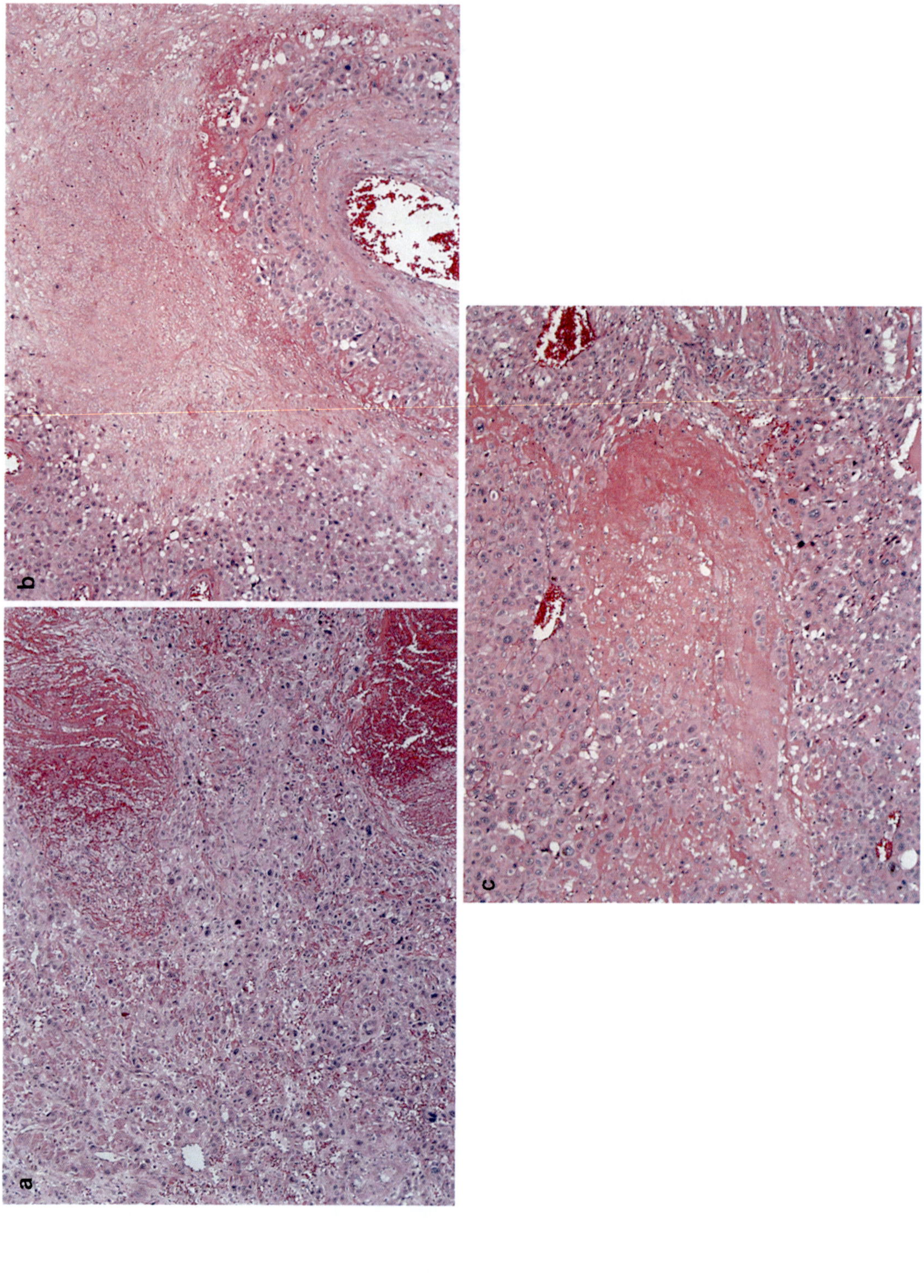

Fig. 6.7 PSTT tumors are frequently associated with tumor hemorrhage (**a**), coagulative tumor cell necrosis (**b**) and focal deposition of fibrin material (**c**)

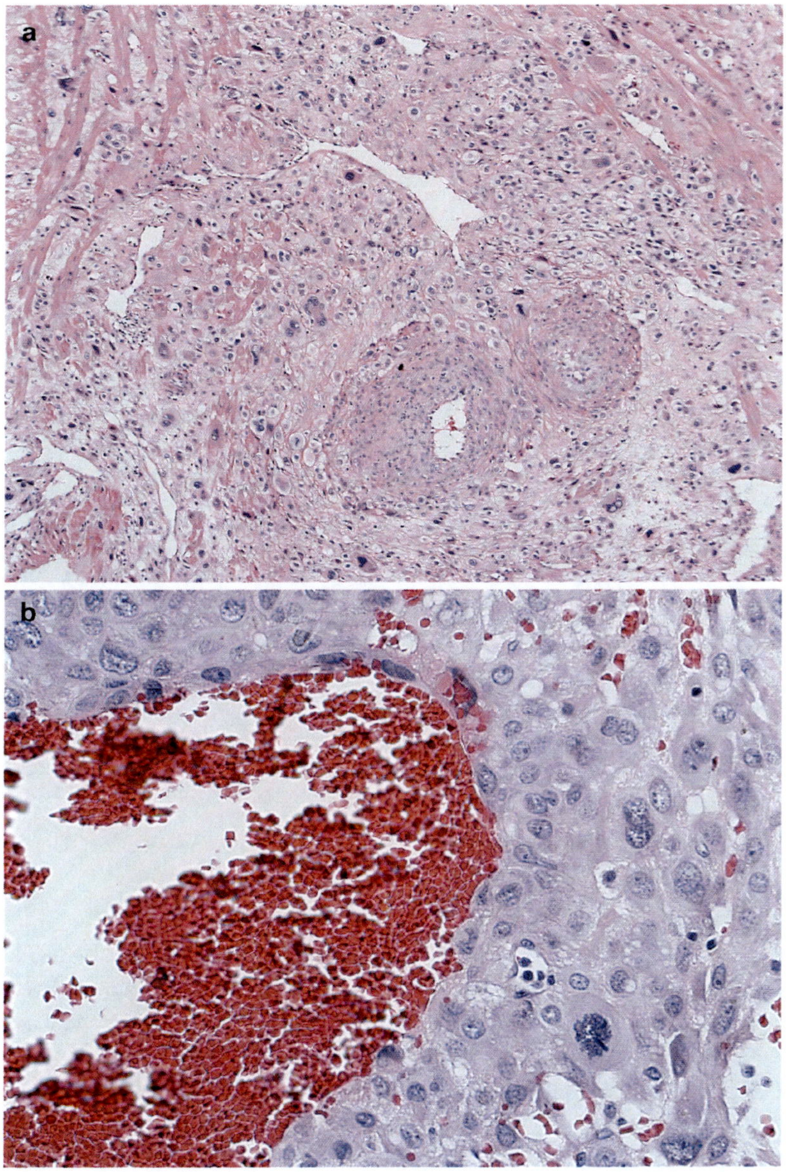

Fig. 6.8 Characteristic vascular invasion by PSTT (**a**), which is frequently complete except leaving the original endothelial cells in place (**b**)

Differential Diagnoses

The differential diagnoses of PSTT include EPS reaction, epithelioid trophoblastic tumor (ETT), poorly differentiated carcinomas, and epithelioid smooth muscle tumors.

EPS reaction may cause a significant diagnostic problem, as it can closely resemble PSTT, particularly in a curettage specimen. It shares many features of PSTT – including the infiltrative growth pattern, vascular invasion by trophoblast, and presence of extracellular fibrin material. However, the time period between the antecedent pregnancy and EPS reaction is mostly concurrent or much shorter than that of PSTT. Moreover, unlike PSTT, EPS reaction does not form a mass lesion and frequently contains chorionic villi and evenly distrib-

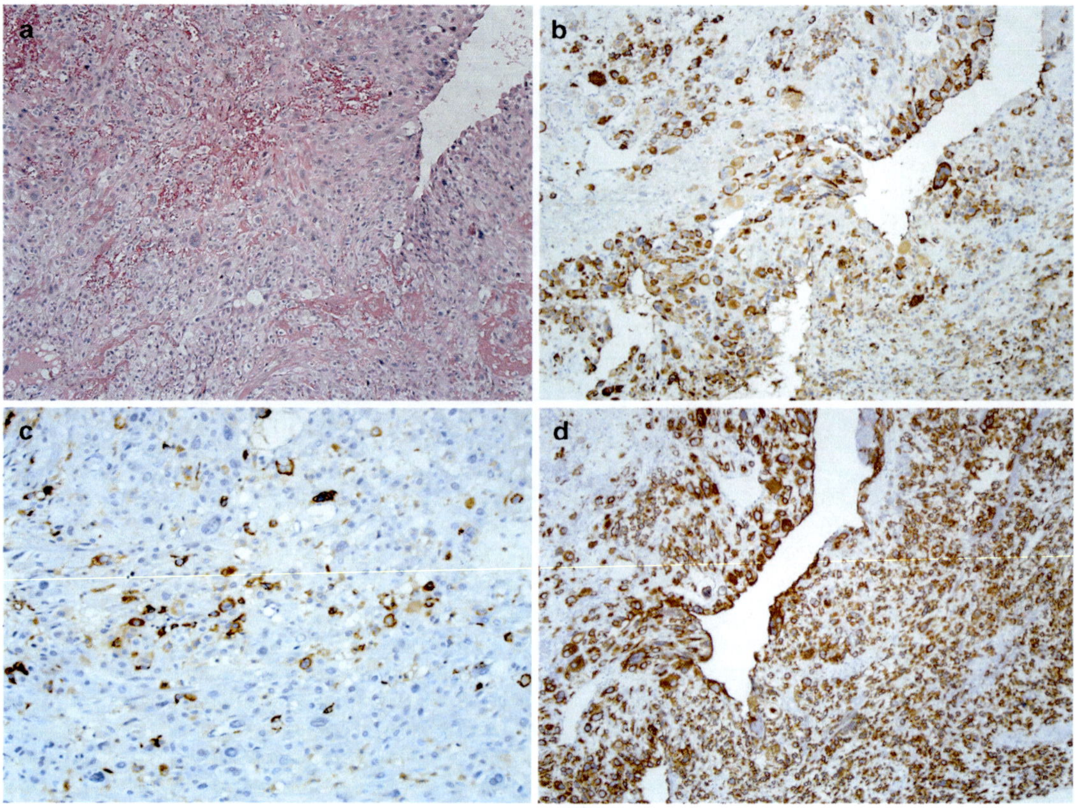

Fig. 6.9 Characteristic immunohistochemistry profiles of PSTT: (**a**) H.E. Stain; (**b**) hPL; (**c**) hCG; and (**d**) cytokeratin

uted, abundant multinucleated intermediate trophoblasts. The mitotic activity is low and the Ki-67 labeling index is less than 1%, as opposed to a higher index (over 10%) in PSTT [43, 44]. Additional discussion can be found in Chap. 10.

Histological features separating ETT from PSTT include a pushing growth margin, a frequent localization in the cervix or lower uterine segment, and the presence of eosinophilic keratin-like material in ETT. Immunohistochemical stains are also helpful: PSTT is diffusely positive for hPL and Mel-CAM (CD146), while ETT is negative or only focally positive for these markers [37, 45, 46]. P63 on the other hand, is strongly positive in ETT and consistently negative in PSTT [47]. Additional differential diagnosis between PSTT and ETT is given in Chap. 7.

Separation of PSTT from poorly differentiated endometrial carcinomas should not be difficult as long as a due suspicion for the presence of trophoblastic tumor is raised by a pathologist. Clinically, a mild elevation of serum hCG supports a diagnosis of PSTT. Trophoblastic markers such as hPL, HLA-G, and hCG should confirm the trophoblastic nature of PSTT and rule out a carcinoma, although focal hCG positive syncytiotrophoblastic differentiation may be present in rare poorly differentiated carcinomas. Recent investigations suggested that the serum free beta-subunit of hCG might be a reliable marker for PSTT [48, 49].

Epithelioid smooth muscle tumors (leiomyoma or leiomyosarcoma) may simulate PSTT due to their infiltrative growth and an epithelioid cytology. Expression of cytokeratin and hPL should confirm a trophoblastic tumor, whereas positivity of muscle markers (desmin and caldesmon) assures a diagnosis of smooth muscle tumor.

Clinicopathological Correlations

Despite its deep myometrial invasion or even perforation at presentation, most PSTTs are apparently cured by simple hysterectomy. However, approximately 25–30% of the patients with PSTT developed recurrent diseases, of whom half died from the tumor and the remaining survived with the disease [19–21, 24]. The most common metastatic sites include the lung, liver, and vagina. Distant metastasis usually occurs after the second or third local tumor recurrence [24]. The overall and recurrence-free survival are 70 and 73%, respectively in patients ten years after initial treatment [50].

Various clinical and pathological parameters have been investigated in the past for prognostic correlations. FIGO staging is the most important predictor of patient survival [22, 24]. Patient age older than 35 years is associated with unfavorable prognosis. Prolonged intervals (over 2 years) between the antecedent gestation and the diagnosis of PSTT have been reported as an independent poor prognostic factor [19, 21, 24, 51–53] and a cut-off of 48 months has been proposed [50]. Prior term pregnancy is also associated with a worse prognosis [22, 24].

Among pathological findings, the presence of tumor cells with clear cytoplasm is associated with a worse prognosis [16, 19]. Other significant histological parameters include the depth of myometrial invasion, tumor necrosis, and size of the tumor. High mitotic count (more than 5 per 10 HPF) is significantly related to tumor metastasis. All five fatal cases of PSTT discussed by Young had seven or more mitoses per HPF [17]. Mitosis of five or more per HPF is significantly associated with a poor survival by other studies [19, 24]. Ki-67 labeling of more than 50% of tumor cells has been suggested to be associated with a malignant course [54]. However, lower mitotic activity does not guarantee a benign clinical outcome. Overall, only the FIGO stage and the presence of tumor cells with clear cytoplasm were found as independent predictors of overall survival, while FIGO stage and the patient's age are the only independent predictors of time to recurrence or disease-free survival [16, 19]. Histological findings that are not correlated with the outcome include cytological atypia, the presence of multinucleated tumor cells, the presence of inflammatory cells, fibrin deposition, hemorrhage, lymphovascular invasion, and abnormal mitotic figures, DNA ploidy, S-phase fraction and expression of immunomarkers (hPL and hCG) [54–56].

Surgery remains the primary treatment of PSTT and patients with the above-mentioned risk factors may benefit from immediate adjuvant combined chemotherapy (see Chap. 12 for details). Although PSTT produces only low levels of hCG, it is still the best available serum maker for monitoring the recurrence and residual disease [57]. More recently, urinary or serum beta-core subunit of hCG has been found to be a better marker for monitoring the treatment effect of PSTT due to its higher percentage in PSTT than other GTDs or somatic malignancies with trophoblastic differentiation [58].

References

1. Marchand F. Uber die sogenannten "decualen" Geschwulste im Anschloss and normale Geburt, Abort Blasenmole and Extrauterin Schwangerschaft. Monatsschr Geburtshilfe Gynaekol. 1895;1:419–38.
2. Reis RA, Decosta EJ. Syncytioma, syncytial endometritis. Am J Obstet Gynecol. 1948;56(3):584–6.
3. Kistner RW. Malignant syncytioma following benign hydatidiform mole. Am J Obstet Gynecol. 1952;63(4):888–92.
4. Acosta-Sison H. Is syncytial endometritis (syncytioma) always benign? J Philipp Med Assoc. 1963;39:720–4.
5. Ewing J. Choriomas: a clinical and pathological study. Surg Gynecol Obstet. 1920;10:366–932.
6. Huber H, Hormann AG. Malignant chorioepithelioma and chorioepitheliosis. Gynecol Prat. 1954;5(1):31–40.
7. Kehrer E. Pathology of trophoblast development; chorioepithelioma malignum and chorioepitheliosis. Z Geburtshilfe Gynakol. 1956;147(2):145–203. concl.
8. Cruz H, Fischer O, Guzman A. Chorioepitheliosis. Rev Chil Obstet Ginecol. 1966;31(4):200–9.
9. Kurman RJ, Scully RE, Norris HJ. Trophoblastic pseudotumor of the uterus: an exaggerated form of "syncytial endometritis" simulating a malignant tumor. Cancer. 1976;38(3):1214–26.
10. Gloor E, Hurlimann J. Trophoblastic pseudotumor of the uterus: clinicopathologic report with immunohistochemical and ultrastructural studies. Am J Surg Pathol. 1981;5(1):5–13.

11. Blackwell JB, Papadimitriou JM. Trophoblastic pseudotumor of the uterus: case report and ultrastructure. Cancer. 1979;43(5):1734–41.
12. Philippe E, Boue J, Boue A. Trophoblastic gestational diseases. Triploid syndrome, perivillous trophoblastic hyperplasia, trophoblastic pseudotumor, trophoblastic microcarcinoma and carcinoma. Ann Anat Pathol (Paris). 1980;25(1):13–38.
13. Wetzel WJ. Trophoblastic pseudotumor: an illustrative case. Diagn Gynecol Obstet. 1980;2(2):147–50.
14. Twiggs LB, Okagaki T, Phillips GL, Stroemer JR, Adcock LL. Trophoblastic pseudotumor-evidence of malignant disease potential. Gynecol Oncol. 1981;12 (2 Pt 1):238–48.
15. Baue G, Hennequin JP. Trophoblastic pseudotumor of the uterus. Unusual 2-stage development. J Gynecol Obstet Biol Reprod (Paris). 1983;12(2):177–82.
16. Scully RE, Young RH. Trophoblastic pseudotumor: a reappraisal. Am J Surg Pathol. 1981;5(1):75–6.
17. Young RH, Scully RE. Placental-site trophoblastic tumor: current status. Clin Obstet Gynecol. 1984; 27(1):248–58.
18. Scully RE, Bonofiglio TA, Kurman RJ, Sliverberg SG, Wilkinson EJ. Histologic typing of female genital tract tumors. 2nd ed. Spinger-Verlag: New York; 1994.
19. Baergen RN, Rutgers JL, Young RH, Osann K, Scully RE. Placental site trophoblastic tumor: a study of 55 cases and review of the literature emphasizing factors of prognostic significance. Gynecol Oncol. 2006; 100(3):511–20.
20. Hassadia A, Gillespie A, Tidy J, Everard RGNJ, Wells M, Coleman R, et al. Placental site trophoblastic tumour: clinical features and management. Gynecol Oncol. 2005;99(3):603–7.
21. Papadopoulos AJ, Foskett M, Seckl MJ, McNeish I, Paradinas FJ, Rees H, et al. Twenty-five years' clinical experience with placental site trophoblastic tumors. J Reprod Med. 2002;47(6):460–4.
22. Chang YL, Chang TC, Hsueh S, Huang KG, Wang PN, Liu HP, et al. Prognostic factors and treatment for placental site trophoblastic tumor-report of 3 cases and analysis of 88 cases. Gynecol Oncol. 1999;73(2): 216–22.
23. Nigam S, Singhal N, Kumar Gupta S, Chhabra D, Manaktala U. Placental site trophoblastic tumor in a postmenopausal female–a case report. Gynecol Oncol. 2004;93(2):550–3.
24. Feltmate CM, Genest DR, Wise L, Bernstein MR, Goldstein DP, Berkowitz RS. Placental site trophoblastic tumor: a 17-year experience at the New England Trophoblastic Disease Center. Gynecol Oncol. 2001;82(3):415–9.
25. Palmieri C, Fisher RA, Sebire NJ, Lindsay I, Smith JR, McCluggage WG, et al. Placental site trophoblastic tumour arising from a partial hydatidiform mole. Lancet. 2005;366(9486):688.
26. Eckstein RP, Paradinas FJ, Bagshawe KD. Placental site trophoblastic tumour (trophoblastic pseudotumour): a study of four cases requiring hysterectomy including one fatal case. Histopathology. 1982;6(2): 211–26.
27. Lambie AT, Baird DT, Thomson D, MacDonald MK, Robson JS. Nephrotic syndrome in association with a trophoblastic neoplasm. Clin Nephrol. 1982;17(3): 160–1.
28. Young RH, Scully RE, McCluskey RT. A distinctive glomerular lesion complicating placental site trophoblastic tumor: report of two cases. Hum Pathol. 1985;16(1):35–42.
29. Bonazzi C, Urso M, Dell'Anna T, Sacco S, Buda A, Cantu MG. Placental site trophoblastic tumor: an overview. J Reprod Med. 2004;49(8):585–8.
30. Piura B, Shaco-Levy R. Placental site trophoblastic tumor. Harefuah. 2007;146(1):62–7. 77.
31. Brewer CA, Adelson MD, Elder RC. Erythrocytosis associated with a placental-site trophoblastic tumor. Obstet Gynecol. 1992;79(5(Pt 2)):846–9.
32. Machtinger R, Gotlieb WH, Korach J, Fridman E, Apter S, Goldenberg M, et al. Placental site trophoblastic tumor: outcome of five cases including fertility preserving management. Gynecol Oncol. 2005;96(1): 56–61.
33. Sakamoto C, Oikawa K, Kashimura M, Egashira K. Sonographic appearance of placental site trophoblastic tumor. J Ultrasound Med. 1990;9(9):533–5.
34. Sumi Y, Ozaki Y, Shindoh N, Katayama H. Placental site trophoblastic tumor: imaging findings. Radiat Med. 1999;17(6):427–30.
35. Hui P, Riba A, Pejovic T, Johnson T, Baergen RN, Ward D. Comparative genomic hybridization study of placental site trophoblastic tumour: a report of four cases. Mod Pathol. 2004;17(2):248–51.
36. Xue WC, Guan XY, Ngan HY, Shen DH, Khoo US, Cheung AN. Malignant placental site trophoblastic tumor: a cytogenetic study using comparative genomic hybridization and chromosome in situ hybridization. Cancer. 2002;94(8):2288–94.
37. Shih IM, Kurman RJ. The pathology of intermediate trophoblastic tumors and tumor-like lesions. Int J Gynecol Pathol. 2001;20(1):31–47.
38. Dotto J, Hui P. Lack of genetic association between exaggerated placental site reaction and placental site trophoblastic tumor. Int J Gynecol Pathol. 2008; 27(4):562–7.
39. Baergen RN, Rutgers J, Young RH. Extrauterine lesions of intermediate trophoblast. Int J Gynecol Pathol. 2003;22(4):362–7.
40. Abdul-Hafeez M, Akhtar M, Ba aqueel HS, Kidess EA. Placental site trophoblastic tumor: report of a case with review of literature. Ann Saudi Med. 1987;7:340–4.
41. Lee Y, Kim KR, McKeon F, Yang A, Boyd TK, Crum CP, et al. A unifying concept of trophoblastic differentiation and malignancy defined by biomarker expression. Hum Pathol. 2007;38(7):1003–13.
42. Shih Ie M. Trophogram, an immunohistochemistry-based algorithmic approach, in the differential diagnosis of trophoblastic tumors and tumorlike lesions. Ann Diagn Pathol. 2007;11(3):228–34.
43. Ichikawa N, Zhai YL, Shiozawa T, Toki T, Noguchi H, Nikaido T, et al. Immunohistochemical analysis of cell cycle regulatory gene products in normal tropho-

blast and placental site trophoblastic tumor. Int J Gynecol Pathol. 1998;17(3):235–40.
44. Shih IM, Kurman RJ. Ki-67 labeling index in the differential diagnosis of exaggerated placental site, placental site trophoblastic tumor, and choriocarcinoma: a double immunohistochemical staining technique using Ki-67 and Mel-CAM antibodies. Hum Pathol. 1998;29(1):27–33.
45. Kalhor N, Ramirez PT, Deavers MT, Malpica A, Silva EG. Immunohistochemical studies of trophoblastic tumors. Am J Surg Pathol. 2009;33(4):633–8.
46. Shih IM, Kurman RJ. Epithelioid trophoblastic tumor: a neoplasm distinct from choriocarcinoma and placental site trophoblastic tumor simulating carcinoma. Am J Surg Pathol. 1998;22(11):1393–403.
47. Shih IM, Kurman RJ. p63 expression is useful in the distinction of epithelioid trophoblastic and placental site trophoblastic tumors by profiling trophoblastic subpopulations. Am J Surg Pathol. 2004;28(9):1177–83.
48. Cole LA, Khanlian SA, Muller CY. Blood test for placental site trophoblastic tumor and nontrophoblastic malignancy for evaluating patients with low positive human chorionic gonadotropin results. J Reprod Med. 2008;53(7):457–64.
49. Cole LA, Khanlian SA, Muller CY, Giddings A, Kohorn E, Berkowitz R. Gestational trophoblastic diseases: 3. Human chorionic gonadotropin-free beta-subunit, a reliable marker of placental site trophoblastic tumors. Gynecol Oncol. 2006;102(2):160–4.
50. Schmid P, Nagai Y, Agarwal R, Hancock B, Savage PM, Sebire NJ, et al. Prognostic markers and long-term outcome of placental-site trophoblastic tumours: a retrospective observational study. Lancet. 2009;374(9683):48–55.
51. Finkler NJ, Berkowitz RS, Driscoll SG, Goldstein DP, Bernstein MR. Clinical experience with placental site trophoblastic tumors at the New England Trophoblastic Disease Center. Obstet Gynecol. 1988;71(6 Pt 1): 854–7.
52. How J, Scurry J, Grant P, Sapountzis K, Ostor A, Fortune D, et al. Placental site trophoblastic tumor. Report of three cases and review of the literature. Int J Gynecol Cancer. 1995;5(4):241–9.
53. Bower M, Paradinas FJ, Fisher RA, Nicholson SK, Rustin GJ, Begent RH, et al. Placental site trophoblastic tumor: molecular analysis and clinical experience. Clin Cancer Res. 1996;2(5):897–902.
54. Shih I, Mazur MT, Kurman RJ. Gestational trophoblastic tumors and related tumor-like lesions. In: Kurman R.J., Hedrick-Ellenson L., Ronnett B.M., editor. 6th ed. Springer; 2011.
55. Fukunaga M, Ushigome S. Malignant trophoblastic tumors: immunohistochemical and flow cytometric comparison of choriocarcinoma and placental site trophoblastic tumors. Hum Pathol. 1993;24(10):1098–106.
56. Fukunaga M, Ushigome S. Metastasizing placental site trophoblastic tumor. An immunohistochemical and flow cytometric study of two cases. Am J Surg Pathol. 1993;17(10):1003–10.
57. Piura B. Placental site trophoblastic tumor–a challenging rare entity. Eur J Gynaecol Oncol. 2006; 27(6):545–51.
58. Cole LA. New discoveries on the biology and detection of human chorionic gonadotropin. Reprod Biol Endocrinol. 2009;7:8.

7 Epithelioid Trophoblastic Tumor

Katja Gwin

Keywords
ETT • Diagnostic features • Differential diagnosis

Introduction

Epithelioid trophoblastic tumor (ETT) is a relatively recently described entity [1], distinct from placental site trophoblastic tumor (PSTT) and choriocarcinoma (CC), with a resemblance to squamous cell carcinoma [2]. With slightly less than 100 cases reported in the literature [1, 3–36], ETT is a rare form of gestational trophoblastic disease (GTD) arising from the chorionic-type intermediate trophoblast. ETT was initially thought to be a variant of choriocarcinoma [37, 38] and is also referred to as "atypical choriocarcinoma." A report by Mazur [37] in 1989, describing persistent lung metastases after intensive chemotherapy in patients with choriocarcinoma, appears to be the first example of ETT in the literature. Similar tumors in the uterus found after hydatidiform mole evacuation were reported in 1993 by Silva et al. [39] as "multiple nodules of intermediate trophoblast." The term "ETT" was first mentioned in the literature in 1994 by Mazur and Kurman [40]. In 1998, Shih and Kurman [1] described the clinicopathological features of 14 ETTs, the largest study of this tumor to date, and suggested based on their findings that ETT is a distinct entity of GTD and not just a treatment-related finding.

ETT can occasionally be found as a component of other gestational trophoblastic lesions. The so-called mixed trophoblastic tumors [3, 11, 39, 41–45] reveal mixed morphologic and immunohistochemical features of ETT, PSTT [45], or choriocarcinoma [21, 22, 46] within the same tumor. Of interest, 5 of the 14 cases initially described as ETT by Shih and Kurman [1] had foci of placental site nodule (PSN), PSTT, or CC [22].

Pathogenesis and Molecular Genetic Aspects

Models of Pathogenesis for GTD, Including ETT

In 2007, Shih [47] proposed a novel model of pathogenesis for GTD. Based on previous studies [1, 2, 51–53] showing that the pattern of differentiation recapitulates the stages of early placental

K. Gwin, MD, PhD (✉)
Department of Pathology, University of Chicago Medical Center, 5841 S. Maryland Ave (MC6101), Chicago, IL 60637, USA
e-mail: Katja.Gwin@uchospitals.edu

P. Hui (ed.), *Gestational Trophoblastic Disease: Diagnostic and Molecular Genetic Pathology*, Current Clinical Pathology, DOI 10.1007/978-1-61779-394-3_7,

development [47], he proposed that trophoblastic stem cells, presumably cytotrophoblastic cells, undergo neoplastic transformation. Subsequently, a specific differentiation program dictates the type of trophoblastic tumor that develops [47]. Variable amounts of neoplastic cytotrophoblasts, syncytiotrophoblasts, and intermediate trophoblasts are the components of CC, which resembles the previllous blastocyst and contains a similar mixture of trophoblastic cells. In PSTT, the neoplastic cytotrophoblast differentiates mainly toward implantation site intermediate trophoblastic cells, whereas in ETT, the neoplastic cytotrophoblast differentiates into chorionic-type intermediate trophoblastic cells in the chorion laeve [47, 48]. According to Shih's model [47], ETT and PSTT would be more differentiated than the most primitive trophoblastic tumor, CC. This novel model also provides a potential explanation for a finding described by Mazur [37]: that ETT occurred after intensive chemotherapy for pulmonary CC metastasis. Chemotherapy may have allowed CC cells to differentiate into a secondary, more chemotherapy-refractory ETT phenotype [47].

Another proposed pathogenesis model for the development of ETT [23, 49] is the transformation of a benign PSN to an atypical PSN, with subsequent progression to a malignant ETT. Morphologic features distinguishing an atypical PSN from a benign PSN include larger size [50], higher cellularity, more cohesive nests and enlarged atypical cells, and a higher mitotic index [23]. Case reports of atypical PSN and cases of observed coexistence of PSN and ETT suggest that PSN has the biologic potential to progress to ETT [1, 23, 44, 50]. Potentially, ETTs could result de novo from neoplastic transformation of PSN-embedded trophoblastic stem cells retained in the uterus [23, 49].

DNA Genotyping

Molecular genetic analysis supports the trophoblastic nature of ETT by demonstrating that this tumor contains new (paternal) alleles not present in adjacent healthy maternal uterine tissue [51]. In 13 informative ETTs, genotyping with microsatellite markers [51] revealed at least one novel, presumably paternal, allele present only in the tumor DNA and not in the adjacent maternal uterine control tissue. Of these 13 ETTS, nine cases revealed a loss of maternal alleles in at least one single-nucleotide polymorphism (SNP) marker, demonstrated by different homozygous alleles in the tumor and the corresponding normal uterine tissue. A certain level of genetic instability was proposed [51] to be present in ETTs, as indicated by their frequent loss of heterozygosity.

DNA genotyping (by short tandem repeat (STR) multiplex polymerase chain reaction (PCR) assay amplifying 15 different tetranucleotide repeat loci) demonstrated unique paternal alleles in all four cases of informative ETTs [52], further supporting their trophoblastic origin.

Additionally, immunohistochemical studies [14, 53] showed that ETTs express the trophoblast-associated markers hydroxyl-δ-5-steroid dehydrogenase (HSD3B1) and human leukocyte antigen G (HLA-G).

Y-Chromosomal Complements in ETT

Conflicting data [51, 54] exist regarding the absence or the presence of Y-chromosomal loci in ETT. If sex chromosomes have no role in the development of GTD and ETT, a similar number of GTD cases with and without a Y chromosome would be expected [54]. In PSTT, however, it has been observed that 85% of patients had a female antecedent gestation [54].

A 2002 study by Oldt et al. [51] used PCR-based identification of the human sex-determining region Y (SRY) to recognize a Y chromosome genetic component, and an X-linked protein to confirm an X-chromosome element. An SRY amplicon was found in 11/19 (58%) ETTs, and the SRY gene was confirmed by nucleotide sequencing of representative PCR products. No SRY amplicons were present in the adjacent normal uterine tissue.

Another genotyping study specifically targeting Y-chromosomal complements was performed by Yap et al. [54] in 2010. They used three independent sex chromosome markers (amelogenin, protein kinase, and zinc finger) with X and Y homologs that are distinguishable by PCR product size. All ETT cases contained an X-chromosomal complement, whereas Y- chromosomal signals were only detected in 3/18 ETTs (18%), demonstrating the absence of a Y chromosome [54] in the majority of cases.

The authors proposed that it is likely that Y-chromosomal deletions have no functional effect on tumor progression [55]. The lack of a Y chromosome may simply reflect that many gestational trophoblastic tumors develop from complete hydatidiform moles. Because 90% of them carry a 46,XX karyotype, due to the fertilization of an anuclear ovum by a single haploid (23x) sperm and subsequent haploid genome duplication [56, 57], the trophoblastic tumors that develop from a complete hydatidiform mole retain this chromosomal assignment and do not harbor a Y chromosome. The fertilization of an empty ovum with two sperms occurs in 10% of complete hydatidiform moles; thus, half of the moles arising from dispermy would be expected to carry a Y chromosome. Subsequently, the predicted percentage of complete hydatidiform moles carrying a Y chromosome would be approximately 5%. This hypothesis does not take into account, however, that the majority of ETTs occur after a normal full-term pregnancy or spontaneous abortion, and only 16% of cases occur after a hydatidiform mole [1].

Another possible explanation for the lack of a Y chromosome [54] in the majority of ETTs is the assumed noncompatibility of a Y chromosome with tumor initiation. This might be related to growth-inhibitory effects caused by products of Y-chromosomal located genes [51].

The second study by Yap et al. [54] comments on the findings of a Y chromosome presence in 50% of ETTs observed in Oldt et al.'s study [51] and provides the higher PCR amplification cycle number, which raises the possibility of nonspecific amplification from contaminants, as a likely explanation for their findings.

Comparative Genomic Hybridization

A recent study [52] screened the genomes of five ETTs for numerical or unbalanced structural chromosomal alterations and found no regional chromosome gains or losses. The balanced chromosomal profile in all three analyzed ETTs [52] suggests that genetic alterations at chromosomal levels are not features of this tumor entity.

Expression of the Transcription Factor p63

The p63 gene is a transcription factor belonging to the p53 family [58–60]. p63 reveals strong homology in structure and function with p53. It occurs in various isoforms, which are classified based on the specific promoter usage in two major groups [61, 62]: the transcription activation (TA) forms and the ΔN isoforms of p63. The TA forms have a p53-like suppressor function and use the upstream (5′) promoter, generating p63 proteins with the TA domain [15]. The ΔNp63 isoforms result from transcription of the downstream (3′) promoter; they lack the TA domain and exert an oncogenic effect. In 2004, Shih and Kurman [15] studied the expression of p63 isoforms in trophoblastic subpopulations and trophoblastic lesions, using immunohistochemistry and reverse transcription (RT)-PCR. Cytotrophoblasts expressed the ΔNp63 isoforms, whereas extravillous (intermediate) trophoblastic cells in the chorion laeve and ETT expressed TAp63. An isoforms switch from ΔNp63 to TAp63, therefore, may play an important role in the transformation of the chorionic-type intermediate trophoblast from cytotrophoblasts [15]. Implantation site intermediate trophoblasts, syncytiotrophoblasts, PSTT, and exaggerated placental sites were devoid of p63 expression. A similar study [63] in 2009 revealed results comparable to those of the 2004 study.

Expression of Cyclin E

An immunohistochemical study by Mao et al. [50] analyzed the expression of the protein cyclin E, which regulates the progression from the G1 to S phase [64] in the cell cycle in ETT, PSN, and cervical squamous cell carcinoma. Cyclin E expression was seen in ETT, but was not present in the extravillous (intermediate) trophoblastic cells of the chorion laeve [50]. Of interest, cyclin E was also expressed in two atypical PSNs [44, 50] with greater cellularity, size, and mitotic activity than typical PSNs. Based on the oncogenic role of cyclin E in other neoplastic diseases, it is possible that cyclin E plays a role in the neoplastic transformation of ETT [47, 50].

Epidermal Growth Factor Receptor (EGFR) Expression

Epidermal growth factor receptor (EGFR), a member of the ErbB-related family, is a transmembrane receptor tyrosine kinase that is overexpressed in many epithelial tumors. High EGFR expression has been observed by immunohistochemistry in CC [65], PSTT [66], and ETT [1, 12]. EGFR immunoreactivity levels in CC and complete hydatidiform moles were significantly higher than in normal placental tissue or partial hydatidiform moles [65]. Additionally, a correlation between strong EGFR expression in the intermediate trophoblastic cells of a complete hydatidiform mole and the development of persistent postmolar gestational trophoblastic neoplasms was observed [65].

K-Ras Oncogene

An analysis of the K-ras oncogene mutational status [51] in 19 ETTs showed no mutation in either codon 12 or 13.

ETT of the Lung

A possible etiology for the development of extrauterine pulmonary ETT includes the de novo transformation of trophoblastic cells that were transmitted to the lung during pregnancy or the spontaneous resolution of an antecedent uterine ETT [21].

Clinical Presentation

Clinical features (Table 7.1)

ETT usually occurs in reproductive-aged women from 15 to 48 years of age [1], with a reported average age of 36.1 years [1]. However, a significant percentage of ETT has also been observed in perimenopausal [10] and postmenopausal women with a distant history of pregnancy. The oldest patient [5] reported in the literature is a 66-year-old Filipino woman, gravida 10, para 8, abortus 1, with a history of hydatidiform mole 17 years earlier that was treated with dilatation and curettage only. She presented with postmenopausal bleeding, a pelvic mass, and slightly elevated β-HCG. The hysterectomy specimen revealed a 4-cm ETT located within the myometrial wall of the left uterine fundus. Similar to other types of GTD, ETT is usually associated with a preceding gestation, but compared with CC, a greater proportion of ETTs appear to develop from a normal pregnancy or spontaneous abortion. Antecedent gestational events of ETT [1, 6, 8] include full-term delivery in 67% and spontaneous abortion in 16% of patients, but hydatidiform moles in only 16% of cases.

Clinically, ETT almost always causes vaginal bleeding or menometrorrhagia, but occasionally, amenorrhea [3] occurs. Patients typically present with normal to slightly elevated (<2,500 mIU/mL) [2, 35, 67] serum hCG, although some cases of high-level serum hCG elevation have been described [18], especially in ETT cases with extrauterine location [8, 12, 28, 68]. The time frame between the antecedent gestation and the presentation of ETT averages 6.2 years [3] but varies tremendously, with reported intervals ranging from 1 year [1] to as long as 25 years after a normal vaginal delivery [10]. Therefore, malignant gestational trophoblastic tumors need to be considered in the work-up of patients with persistent vaginal bleeding months or even years after a gestation.

The uterus is the most common site for ETT. In contrast with other types of GTD, approximately 50% of ETT arise from the uterine cervix

Table 7.1 Clinical features of ETT

Age range	15–66 years (average: 36.1 years)
Menstrual status	Mostly premenopausal Peri- or postmenopausal possible
Antecedent gestation	Full-term delivery (67%) Spontaneous abortion (16%) Hydatidiform mole (16%)
Time frame from antecedent gestation to ETT	1–25 years (average: 6.2 years)
Clinical complaint	Vaginal bleeding/menometrorrhagia Postmenopausal bleeding (rare) Amenorrhea (rare)
Serum hCG	Slightly elevated (<2,500 mIU/mL) Normal Strongly elevated (>2,500 mIU/mL) (rare)
Clinical exam	Cervical mass Uterine enlargement/mass No abnormalities on pelvic exam
PAP smear	Atypical cells Malignant cells Normal

or lower uterine segment [1, 3]. The cervical predilection of ETT and its histological resemblance to a carcinoma can cause a potential pitfall in the differential diagnosis of ETT and keratinizing squamous cell carcinoma. Multiple cases of ETT have been initially misdiagnosed as carcinoma [13, 14, 16, 21] on cervical biopsies and treated as cervical cancer. In addition, ETT can exhibit focal replacement of the cervical glandular epithelium with stratified neoplastic cells [2, 3], which simulates squamous intraepithelial neoplasia. The myometrial wall of the uterine corpus is another common site of ETT. Common clinical findings are summarized in Table 7.1.

Rarely, ETT can occur in isolated extrauterine sites without evidence of cervical or uterine disease. To date, seven cases of isolated ETT of the lung have been reported [1, 6, 21, 32]. Clinical presentations included irregular vaginal bleeding [21], incidentally discovered preoperative HCG elevation [21], incidental lesions [6] found on a chest X-ray, and hemoptysis and cough [6]. Distinguishing ETT of the lung from primary pulmonary carcinoma is important because the therapy and prognosis of the two diseases differ significantly [21]. Extrauterine ETT has also presented as a tubal mass [12], most likely arising from an unidentified ectopic pregnancy, as an ovarian mass [27] and as a well-circumscribed mass in the broad ligament near the right ovary [8]. Other extrauterine sites include the paracervix, parametrium, periadnexal soft tissue [30], small bowel [1], and gallbladder [28].

Metastases are seen in 25% of patients [35, 69] and can be present at the initial diagnosis. Common sites of metastatic disease include the lungs, liver, gallbladder, kidney, pancreas, spine [26, 28], vagina [11], bladder surface [3], bladder wall, and ureter [3]. Choroidal infiltration by metastatic ETT [31] at the lower border of the maculae caused a superior field defect in the left eye of a 37-year-old woman.

Lymphovascular invasion [3] can be present in ETT, and lymph node metastases have been observed to pelvic [3, 23] and neck [27] lymph nodes.

ETT is generally regarded as a gestational tumor and has, therefore, only been reported in women. Recently, however, a case of mixed metastatic ETT and teratoma in a paraaortic lymph node was described in a 39-year-old male [70]. He had a history of a testicular malignant mixed germ cell tumor with a CC component that had been treated by orchiectomy and chemotherapy 2 years earlier. The morphology and immunohistochemical profile [70] of the metastasis supported the diagnosis of ETT, and the authors proposed that ETT can be one of the histologic features of a recurrent testicular germ cell tumor.

Imaging Studies

On ultrasonography, ETT is visible as well-circumscribed, solid, single hyperechogenic [20, 71] lesions of variable size with heterogeneity, containing cystic components [71]. The different patterns of myometrial invasion seen on ultrasonography can be useful for the differential diagnosis of ETT and PSTT [20]. ETT normally reveals solitary nodules with a sharp tumor border, deeply invading the cervix and myometrium in a pushing, expansive manner that is well-defined

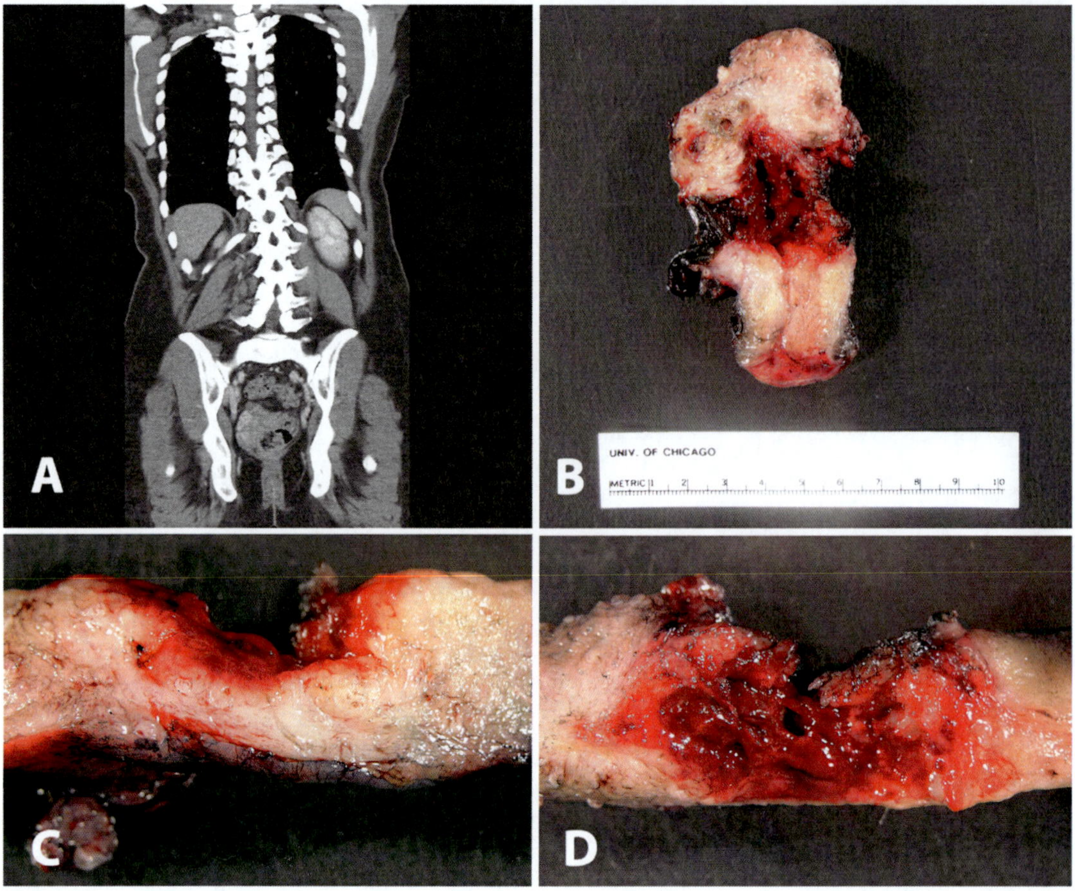

Fig. 7.1 CT imaging study and gross pathological features of ETT. (**a**) The coronal CT image shows an enlarged and heterogeneous uterus with areas of low attenuation, consistent with tumor necrosis of the ETT. Prior to hysterectomy, this patient was treated with chemotherapy based on an outside biopsy diagnosis of choriocarcinoma (which was revised on review). Clinical response to chemotherapy was minimal. (**b**) Gross image of the hysterectomy specimen with a 3 × 1.6 cm ETT involving the lower uterine segment and endometrial cavity. The tumor is a hemorrhagic solid and cystic mass. (**c**) Solid and cystic hemorrhagic tumor components are extending to the inked serosa. (**d**) A sagittal image shows well-circumscribed tan solid nodules invading deep into the myometrium

from the myometrium, whereas PSTT shows infiltrating growth between individual muscle fibers. Intratumoral blood flow assessment by transvaginal color-pulsed Doppler sonography [71], which shows a high-velocity, low-impedance blood flow pattern in ETT, can also be of value. On computed tomography (CT), ETT can exhibit an enlarged and heterogeneous uterus with areas of low attenuation consistent with necrosis (Fig. 7.1a). Magnetic resonance imaging (MRI) can also detect ETTs as well-circumscribed lesions [20]. However, none of the image findings is diagnostic by itself; clinical correlation and pathologic confirmation are required.

Pathology

Macroscopic Findings (Figs. 7.1 and 7.2)

Grossly, ETT forms solitary, circumscribed, discrete nodules or cystic hemorrhagic mass deeply invading the cervix or myometrial wall (Fig. 7.1). The tumor can communicate with the uterine cavity or be confined to the myometrium. In approximately half of the cases, ETT is located in the lower uterine segment, endocervical canal [9] or cervix [1, 3]. The tumor has a solid and cystic cut

Table 7.2 Histopathological features of ETT

Macroscopic findings
Located in cervix (~50%), uterine corpus (~50%), or extrauterine (rare)
Grossly solitary circumscribed nodules, usually 0.5–5 cm in size
Solid and cystic, brown-tan and hemorrhagic cut surface
Deep invasion of cervix or myometrium
Microscopic findings
Nodular, expansile growth pattern with pushing borders
Mononucleate intermediate trophoblastic cells
Moderate amount of fine granular pale or eosinophilic cytoplasm
Medium to large oval tumor nuclei with distinct nucleoli
Tumor cells form nests, cords and solid masses
Nests of tumor cells surrounded by necrosis and hyaline-like matrix
Tumor necrosis creates a geographic pattern
Small vessels in tumor cell nests surrounded by hyalinized necrosis
Adjacent decidualized endocervical or endometrial stromal cells
Neoplastic cells can focally replace endocervical epithelium

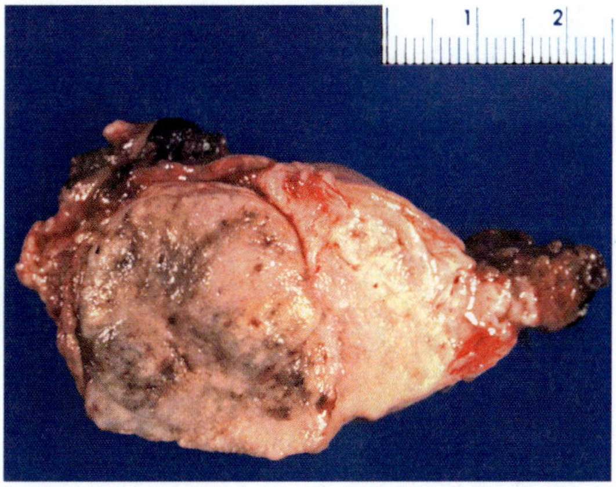

Fig. 7.2 Gross pathological features (cross-section) of an ETT involving the lower uterine segment [3]

surface. The solid component is tan-brown, with varying amounts of hemorrhage and necrosis (Fig. 7.2) and occasionally dystrophic calcifications [72]. Ulceration and fistulous tract formation have been described in ETTs [3]. The tumor size of cervical and uterine ETTs ranges from 0.5 to 5 cm [1, 73]. An extrauterine ETT presented in the broad ligament as an 8.5-cm, well-circumscribed, spongy-looking, tanned to dark-brown mass [8].

Histologic Findings (Table 7.2, Fig. 7.3)

ETT displays a relatively uniform population of mononucleate chorion laeve-type intermediate trophoblastic cells with a moderate amount of partially fine granular, eosinophilic, or clear cytoplasm. The tumor grows in a nodular, expansile fashion with well-circumscribed pushing borders, forming nests, cords, and solid masses [1, 74], but infiltrative areas can be present in the periphery [73]. Medium to large tumor cell nuclei are oval-shaped to round, with slight nuclear membrane irregularities and distinct nucleoli. Nuclear pleomorphism [1] is mild to moderate. Scattered multinucleated giant cells [3] can be admixed with the mononucleate intermediate trophoblastic cells. Characteristic of ETT, nests of intermediate trophoblastic cells are surrounded by extensive necrosis, hyaline-like matrix, or eosinophilic debris, resembling the keratinous material in squamous cell carcinoma [3]. The extensive tumor necrosis of ETT surrounded by island of viable cells creates the geographical pattern [1] typical of ETT. Foci of dystrophic calcifications may be seen [1, 72] in the tumor necrosis [5, 74]. Aggregates of decidualized endometrial [1] or endocervical [3] stromal cells may be present in the adjacent areas, along with peritumoral lymphoplasmacytic infiltrates [5, 18]. Mitotic activity [1, 18, 69, 73] usually ranges from 0 to 9/10 high-power fields, with a mean of 2/10 high-power fields, but has been reported in a single case at 48/10 high-power fields [3]. Small vessels in tumor cell nests are often surrounded by hyalinized necrosis [72], but in contrast to PSTT, the vascular architecture is normally preserved. The occasional vascular deposition of amorphous fibrinoid material has been described [1]. In ETTs with cervical/endocervical involvement, neoplastic cells can focally replace the endocervical glands with stratified neoplastic cells, thus simulating high-grade squamous intraepithelial lesions [2, 3]. Lymphovascular invasion can present in ETT [3].

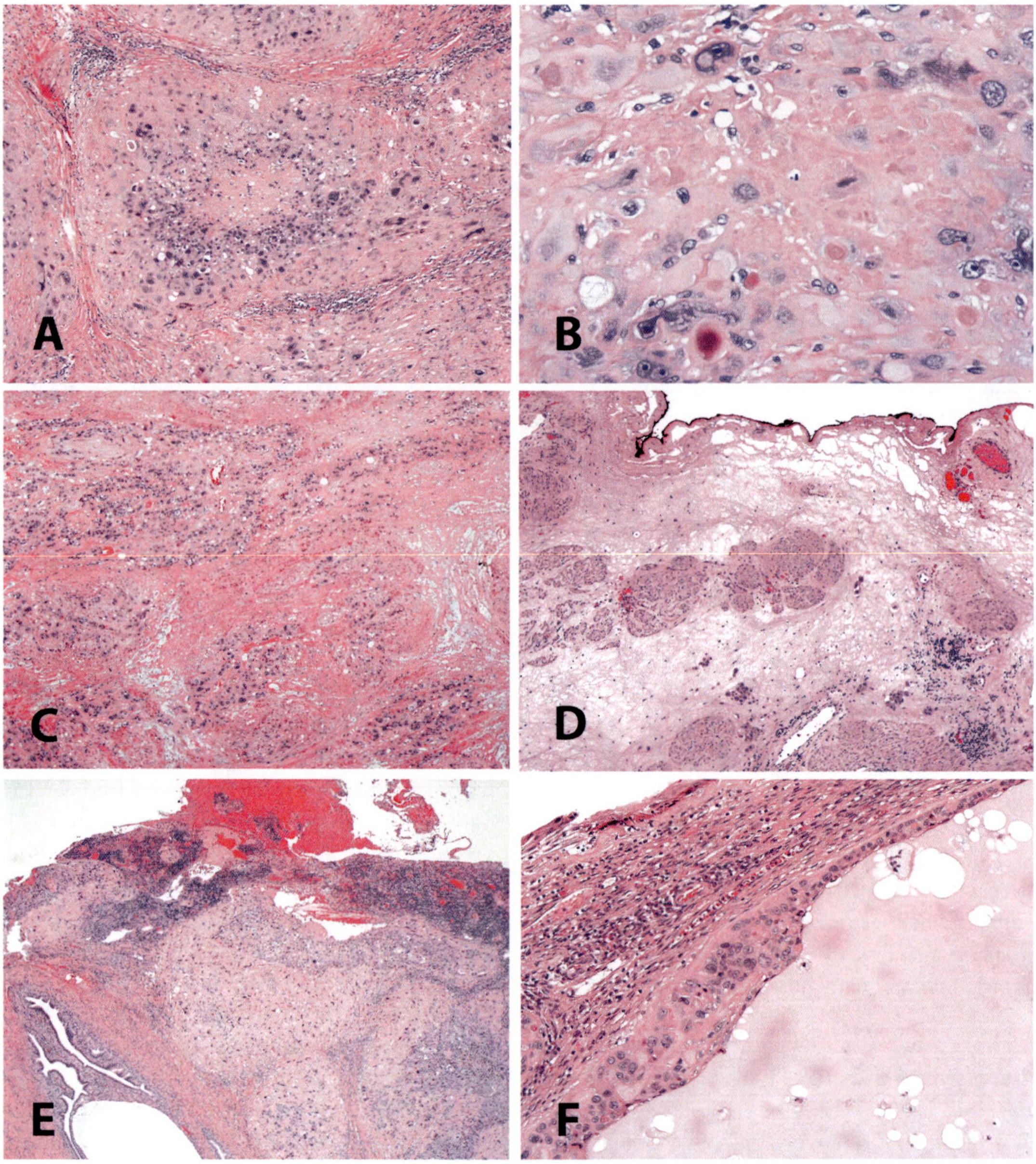

Fig. 7.3 Histological features of ETT. (**a**) Nodular, expansile growth pattern with pushing borders. (**b**) Mononucleate intermediate trophoblast cells surrounded by hyaline-like matrix and eosinophilic debris resembling the keratinous material in squamous cell carcinoma. (**c**) Extensive tumor necrosis surrounded by island of viable cells, causing the geographical pattern typical for ETT. (**d**) Infiltrative area at the periphery of the tumor. Tumor cell cords and small nests are present <1 mm from the inked uterine serosa. (**e**) Endocervical involvement by ETT. (**f**) Focal replacement of endocervical gland epithelium with stratified neoplastic cells resembling squamous intraepithelial neoplasia ((**f**) Courtesy of Pei Hui, MD, PhD, Yale University, New Haven, CT)

ETT may be deeply invasive and can extend into adjacent anatomic structures including vagina and bladder and ureter (Fig. 7.4). Common sites of metastatic disease include the lungs (Fig. 7.5), liver, gallbladder, kidney, pancreas, spine [26, 28], and vagina [11].

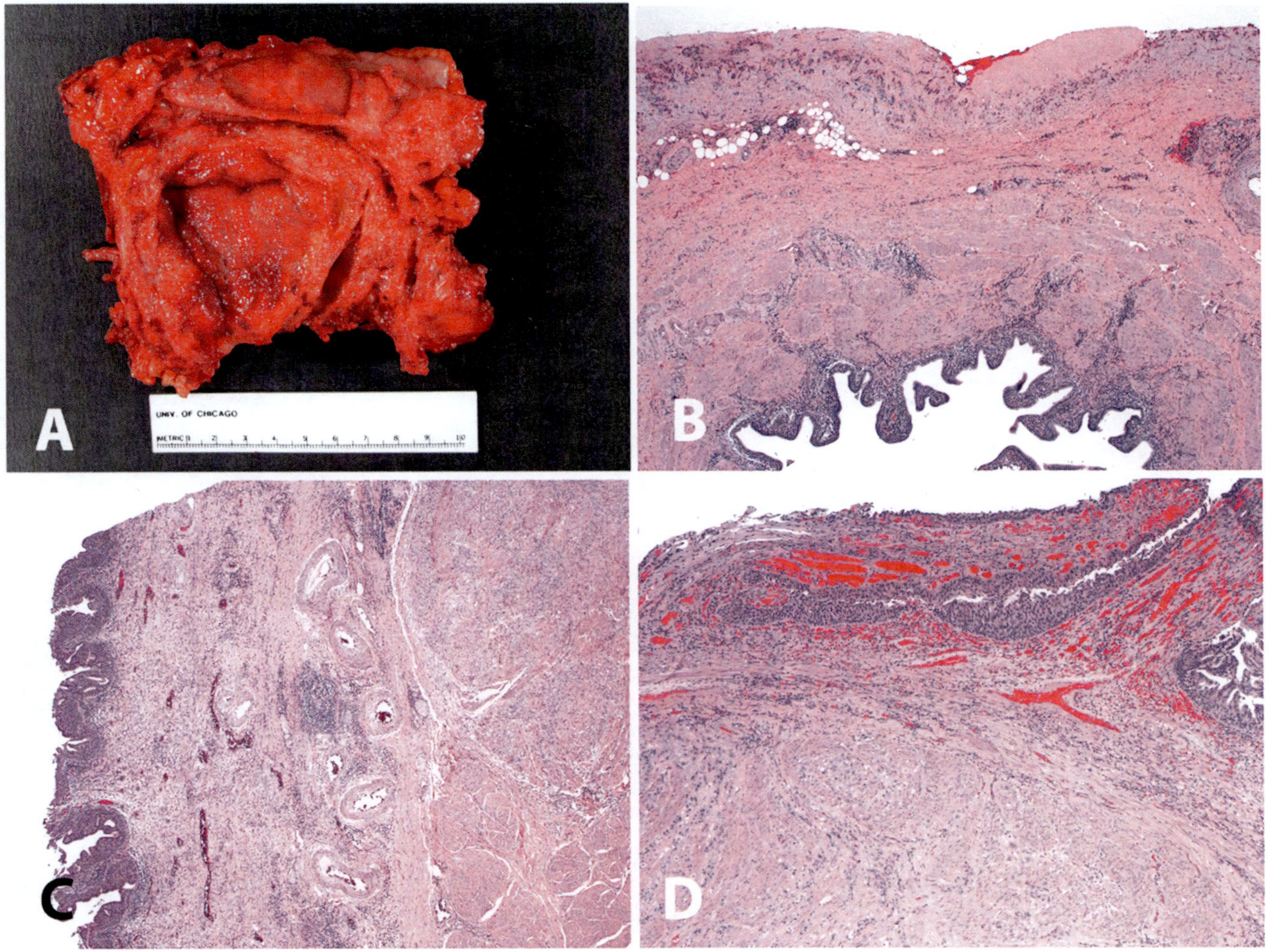

Fig. 7.4 ETT with extrauterine extension into adjacent structures (bladder and ureter). (**a**) Gross image of a cystectomy specimen with attached anterior vaginal wall. A 5×4×2 cm recurrent ETT is located in the dome, anterior and right lateral wall of the bladder. The patient previously underwent a hysterectomy and chemotherapy. (**b**) ETT tumor cells invade the adventitia of the ureter wall. (**c**) Infiltration of the tunica muscularis propria, showing the typical nodular growth pattern of ETT. (**d**) The tumor infiltrates the bladder wall transmurally into the tunica submucosa and mucosa

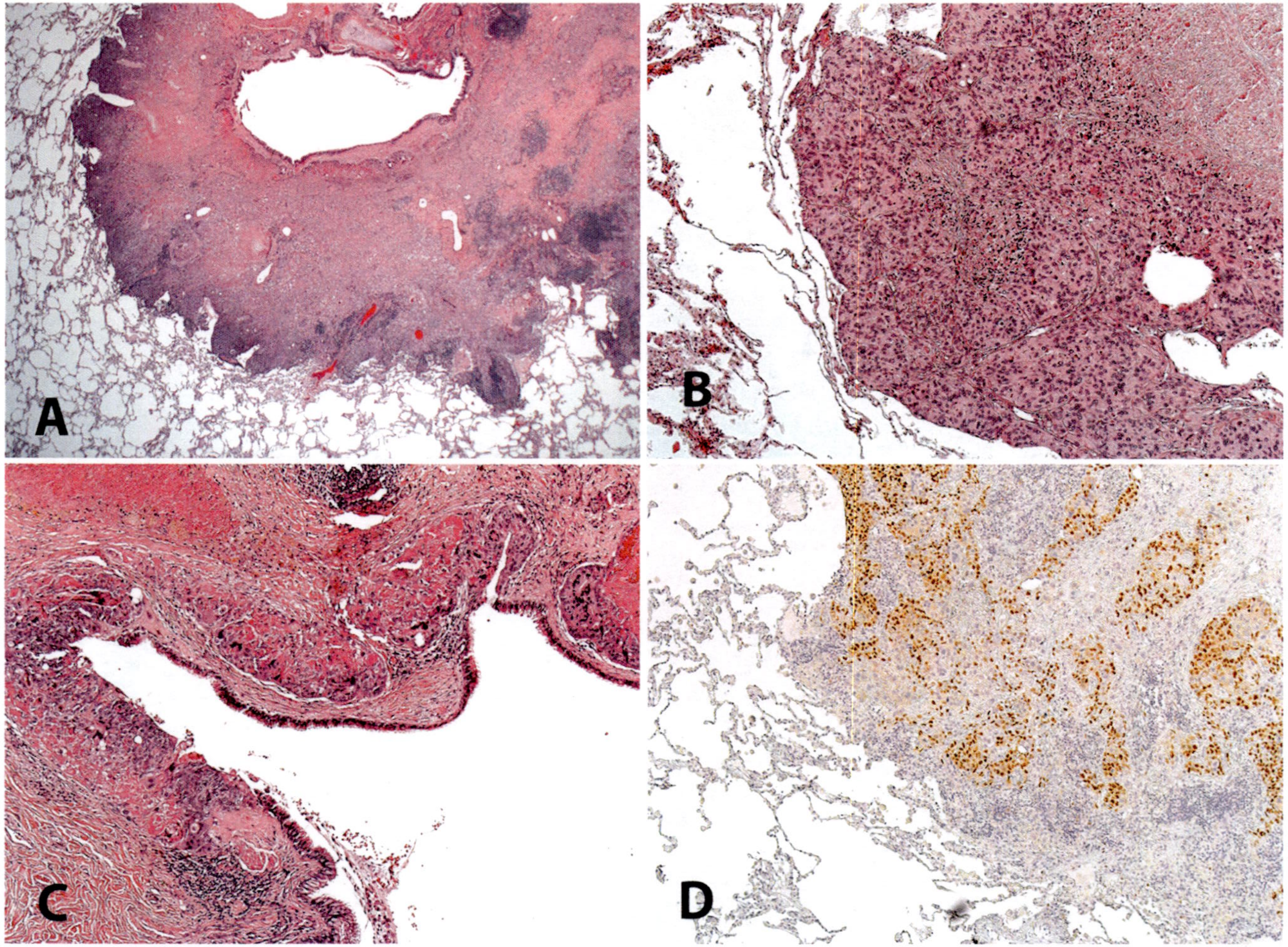

Fig. 7.5 Metastatic ETT involving lungs. (**a**) Peribronchiolar metastasis of an ETT. (**b**) A pulmonary metastasis shows nests of mononuclear chorion laeve-like tumor cells with eosinophilic cytoplasm and abundant necrosis. (**c**) The tumor cells colonize the lamina propria of the bronchial wall and partially replace the respiratory epithelium. (**d**) Immunohistochemical stain for p63 reveals diffuse nuclear staining in the pulmonary metastasis ((**a–d**) Courtesy of Pei Hui, MD, PhD, Yale University, New Haven, CT)

Cytological Findings

Cytologic features of ETT are only described in two case reports [7, 16]. One patient [16] was initially diagnosed with squamous cell carcinoma of the cervix, until the hysterectomy specimen was available for examination. In the other case [7], the cells were originally interpreted as regenerative or metaplastic changes. In a 35-year-old female with a clinical history of 2 months of vaginal bleeding, a preoperative conventional cervical Papanicolaou (PAP) smear [16] reveled a few scattered, solitary or small clusters of polygonal, atypical giant cells in a background of inflammation. The large polygonal cells had abundant, thin cytoplasm with a distinct cell membrane, and occasionally, eosinophilic granules or cytoplasmic vacuolation was present. Most cells were mononucleate and exhibited ovoid, hyperchromatic and irregularly enlarged nuclei with one or more conspicuous nucleoli. Multinucleated giant cells, necrosis, or hyaline material was not observed. Preoperative PAP smears [7] from a 36-year-old female with complaints of heavy menstruation and lower abdominal pain showed no abnormalities of the ecto- and endocervix, but the endometrial brushings revealed atypical giant cells scattered alone or in clusters in the background of a secretory endometrium.

The cells revealed abundant thick cytoplasm with occasional vacuolation and ill-defined cytoplasmic borders. The majority of the cells were mononucleate, with irregularly enlarged and hyperchromatic nuclei and one or two inconspicuous nucleoli.

Especially, in cervical or uterine lesions with an unusual clinical appearance, the presence of large, polygonal cells with abundant cytoplasm in cervical [16] or endometrial [7] cytology specimens should raise concern about a possible intermediate trophoblastic lesion, such as ETT. However, it is not possible to differentiate between ETT, PSTT, and PSN [7, 16] on the basis of cytologic features alone.

Ancillary Studies

Electron Microscopy

Ultrastructurally [6, 11, 32, 75], ETTs reveal mononuclear cells with one or two conspicuous nucleoli, abundant euchromatin, moderate to abundant cytoplasm, and polygonal outlines. The cells are joined by multiple well-formed desmosomes. Perinuclearly, abundant organella (numerous mitochondria, free ribosomes, and rough endoplasmic reticulum), bundles of intermediate-type filament and glycogen granules can be found.

Cells at the periphery of the nests can be focally invested by a thick basement membrane [6], and rarely, cells may present a few short microvilli at the surface [6]. Multinucleated giant cells with increased cytoplasmic electron density, pleomorphic nuclei, abundant heterochromatin and inconspicuous nucleoli, have been described as a second cell type mixed with the mononuclear cells [6] forming desmosomes between the two tumor cell types. The multinucleated giant cells contain abundant cytoplasmic organella and vesicles [6] and, if they face an open space, exhibit abundant microvilli [6].

Ultrastructural findings of ETT in cases with [6, 75] and without prior chemotherapy for gestational choriocarcinoma or an invasive mole were compatible [11]. ETT cannot be distinguished from PSTT [41] by electron microscopy, as they exhibit similar features.

Immunohistochemistry Fig. 7.6

The trophoblastic cells of ETT generally express various trophoblastic markers including H3D3B1, HLA-G, hPL, Inhibin-alpha, and Mel-CAM. Cytokeratin proteins are also expressed in the tumor cells, including CK18, CK, AE1/AE3, and p63.

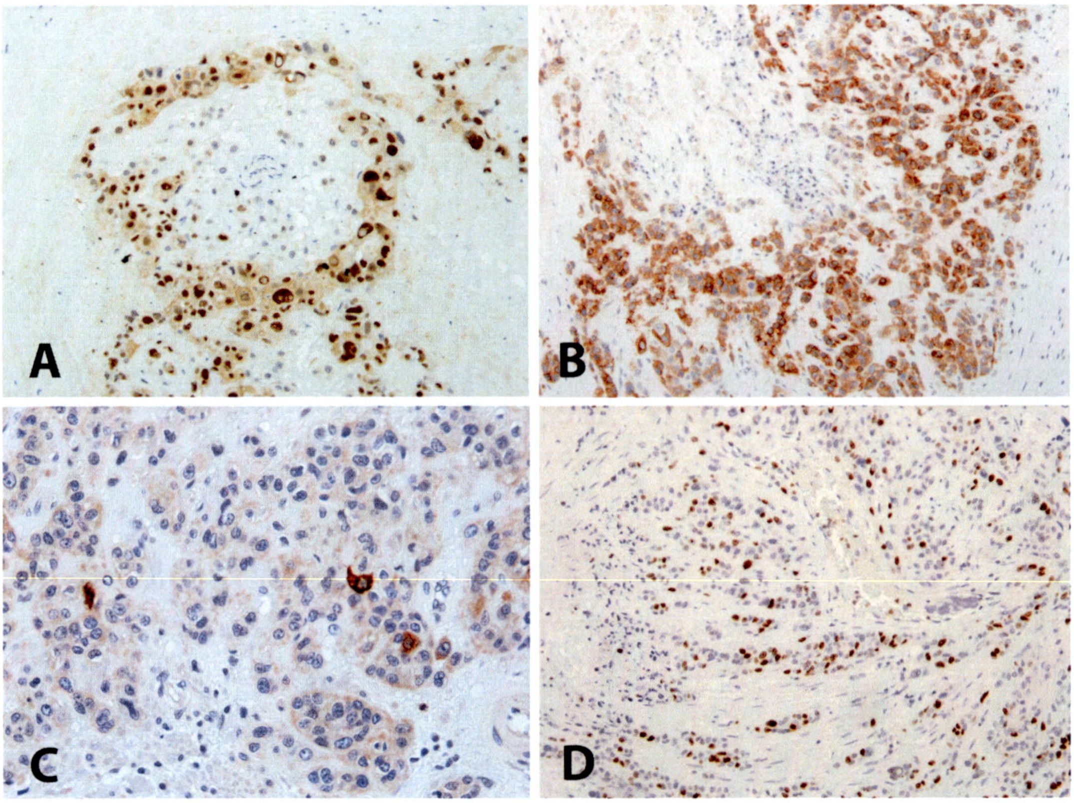

Fig. 7.6 Immunohistochemistry features of ETT. (**a**) The majority of tumor cells exhibit diffuse nuclear expression of p63. (**b**) Strong diffuse immunoreactivity for inhibin-α in the tumor cells. (**c**) hPL expression in ETT is typically limited to individual cells. (**d**) The Ki-67 proliferation index is >10% in ETT

Hydroxyl-δ-5-Steroid Dehydrogenase (HSD3B1) (Diagram 7.1)

The enzyme hydroxyl-δ-5-steroid dehydrogenase (HSD3B1) is involved in steroid hormone synthesis [76] by catalyzing the oxidative conversion of δ-5-3 β hydroxy steroids into the δ-4-3-keto configuration. A review [53] of HSD3B1 expression in silica by serial analysis of gene expression (SAGE) revealed no HSD3B1 expression in 159 libraries of lung, colorectal, pancreatic and ovarian carcinomas, and other types of adult and fetal tissue. Immunohistochemistry results [53] from a commercially available monoclonal anti-HSD3B1 antibody (clone 3C11-D4) show that HSD3B1 is intensively and diffusely expressed in intermediate and syncytiotrophoblasts from normal placental tissue, hydatidiform moles, trophoblastic tumors, and tumor-like lesions, with the exemption of a few CCs. In <1% [53] of non-trophoblastic carcinomas, HSD3B1 shows weak and focal expression. HSD3B1 is therefore accepted as a specific and sensitive trophoblastic marker [53].

Human Leukocyte Antigen G (Diagram 7.1)

HLA-G is a nonclassical, major histocompatibility complex (MHC) Class I antigen that appears to contribute to maternal tolerance of fetal tissue [14]. Isoforms of HLA-G have been identified [77–79] in the intermediate trophoblasts of normal placenta samples and hydatidiform moles, as well as in the CC cell line JEG-3. HLA-G immunoreactivity [14], assessed with a commercially available antibody (clone 4H84), is present in at least 70%

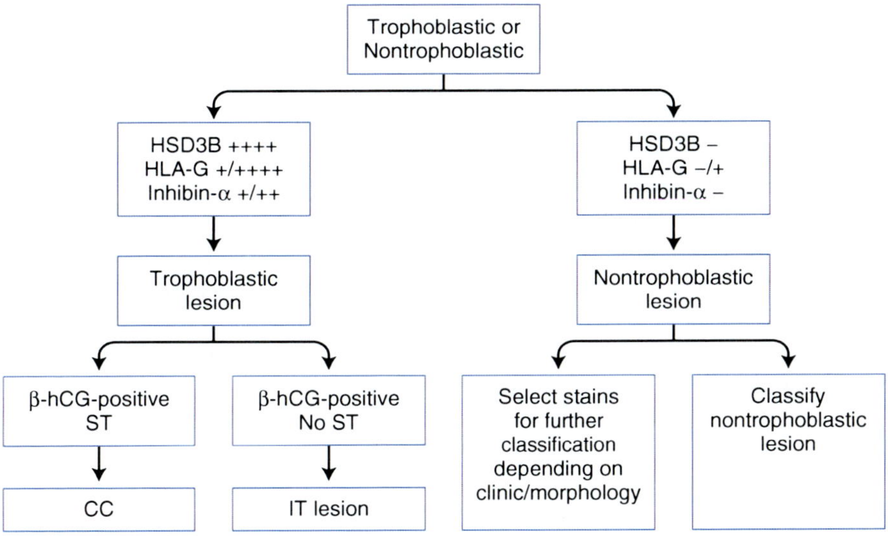

Diagram 7.1 Immunohistochemical approach for potential trophoblastic lesions [14, 22, 53, 82]. *CC* choriocarcinoma; *IT* intermediate trophoblast; *ST* syncytiotrophoblast

of intermediate trophoblastic cells from normal placentas, hydatidiform moles, trophoblastic tumors, and tumor-like lesions. HLA-G is not expressed in uterine neoplasms [14]. Rare expression in cervical carcinoma has been observed [22] using a different, possibly less specific [22] antibody (clone 3H2680). HLA-G appears to be a specific marker for intermediate trophoblasts and is useful in the differential diagnosis of nontrophoblastic lesions.

Inhibin-α (Diagram 7.1)

Another valuable marker, which is less specific but more widely available even in a smaller laboratory setting, is inhibin-α, the α-subunit of the heterodimeric gonadal peptide hormone inhibin. Inhibin-α is expressed in the intermediate trophoblast and the syncytiotrophoblast of all types of GTD [80]. In normal placental tissue, the expression pattern depends on gestational age [80]. Inhibin-α is not expressed by uterine tumors [80], but by sex-cord stromal tumors of the ovary [81]. Therefore, inhibin-α is a useful and generally readily available marker for identifying trophoblastic lesions.

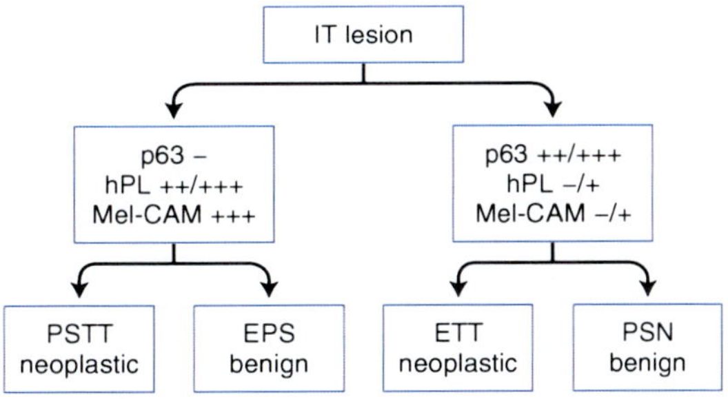

Diagram 7.2 Immunohistochemical differentiation of intermediate trophoblastic lesions [15, 22, 69, 82]. *IT* intermediate trophoblast; *PSTT* placental site trophoblastic tumor; *EPS* exaggerated implantation site; *ETT* epithelioid trophoblastic tumor; *PSN* placental site nodule

P63 (Diagram 7.2)

The analysis of p63 gene expression, a transcription factor belonging to the p53 family [58–60], is useful in discriminating p63-negative intermediate trophoblastic lesion from p63-positive chorion-type intermediate trophoblastic lesions. In ETT, p63 usually exhibits a highly specific, diffuse nuclear staining [3]. It is important, however, to select an antibody that recognizes TAp63 (see also Fig. 7.6a), like 4A4, because the ΔNp63 form will not stain ETT or PSN [15].

Human Placental Lactogen (Diagram 7.2)

Human placental lactogen (hPL), a polypeptide placental hormone normally produced in syncytiotrophoblasts and intermediate trophoblasts at the implantation site of the placenta, is another highly valuable marker in the differential diagnosis of implantation site and chorionic-type intermediate trophoblast-related lesions [82]. PSTT and EPS diffusely express hPL in the majority of trophoblastic cells [3, 83], whereas hPL expression in ETTs is normally limited to individual cells (<5%) [1, 3, 69, 82].

Melanoma Cell Adhesion Molecule (Diagram 7.2)

The melanoma cell adhesion molecule (Mel-CAM, also known as CD146) is a membrane glycoprotein belonging to the immunoglobulin supergene family that is involved in cell adhesions [84]. Immunohistochemistry results show that Mel-CAM (monoclonal mouse antibody MN-4 [85]) is strongly expressed in implantation site intermediate trophoblasts, but is expressed in only a few cells of chorionic-type intermediate trophoblasts of ETT.

Other Immunohistochemical Marker

Other markers expressed in ETTs, mostly reported in case reports, include CKAE1/AE3 [3], CK18 [18], placental alkaline phosphatase (PLAP), CK7 [12], and CD117 (c-kit) (nuclear). No staining was found for CK20, CK 5/6, TTF-1 [21], S100, CA-125, or calretinin. Variable staining patterns for epithelial membrane antigen (EMA) [2, 12] have been observed.

Differential Diagnosis

ETT vs. Squamous Cell Carcinoma Table 7.3

The most common diagnostic pitfall in the differential diagnosis of ETT is keratinizing squamous cell carcinoma of the cervix [13, 14, 16, 21], especially if the ETT arises from the cervix or lower uterine segment [2, 3]. A typical clinical history (women of reproductive age with an antecedent gestation and slightly elevated serum hCG) can be extremely helpful; however, it is important to consider ETT generally as a differential diagnosis for squamous cell carcinoma of the cervix, as ETT can occur many years after a remote gestation and even in peri- [10] and postmenopausal [5] women. Morphological features supporting ETT include the absence of definitive squamous intraepithelial neoplasia, lack of cell bridges, the presence of decidualized stromal cells, and nodular proliferation with hyalinizing matrix as opposed to true squamous carcinoma nests with keratin [3].

Table 7.3 Immunohistochemical expression of cervical lesions resembling ETT [2, 3, 14, 28, 53, 82]

Stain	Epithelioid trophoblastic tumor	Squamous cell carcinoma	Epithelioid leiomyosarcoma
HSD3B1	+	–	–
HLA-G	+	–	–
Mel-Cam	+ (individual cells)	–	–
hPL	+ (individual cells)	–	–
Inhibin-α	+	–	–
CK 18	+	–	–
Cyclin E	+	–	–
CK AE1/AE7	+	+	–
P63	+	+	–
Desmin	–	–	+
Smooth muscle actin	–	–	+
Caldesmon	–	–	+

Immunohistochemical panel (Table 7.3): HSD3B1, HLA-G, inhibin-a, CK18 (all expressed in ETT); p16[50] *(expressed in squamous cell carcinoma).*

ETT vs. PSTT (Table 7.4)

ETT reveals a nodular growth pattern with a pushing tumor border and central hyalinization, which is usually not seen in PSTT. The tumor cells in ETT display less nuclear pleomorphism than in PSTT. ETT and PSTT also reveal a different vascular morphology [72]; in ETT, small vessels located in tumor cell nests preserve their regular architecture and are surrounded by hyalinized necrosis, whereas in PSTT, tumor cells invade, migrate through, or replace vessel walls.

Immunohistochemical panel: p63 (expressed in ETT); hPL, Mel-CAM (expressed in PSTT; only single cells in ETT).

ETT vs. Choriocarcinoma

ETT does not reveal the bilaminar growth pattern of CC and usually presents clinically only with mild serum hCG elevation. The presence of β-hCG-expressing syncytiotrophoblasts confirms the diagnosis of CC and distinguishes it from other types of intermediate trophoblastic tumors, including ETT.

Immunohistochemical panel: β-hCG (expression in syncytiotrophoblast of CC).

Caveat: Multinucleated intermediate trophoblastic β-hCG expressing cells can be present in ETT and should not be confused with syncytiotrophoblastic cells.

ETT vs. PSN

It has been proposed that PSN could be the precursor lesion of ETT by transforming into an atypical PSN and subsequently ETT [23, 50]. Although certain histologic features (hypercellularity, geographic necrosis, and proliferation) can be useful in the differential diagnosis, distinguishing a PSN from an ETT can be difficult in a biopsy or curettage specimen [50]. A PSN represents the remnants of the intermediate trophoblast from a prior gestation that has failed to completely involute. It is typically an incidental finding in a biopsy or hysterectomy specimen [86, 87]. Most PSNs are solitary, small (<5 mm) nodules within the uterine cavity; however, multiple lesions and cervical, ovarian, fallopian tube and broad ligament involvement have been reported [44, 88]. Microscopically, PSNs represent hyalinized nodules containing regressed,

Table 7.4 Differential diagnosis of ETT vs. PSTT [1–3, 82]

	ETT	PSTT
Uterine location	Cervix (50%) Uterine corpus (50%)	Uterine corpus
Growth	Nodular growth pattern	Between muscle bundles
Circumscription	Pushing borders	Myometrial infiltration
Material	Hyalinized material Eosinophilic debris	Usually not present
Necrosis	Geographic necrosis	Focal necrosis
Nuclear pleomorphism	Mild-moderate	Moderate-severe
Multinucleated cells	Rare	Common
Relationship of TC to vessel	TC around vessels	TC invade vessels TC replace vessels
Type of IT	Chorion-type IT	Implantation-site IT
p63 IHC	Diffusely positive	Negative
hPL IHC	Only individual cells	Diffusely positive
Mel-CAM	Only individual cells	Diffusely positive

TC tumor cells; *IT* intermediate trophoblast; *IHC* immunohistochemistry degenerated chorionic-type intermediate trophoblasts [82] with a noninvasive growth pattern. PSNs exhibit low cellularity and minimal proliferation. Based on these features, PSN can normally be distinguished from ETT; however, some rare cases exhibit size, cellularity, and proliferation [23, 44, 50] that fall between those of typical PSN and ETT. These cases have been termed "atypical PSN." Especially for a small specimen, immunohistochemical stains for cyclin E and Ki-67 may be of value. Cyclin E is involved in cell cycle regulation and is diffusely expressed in ETT and in atypical PSN, but usually not in PSN [50]. Additionally, the proliferation marker Ki-67 (Mib1) is useful for discriminating between PSN and ETT:

Cyclin E (expressed in ETT and atypical PSN), Ki-67 (labeling index >10% in ETT and <8% in PSN [82]*). Importantly, normal inflammatory cells may be present in the endomyometrium and label for Ki-67; however, these cells may not be included in the tumor proliferation count* [82].

Further differential diagnosis can be found in Chap. 10.

ETT vs. Epithelioid Leiomyosarcoma Table 7.3

The distinction of epithelioid leiomyosarcoma [28] and other smooth muscle neoplasms from ETT can easily be made by immunohistochemistry on the basis of a lack of smooth muscle marker expression.

Immunohistochemical panel (Table 7.3): HSD3B1, HLA-G, inhibin-a, CK18 (all expressed in ETT); desmin, smooth muscle actin, caldesmon (all expressed smooth muscle neoplasms).

Rare Differential Diagnosis of ETT

A rare, differential diagnosis for ETT is lymphoepithelioma-like carcinoma of the cervix (LELC) [89] with ectopic β-human chorionic gonadotropin production [90], a subtype of squamous cell carcinoma. Intense lymphoplasmacytic infiltrates surrounding sheets, islands, and nests of tumor cells can provide diagnostic clues.

Immunohistochemical panel (based on a case report [90]*) : inhibin-a, CK18 (expressed in ETT); hPL (individual cells in ETT, negative in LELC); β-hCG (focal reactivity in LELC).*

Another rare, differential diagnosis for ETT is poorly differentiated endometrioid carcinoma with focal syncytiotrophoblastic cell differentiation [2]. An appropriate immunohistochemical panel is necessary to confirm this diagnosis. As a first step, it should include markers to distinguish a trophoblastic from a nontrophoblastic lesion.

Metastatic Disease and Extrauterine ETT, Especially Lung Lesions

The first and most important step in accurately diagnosing metastatic or extrauterine ETT is actually a high level of suspicion to initiate a work-up for GTD. In the lung, ETT can resemble pulmonary non-small cell carcinoma [6], such as squamous cell carcinoma or pleomorphic carcinoma [21], as well as primary or metastatic germ cell tumors with trophoblastic differentiation or CC.

The patient's age, smoking status, a clinical history of β-hCG elevation, and imaging findings all contribute to the differential diagnosis. Like cervical and uterine ETTs, trophoblastic lesions can be disguised from nontrophoblastic lesions by applying the immunohistochemical panel [82] of HSD3B1, HLA-G, and inhibin-α. If the lesion is of trophoblastic origin, CC can be excluded by the absence of β-hCG staining syncytiotrophoblastic cells, and ETT can be distinguished from PSTT with p63, hPL, and Mel-CAM. If the lesion is not of trophoblastic origin, other markers are needed for further classification. Squamous cell carcinoma reveals immunoreactivity for CK5/6, which is not seen in ETT, whereas pleomorphic carcinoma of the lung usually expresses TTF-1 [21], which is not expressed in ETT. In the differential diagnosis of potential germ cell neoplasms, it is important to consider that ETTs can express PLAP, certain cytokeratins, and CD117 (c-kit).

Clinicopathological Correlations

Clinical Staging

ETT is staged according to the FIGO staging system for GTD [91]. The WHO scoring system cannot be used for ETT [91] (see also Chap. 11).

Clinical Management

In contrast to CC, ETT shows relative resistance to chemotherapy [92] and is therefore primarily treated surgically. The recommended procedure is a hysterectomy with pelvic lymph node dissection [92] due to possible lymphatic spread and lymph node metastasis [3, 23]. Chemotherapy is suggested [92] in patients with metastatic disease and in cases of nonmetastatic disease with unfavorable prognostic factors, which include the following: interval from last known antecedent gestation to diagnosis >2 years; deep invasion of the myometrium; tumor necrosis; and >6 mitoses/10 high-point power fields. Currently, a platinum-containing regimen, such as EMA-EP or a paclitaxel/cisplatin–paclitaxel/etoposide doublet, is recommended [92] (see also Table 11.8).

Successful treatment of a relapsed ETT with a focal CC component by a high-dose chemotherapy regimen and autologous stem cell support has been reported [93]. After ETT treatment and subsequent hCG regression to normal, serum hCG levels should be monitored monthly for 1 year [92].

Prognosis and Prognostic Markers

Although the majority of patients with ETT have a favorable outcome, metastases occur in 25% of cases [35, 69], and 10% of patients [35, 69] die of ETT. The survival rate for ETT appears to be similar to that of PSTT; in nonmetastatic disease, it is estimated as near 100% and in metastatic disease as approximately 50–60% [92, 94–96].

So far, however, neither the analysis of morphologic features nor evaluation for specific molecular characteristics has provided any reliable markers to predict long-term clinical behavior [47]. High mitotic activity has been proposed as an adverse prognostic factor [3, 5], but a well-defined cut-off has yet to be established. A mitotic index of >6/10 high point-power fields is considered unfavorable in decisions about possible adjuvant chemotherapy [92].

Future Molecular Targets

In CC and PSTT, several molecular markers, such as c-MYC proto-oncogene, mitogen-activated protein kinase (MAPK), mammalian target of rapamycin (mTOR), and matrix metalloproteinase (MMP), have been identified [47] as potential future treatment options. The only therapeutic target for ETT that has been demonstrated to date is the transmembrane receptor tyrosine kinase EGFR, which is expressed [1, 12] by immunohistochemistry. Hypothetically, patients might benefit from treatment with EGFR tyrosine inhibitors [47, 65, 66] including cetuximab, gefitinib, and erlotinib [47]; however, a major problem is the absence of definitive predictive markers for the response to EGFR inhibition. EGFR-activating mutations in exons 18, 19, and 21, which can predict gefitinib response in non-small cell carcinoma of the lung [97, 98], have not yet been demonstrated in ETTs.

References

1. Shih IM, Kurman RJ. Epithelioid trophoblastic tumor: a neoplasm distinct from choriocarcinoma and placental site trophoblastic tumor simulating carcinoma. Am J Surg Pathol. 1998;22(11):1393–403.
2. Hui P, Martel M, Parkash V. Gestational trophoblastic diseases: recent advances in histopathologic diagnosis and related genetic aspects. Adv Anat Pathol. 2005;12(3):116–25.
3. Fadare O, Parkash V, Carcangiu ML, Hui P. Epithelioid trophoblastic tumor: clinicopathological features with an emphasis on uterine cervical involvement. Mod Pathol. 2006;19(1):75–82.
4. Bouchet-Mishellany F, Ledoux-Pilon A, Darcha C, Dechelotte P. Trophoblastic gestational disease: a placental site trophoblastic tumor and an epithelioid trophoblastic tumor. Ann Pathol. 2004;24(2):167–71.

5. Coulson LE, Kong CS, Zaloudek C. Epithelioid trophoblastic tumor of the uterus in a postmenopausal woman: a case report and review of the literature. Am J Surg Pathol. 2000;24(11):1558–62.
6. Hamazaki S, Nakamoto S, Okino T, Tsukayama C, Mori M, Taguchi K, et al. Epithelioid trophoblastic tumor: morphological and immunohistochemical study of three lung lesions. Hum Pathol. 1999;30(11): 1321–7.
7. Kamoi S, Ohaki Y, Mori O, Yokoyama M, Kawamoto Y, Kawamura T, et al. Epithelioid trophoblastic tumor of the uterus: cytological and immunohistochemical observation of a case. Pathol Int. 2002;52(1):75–81.
8. Kuo KT, Chen MJ, Lin MC. Epithelioid trophoblastic tumor of the broad ligament: a case report and review of the literature. Am J Surg Pathol. 2004;28(3):405–9.
9. Meydanli MM, Kucukali T, Usubutun A, Ataoglu O, Kafkasli A. Epithelioid trophoblastic tumor of the endocervix: a case report. Gynecol Oncol. 2002;87(2): 219–24.
10. Narita F, Takeuchi K, Hamana S, Ohbayashi C, Ayata M, Maruo T. Epithelioid trophoblastic tumor (ETT) initially interpreted as cervical cancer. Int J Gynecol Cancer. 2003;13(4):551–4.
11. Ohira S, Yamazaki T, Hatano H, Harada O, Toki T, Konishi I. Epithelioid trophoblastic tumor metastatic to the vagina: an immunohistochemical and ultrastructural study. Int J Gynecol Pathol. 2000;19(4): 381–6.
12. Parker A, Lee V, Dalrymple C, Valmadre S, Russell P. Epithelioid trophoblastic tumour: report of a case in the fallopian tube. Pathology. 2003;35(2):136–40.
13. Shen DH, Khoo US, Ngan HY, Ng TY, Chau MT, Xue WC, et al. Coexisting epithelioid trophoblastic tumor and choriocarcinoma of the uterus following a chemoresistant hydatidiform mole. Arch Pathol Lab Med. 2003;127(7):e291–3.
14. Singer G, Kurman RJ, McMaster MT, Shih Ie M. HLA-G immunoreactivity is specific for intermediate trophoblast in gestational trophoblastic disease and can serve as a useful marker in differential diagnosis. Am J Surg Pathol. 2002;26(7):914–20.
15. Shih IM, Kurman RJ. p63 expression is useful in the distinction of epithelioid trophoblastic and placental site trophoblastic tumors by profiling trophoblastic subpopulations. Am J Surg Pathol. 2004;28(9):1177–83.
16. Takekawa Y, Yamamoto T, Sakakibara M, Kimura M, Yoshii R, Yamashita Y. Cytologic findings of epithelioid trophoblastic tumor of the uterus: a case report. Acta Cytol. 2010;54(3):345–8.
17. Phippen NT, Lowery WJ, Leath III CA, Kost ER. Epithelioid trophoblastic tumor masquerading as invasive squamous cell carcinoma of the cervix after an ectopic pregnancy. Gynecol Oncol. 2010;117(2):387–8.
18. Li J, Shi Y, Wan X, Qian H, Zhou C, Chen X. Epithelioid trophoblastic tumor: a clinicopathological and immunohistochemical study of seven cases. Med Oncol. 2011;28(1):294–9.
19. Liang Y, Chen XD, Lu BJ, Shi HY, Zhang XF. Clinicopathologic analysis of uterine epithelioid trophoblastic tumor. Zhonghua Bing Li Xue Za Zhi. 2009;38(9):590–3.
20. Okumura M, Fushida K, Rezende WW, Schultz R, Zugaib M. Sonographic appearance of gestational trophoblastic disease evolving into epithelioid trophoblastic tumor. Ultrasound Obstet Gynecol. 2010;36(2): 249–51.
21. Lewin SN, Aghajanian C, Moreira AL, Soslow RA. Extrauterine epithelioid trophoblastic tumors presenting as primary lung carcinomas: morphologic and immunohistochemical features to resolve a diagnostic dilemma. Am J Surg Pathol. 2009;33(12):1809–14.
22. Kalhor N, Ramirez PT, Deavers MT, Malpica A, Silva EG. Immunohistochemical studies of trophoblastic tumors. Am J Surg Pathol. 2009;33(4):633–8.
23. Tsai HW, Lin CP, Chou CY, Li CF, Chow NH, Shih IM, et al. Placental site nodule transformed into a malignant epithelioid trophoblastic tumour with pelvic lymph node and lung metastasis. Histopathology. 2008;53(5):601–4.
24. Cheng XD, Lu WG, Wan XY, Chen XD, Xie X. Case report and literature review of epithelioid trophoblastic tumor. Zhonghua Fu Chan Ke Za Zhi. 2008;43(4): 281–5.
25. Eiholm S, Langhoff JL, Palle C. Epithelioid trophoblastic tumour. Ugeskr Laeger. 2010;172(42):2904–5.
26. Chohan MO, Rehman T, Cerilli LA, Devers K, Medina-Flores R, Turner P. Metastatic epithelioid trophoblastic tumor involving the spine. Spine. 2010;35(20):E1072–5.
27. Shet T, Parage M, Maheshwari A, Nair R, Gupta S, Tongaonkar H, et al. Epithelioid trophoblastic tumor of uterus presenting as an ovarian mass: a diagnostic and therapeutic dilemma. Indian J Pathol Microbiol. 2008;51(2):242–4.
28. Macdonald MC, Palmer JE, Hancock BW, Tidy JA. Diagnostic challenges in extrauterine epithelioid trophoblastic tumours: a report of two cases. Gynecol Oncol. 2008;108(2):452–4.
29. Gan MF, Yu CK, Lu HS, Yang PN. Uterine epithelioid trophoblast tumor: report of a case. Zhonghua Bing Li Xue Za Zhi. 2007;36(8):570–1.
30. Noh HT, Lee KH, Lee MA, Ko YB, Hwang SH, Son SK. Epithelioid trophoblastic tumor of paracervix and parametrium. Int J Gynecol Cancer. 2008;18(4): 843–6.
31. Theodossiadis P, Rouvas A, Nakopoulou L, Halvatziotis P, Magkou C, Vergados I. Epithelioid trophoblastic tumor. Ophthalmology. 2007;114(7):1421.
32. Urabe S, Fujiwara H, Miyoshi H, Arihiro K, Soma H, Yoshihama I, et al. Epithelioid trophoblastic tumor of the lung. J Obstet Gynaecol Res. 2007;33(3):397–401.
33. Liu Q, Shi QL, Zhang JM, Li Y, Du YM, Shen SM, et al. Epithelioid trophoblastic tumor of the uterus: a report of. China Med J (Engl). 2007;120(8):729–30.
34. Vencken PM, Ewing PC, Zweemer RP. Epithelioid trophoblastic tumour: a case report and review of the literature. J Clin Pathol. 2006;59(12):1307–8.
35. Lo C, Low I, Tan AL, Baranyai J. Epithelioid trophoblastic tumor: a case report. Int J Gynecol Cancer. 2006;16(3):1473–6.

36. Zavadil M, Feyereisl J, Safar P, Pan M. Undifferentiated choriocarcinoma–epithelioid trophoblastic tumors treated at the Center for Trophoblastic Diseases in the Czech Republic 1955–2003. Ceska Gynekol. 2003; 68(6):420–6.
37. Mazur MT. Metastatic gestational choriocarcinoma. Unusual pathologic variant following therapy. Cancer. 1989;63(7):1370–7.
38. Jones WB, Romain K, Erlandson RA, Burt ME, Lewis Jr JL. Thoracotomy in the management of gestational choriocarcinoma. A clinicopathologic study. Cancer. 1993;72(7):2175–81.
39. Silva EG, Tornos C, Lage J, Ordonez NG, Morris M, Kavanagh J. Multiple nodules of intermediate trophoblast following hydatidiform moles. Int J Gynecol Pathol. 1993;12(4):324–32.
40. Mazur MT, Kurman RJ. Gestational trophoblastic disease and related lesions. In: Kurman RJ, editor. Blaustein's pathology of the female genital tract. 4th ed. New York: Springer; 1994. p. 1049–93.
41. Duncan DA, Mazur MT. Trophoblastic tumors: ultrastructural comparison of choriocarcinoma and placental-site trophoblastic tumor. Hum Pathol. 1989;20(4): 370–81.
42. Fukunaga M, Ushigome S. Malignant trophoblastic tumors: immunohistochemical and flow cytometric comparison of choriocarcinoma and placental site trophoblastic tumors. Hum Pathol. 1993;24(10):1098–106.
43. Ramondetta LM, Silva EG, Levenback CF, Burke TW. Mixed choriocarcinoma in a postmenopausal patient. Int J Gynecol Cancer. 2002;12(3):312–6.
44. Sebire NJ, Lindsay I. Current issues in the histopathology of gestational trophoblastic tumors. Fetal Pediatr Pathol. 2010;29(1):30–44.
45. Cole ME, Broaddus R, Thaker P, Landen C, Freedman RS. Placental-site trophoblastic tumors: a case of resistant pulmonary metastasis. Nat Clin Pract Oncol. 2008;5(3):171–5.
46. Zavadil M, Feyereisl J, Safar P, Pan M. Malignant trophoblastic tumors (MTT) treated in the years 1955–2004 in trophoblastic disease center in the Czech Republic (TDC-CZ): clinical-pathological features, curability, typing, pathogenesis. Ceska Gynekol. 2004;69 Suppl 1:9–15.
47. Shih Ie M. Gestational trophoblastic neoplasia – pathogenesis and potential therapeutic targets. Lancet Oncol. 2007;8(7):642–50.
48. Mao TL, Kurman RJ, Huang CC, Lin MC, Shih Ie M. Immunohistochemistry of choriocarcinoma: an aid in differential diagnosis and in elucidating pathogenesis. Am J Surg Pathol. 2007;31(11):1726–32.
49. Horn LC, Einenkel J, Vogel M. Histopathology of gestational trophoblastic disease. An update. Pathologe. 2009;30(4):313–23.
50. Mao TL, Seidman JD, Kurman RJ, Shih Ie M. Cyclin E and p16 immunoreactivity in epithelioid trophoblastic tumor – an aid in differential diagnosis. Am J Surg Pathol. 2006;30(9):1105–10.
51. Oldt III RJ, Kurman RJ, Shih Ie M. Molecular genetic analysis of placental site trophoblastic tumors and epithelioid trophoblastic tumors confirms their trophoblastic origin. Am J Pathol. 2002;161(3): 1033–7.
52. Xu ML, Yang B, Carcangiu ML, Hui P. Epithelioid trophoblastic tumor: comparative genomic hybridization and diagnostic DNA genotyping. Mod Pathol. 2009;22(2):232–8.
53. Mao TL, Kurman RJ, Jeng YM, Huang W, Shih Ie M. HSD3B1 as a novel trophoblast-associated marker that assists in the differential diagnosis of trophoblastic tumors and tumorlike lesions. Am J Surg Pathol. 2008;32(2):236–42.
54. Yap KL, Hafez MJ, Mao TL, Kurman RJ, Murphy KM, Shih Ie M. Lack of a y-chromosomal complement in the majority of gestational trophoblastic neoplasms. J Oncol. 2010;2010:364508.
55. Bianchi NO. Y chromosome structural and functional changes in human malignant diseases. Mutat Res. 2009;682(1):21–7.
56. Li HW, Tsao SW, Cheung AN. Current understandings of the molecular genetics of gestational trophoblastic diseases. Placenta. 2002;23(1):20–31.
57. Garner EI, Goldstein DP, Feltmate CM, Berkowitz RS. Gestational trophoblastic disease. Clin Obstet Gynecol. 2007;50(1):112–22.
58. Yang A, Kaghad M, Wang Y, Gillett E, Fleming MD, Dotsch V, et al. p63, a p53 homolog at 3q27-29, encodes multiple products with transactivating, death-inducing, and dominant-negative activities. Mol Cell. 1998;2(3):305–16.
59. Yang A, Kaghad M, Caput D, McKeon F. On the shoulders of giants: p63, p73 and the rise of p53. Trends Genet. 2002;18(2):90–5.
60. Flores ER, Tsai KY, Crowley D, Sengupta S, Yang A, McKeon F, et al. p63 and p73 are required for p53-dependent apoptosis in response to DNA damage. Nature. 2002;416(6880):560–4.
61. Little NA, Jochemsen AG. p63. Int J Biochem Cell Biol. 2002;34(1):6–9.
62. Patturajan M, Nomoto S, Sommer M, Fomenkov A, Hibi K, Zangen R, et al. DeltaNp63 induces beta-catenin nuclear accumulation and signaling. Cancer Cell. 2002;1(4):369–79.
63. Zhang HJ, Xue WC, Siu MK, Liao XY, Ngan HY, Cheung AN. P63 expression in gestational trophoblastic disease: correlation with proliferation and apoptotic dynamics. Int J Gynecol Pathol. 2009;28(2): 172–8.
64. Ohtsubo M, Theodoras AM, Schumacher J, Roberts JM, Pagano M. Human cyclin E, a nuclear protein essential for the G1-to-S phase transition. Mol Cell Biol. 1995;15(5):2612–24.
65. Tuncer ZS, Vegh GL, Fulop V, Genest DR, Mok SC, Berkowitz RS. Expression of epidermal growth factor receptor-related family products in gestational trophoblastic diseases and normal placenta and its relationship with development of postmolar tumor. Gynecol Oncol. 2000;77(3):389–93.
66. Muller-Hocker J, Obernitz N, Johannes A, Lohrs U. P53 gene product and EGF-receptor are highly

expressed in placental site trophoblastic tumor. Hum Pathol. 1997;28(11):1302–6.
67. Palmer JE, Macdonald M, Wells M, Hancock BW, Tidy JA. Epithelioid trophoblastic tumor: a review of the literature. J Reprod Med. 2008;53(7):465–75.
68. Baergen RN, Rutgers J, Young RH. Extrauterine lesions of intermediate trophoblast. Int J Gynecol Pathol. 2003;22(4):362–7.
69. Shih IM, Kurman RJ. The pathology of intermediate trophoblastic tumors and tumor-like lesions. Int J Gynecol Pathol. 2001;20(1):31–47.
70. Allan RW, Algood CB, Shih Ie M. Metastatic epithelioid trophoblastic tumor in a male patient with mixed germ-cell tumor of the testis. Am J Surg Pathol. 2009;33(12):1902–5.
71. Li J, Shi Y, Wan X, Yao W, Zhou C, Qian H. Intratumoral blood flow analysis in epithelioid trophoblastic tumors. J Ultrasound Med. 2009;28(12): 1709–14.
72. Horn LC, Vogel M. Gestational trophoblastic disease. Non-villous forms of gestational trophoblastic disease. Pathologe. 2004;25(4):281–91.
73. Allison KH, Love JE, Garcia RL. Epithelioid trophoblastic tumor: review of a rare neoplasm of the chorionic-type intermediate trophoblast. Arch Pathol Lab Med. 2006;130(12):1875–7.
74. Cheung AN. Pathology of gestational trophoblastic diseases. Best Pract Res Clin Obstet Gynaecol. 2003;17(6):849–68.
75. Soma H, Osawa H, Oguro T, Yoshihama I, Fujita K, Mineo S, et al. P57kip2 immunohistochemical expression and ultrastructural findings of gestational trophoblastic disease and related disorders. Med Mol Morphol. 2007;40(2):95–102.
76. Simard J, Ricketts ML, Gingras S, Soucy P, Feltus FA, Melner MH. Molecular biology of the 3beta-hydroxysteroid dehydrogenase/delta5-delta4 isomerase gene family. Endocr Rev. 2005;26(4):525–82.
77. Blaschitz A, Hutter H, Leitner V, Pilz S, Wintersteiger R, Dohr G, et al. Reaction patterns of monoclonal antibodies to HLA-G in human tissues and on cell lines: a comparative study. Hum Immunol. 2000; 61(11):1074–85.
78. Goldman-Wohl D, Ariel I, Greenfield C, Hochner-Celnikier D, Lavy Y, Yagel S. A study of human leukocyte antigen G expression in hydatidiform moles. Am J Obstet Gynecol. 2001;185(2):476–80.
79. Rabreau M, Rouas-Freiss N, Landi M, Le Danff C, Carosella ED. HLA-G expression in trophoblast cells is independent of embryonic development. Hum Immunol. 2000;61(11):1108–12.
80. Shih IM, Kurman RJ. Immunohistochemical localization of inhibin-alpha in the placenta and gestational trophoblastic lesions. Int J Gynecol Pathol. 1999; 18(2):144–50.
81. Kommoss F, Oliva E, Bhan AK, Young RH, Scully RE. Inhibin expression in ovarian tumors and tumor-like lesions: an immunohistochemical study. Mod Pathol. 1998;11(7):656–64.
82. Shih Ie M. Trophogram, an immunohistochemistry-based algorithmic approach, in the differential diagnosis of trophoblastic tumors and tumorlike lesions. Ann Diagn Pathol. 2007;11(3):228–34.
83. Kurman RJ, Young RH, Norris HJ, Main CS, Lawrence WD, Scully RE. Immunocytochemical localization of placental lactogen and chorionic gonadotropin in the normal placenta and trophoblastic tumors, with emphasis on intermediate trophoblast and the placental site trophoblastic tumor. Int J Gynecol Pathol. 1984;3(1):101–21.
84. Shih IM, Kurman RJ. Expression of melanoma cell adhesion molecule in intermediate trophoblast. Lab Invest. 1996;75(3):377–88.
85. Shih IM, Nesbit M, Herlyn M, Kurman RJ. A new Mel-CAM (CD146)-specific monoclonal antibody, MN-4, on paraffin-embedded tissue. Mod Pathol. 1998;11(11):1098–106.
86. Jacob S, Mohapatra D. Placental site nodule: a tumor-like trophoblastic lesion. Indian J Pathol Microbiol. 2009;52(2):240–1.
87. Young RH, Kurman RJ, Scully RE. Placental site nodules and plaques. A clinicopathologic analysis of 20 cases. Am J Surg Pathol. 1990;14(11):1001–9.
88. Kouvidou C, Karayianni M, Liapi-Avgeri G, Toufexi H, Karaiossifidi H. Old ectopic pregnancy remnants with morphological features of placental site nodule occurring in fallopian tube and broad ligament. Pathol Res Pract. 2000;196(5):329–32.
89. Mills SE, Austin MB, Randall ME. Lymphoepithelioma-like carcinoma of the uterine cervix. A distinctive, undifferentiated carcinoma with inflammatory stroma. Am J Surg Pathol. 1985;9(12):883–9.
90. Coleman RL, Lindberg G, Muller CY, Miller DS, Hameed A. Ectopic production and localization of beta-human chorionic gonadotropin in lymphoepithelioma-like carcinoma of the cervix: a case report. Int J Gynecol Pathol. 2000;19(2):179–82.
91. Behtash N, Karimi Zarchi M. Placental site trophoblastic tumor. J Cancer Res Clin Oncol. 2008; 134(1):1–6.
92. Lurain JR. Gestational trophoblastic disease II: classification and management of gestational trophoblastic neoplasia. Am J Obstet Gynecol. 2011; 204(1):118.
93. Knox S, Brooks SE, Wong-You-Cheong J, Ioffe O, Meisenberg B, Goldstein DP. Choriocarcinoma and epithelial trophoblastic tumor: successful treatment of relapse with hysterectomy and high-dose chemotherapy with peripheral stem cell support: a case report. Gynecol Oncol. 2002;85(1):204–8.
94. Papadopoulos AJ, Foskett M, Seckl MJ, McNeish I, Paradinas FJ, Rees H, et al. Twenty-five years' clinical experience with placental site trophoblastic tumors. J Reprod Med. 2002;47(6):460–4.
95. Hassadia A, Gillespie A, Tidy J, Everard RGNJ, Wells M, Coleman R, et al. Placental site trophoblastic tumour: clinical features and management. Gynecol Oncol. 2005;99(3):603–7.

96. Schmid P, Nagai Y, Agarwal R, Hancock B, Savage PM, Sebire NJ, et al. Prognostic markers and long-term outcome of placental-site trophoblastic tumours: a retrospective observational study. Lancet. 2009;374(9683):48–55.
97. Lynch TJ, Bell DW, Sordella R, Gurubhagavatula S, Okimoto RA, Brannigan BW, et al. Activating mutations in the epidermal growth factor receptor underlying responsiveness of non-small-cell lung cancer to gefitinib. N Engl J Med. 2004;350(21):2129–39.
98. Paez JG, Janne PA, Lee JC, Tracy S, Greulich H, Gabriel S, et al. EGFR mutations in lung cancer: correlation with clinical response to gefitinib therapy. Science. 2004;304(5676):1497–500.

Gestational Choriocarcinoma

8

Pei Hui

Keywords
Choriocarcinoma • Diagnostic features • Differential diagnosis

Introduction

Gestational choriocarcinoma is the most aggressive form of trophoblastic disease with tumor cells morphologically recapitulating the trophoblast of developing placenta at its previllous stage. The tumor has a high propensity for hematogenous spread, and in fact, is one of the most malignant tumors in humans if untreated. Being a disease of long historical recognition (see Chap. 1), various names were used in the past including *sarcoma uteri deciduocellulare* as a malignant tumor derived from the decidua of pregnancy [1], "deciduoma malignum" or "chorio-deciduocellular sarcoma," "sarcoma of the chorial villi," and "chorioepithelioma" [1, 2]. The term "choriocarcinoma" was eventually introduced by Ewing [3, 4]. The inception of chemotherapy management in late 1950s marked the beginning of the era of dramatic decrease in mortality of patients with gestational choriocarcinoma [5]. Once an invariably fatal malignancy, the tumor can be treated with over 90% survival or cure rate by methotrexate-based chemotherapy [5, 6].

P. Hui, MD, PhD (✉)
Department of Pathology,
Yale University School of Medicine, 310 Cedar Street,
254B New Haven, CT 06520-8023, USA
e-mail: pei.hui@yale.edu

Clinical Presentation

Vaginal bleeding is the most common symptom, and extrauterine hemorrhagic events may be the first presentation in those with extrauterine spread: lung (60–75%), liver (15–20%), central nerve system (15–20%), and gastrointestinal tract (10–20%) [7–11]. The tumor may arise from any types of prior gestational events: normal pregnancy, spontaneous abortion, but more frequently complete hydatidiform mole, regardless of its intrauterine or ectopic location (see an example in Chap. 12, Fig. 12.2). The age range of the presentation is wide but mainly in the reproductive years with a mean of 29–31 years. Gestational choriocarcinoma may develop after menopause [12–14]. The oldest patient was a 73-year-old woman who developed a choriocarcinoma 38 years after her last pregnancy and 23 years after her last menstrual period [15]. The tumor occurs after a CHM in approximately 50% of cases and after an abortion, a normal gestation or an ectopic pregnancy in 25, 22.5, and 2.5% of the cases, respectively [16].

P. Hui (ed.), *Gestational Trophoblastic Disease: Diagnostic and Molecular Genetic Pathology*, Current Clinical Pathology, DOI 10.1007/978-1-61779-394-3_8,

The risk of developing choriocarcinoma following CHM is approximately 2–3%. There is a very low but definitive risk of developing choriocarcinoma from a partial mole. In general, less than 0.5% of partial moles were complicated with choriocarcinoma [17] with inclusion of patients with current or recent diagnosis of partial moles [18, 19]. Possible partial moles with a coexisting choriocarcinoma were reported and confirmed by the presence of triploidy in the molar tissue [20–22]. However, triploid non-molar gestations cannot be ruled out in these cases. One case of subsequent possible choriocarcinoma was reported in a true partial mole that was confirmed to have one maternal and two paternal chromosome complements by chromosomal heteromorphisms analysis, but the genetic makeup of the choriocarcinoma was not analyzed [23]. Up to now, the only well-documented cases of gestational choriocarcinoma arising from a true partial mole were reported by Seckl et al. [24], in which among 3,000 cases of partial mole, three patients developed choriocarcinoma in subsequent uterine biopsies. DNA microsatellite genotyping comparison between the moles and subsequent choriocarcinomas confirmed the presence of identical dispermic monogynic genetic profiles in both, confirming a direct malignant transformation [24].

The latency period between the antecedent pregnancy and choriocarcinoma may be several months to as long as 14 years in rare cases [9, 25]. In most patients with choriocarcinoma following term delivery, the pathology diagnosis is made by evaluation of uterine curettage specimens 1–3 months after delivery [9]. Postmolar choriocarcinoma is diagnosed by histology in an average of 13 months (1–48 months) after the evacuation of hydatidiform mole [9]. Gestational choriocarcinoma transmission to organ recipients has been reported [26–30], the most recent of which was documented in a 26-year-old pregnant woman who died of metastatic gestational choriocarcinoma and the donor organs developed choriocarcinoma in all four recipients. All were treated with chemotherapy. Two patients had a complete remission. Another two organ recipients developed metastasis, one of the two died of the tumor [28].

Pathogenesis

Genotyping studies demonstrated various genomic compositions of gestational choriocarcinomas, some being androgenetic while others being biparental, consistent with different forms of antecedent gestations [31]. Similar to PSTT, the majority of gestational choriocarcinomas have been found to have an XX genome [32], suggesting a growth advantage provided by the paternal X chromosome according to placental imprinting theory (see Chap. 3). In addition, cytogenetic studies revealed highly complex karyotypical changes irrespective of the associated prior term pregnancy, hydatidiform mole, or spontaneous abortion [33–36]. Chromosomal 7p amplification and 8p deletion were observed in a series of gestational choriocarcinomas, suggesting a causal relationship involving possible oncogene(s) and tumor suppressor gene(s) in these chromosomal regions [37]. NECC1, a candidate tumor suppressor gene on chromosome 4q11-q12, was specifically silenced in choriocarcinoma cell lines and transfection–expression of NECC1 into these cell lines inhibited the cell growth along with an altered cell morphology, suggesting a loss of NECC1 expression may be involved in malignant transformation of placental trophoblast [38]. Studies of H19 and IGF2 imprinting expression in choriocarcinoma have indicated that deregulation/relaxation of imprinting of these genes may play a significant role in the development of the tumor, particularly for those following a hydatidiform mole [39, 40]. Additional discussion of imprinting alterations in the pathogenesis of choriocarcinoma can be found in Chap. 3.

Rare cases of intraplacental choriocarcinoma with coexisting intrauterine pregnancy have been reported, with implication as the origin of choriocarcinoma occurring after a term pregnancy [41–44]. In those after a term pregnancy, fetal sex distribution showed no sex preference [9]. No significant difference in risk was found by comparing the number of pregnancies following hydatidiform mole with the number of pregnancies following term delivery or non-molar abortion [9].

Pathology

Gross Pathology

Choriocarcinoma has a characteristic gross presentation as bulky, destructive masses that are dark red, shaggy, extensively hemorrhagic with variable amount of necrosis [8, 9, 45, 46]. There may be single to multiple nodules involving the endomyometrium. The tumor may deeply invade the myometrium, leading to uterine perforation. Primary gestational choriocarcinoma may arise from the cervix [47], fallopian tube in association with a tubal pregnancy [48–50], or sites involved by ectopic pregnancy (ovary, cornu of the uterus, or other extrauterine sites) [51–55]. In some cases, the tumor may consist of predominantly blood or blood clots with only viable tumor tissue at the periphery [46]. Similar findings may be seen in a metastatic lesion. Occasionally, a curettage specimen may contain only blood, and the tumor cells can only be found after submitting the remaining specimen for histological evaluation.

Histological Pathology

Table 8.1 summarizes histological features of gestational choriocarcinoma. Microscopically, gestational choriocarcinomas present either as a diffusely infiltrative or a solid mass involving the endomyometrium with histological features resembling proliferation of the previllous trophoblast during early implantation. The tumor displays a biphasic growth pattern of sheets or cords of mononuclear tumor cells rimmed by layers of multinuclear syncytiotrophoblastic cells (Fig. 8.1 and Fig. 8.2), but sometimes more haphazard arrangements of the components may be seen. Although traditionally

Table 8.1 Histological features of choriocarcinoma

Destructive mass lesion with marked hemorrhage and necrosis
Bilamellar growth pattern: inner mononuclear cells rimmed by multinuclear syncytiotrophoblastic cells
Marked cytological atypia
Absence of chorionic villi
Diffuse staining for hCG

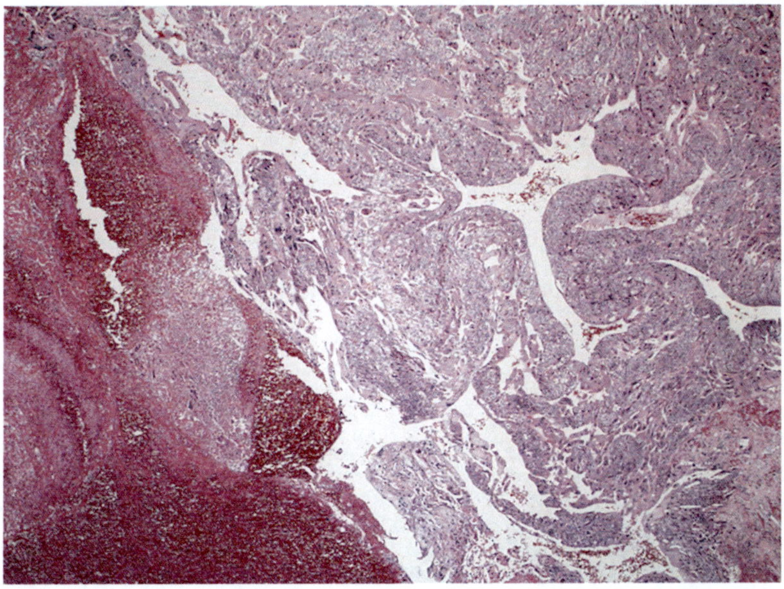

Fig. 8.1 Gestational choriocarcinoma at low magnification. Note the characteristic destructive mass with the presence of marked hemorrhage

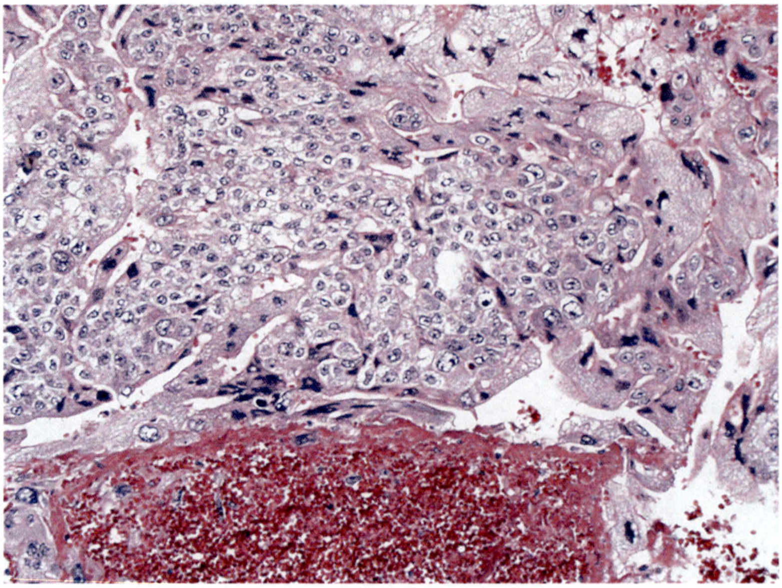

Fig. 8.2 Gestational choriocarcinoma with characteristic bilamellar growth pattern consisting of mononuclear intermediate trophoblastic cells in sheets or cords surrounded by multinuclear syncytiotrophoblastic tumor cells

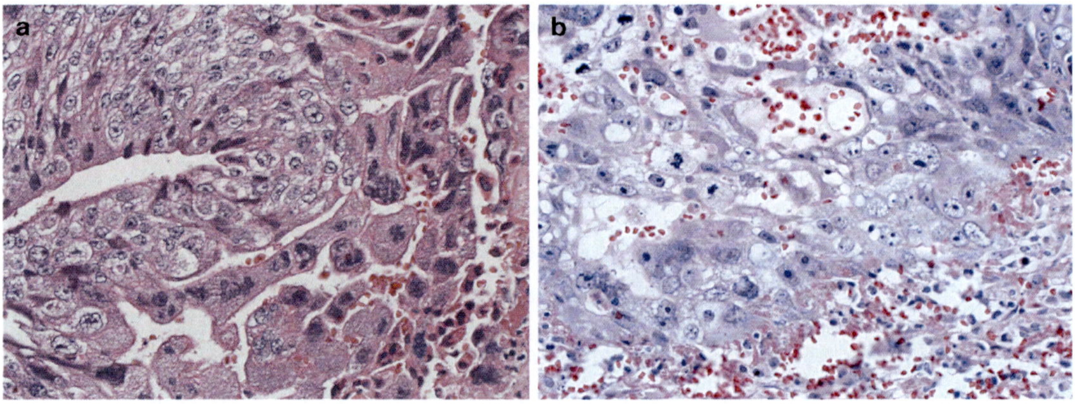

Fig. 8.3 Gestational choriocarcinoma with marked cytological atypia present in both mononuclear and syncytiotrophoblastic cells (**a**) and high mitotic activity (**b**)

considered as neoplastic cytotrophoblasts, the nature of the mononuclear cells in choriocarcinoma is now considered to be neoplastic cells resembling intermediate trophoblast at either the trophoblastic column or implantation site [56] (Fig. 8.2). These cells are large with abundant amphophilic to eosinophilic cytoplasm. Relatively smaller mononuclear cells may be of cytotrophoblastic nature, and they represent a minor proportion in choriocarcinoma [56]. Choriocarcinoma cells generally demonstrate significant cytological atypia. Cytological pleomorphism and nuclear atypia may be extreme, often bizarre in shape (Fig. 8.3a), and mitoses are numerous with frequent atypical forms (Fig. 8.3b). Unlike all other types of epithelial malignancies, choriocarcinoma does not have intrinsic stromal and vascular elements. Extensive tumor necrosis and hemorrhage are characteristic (Fig. 8.4). Frequently, central areas of hemorrhage and necrosis are rimmed by viable tumor cells at

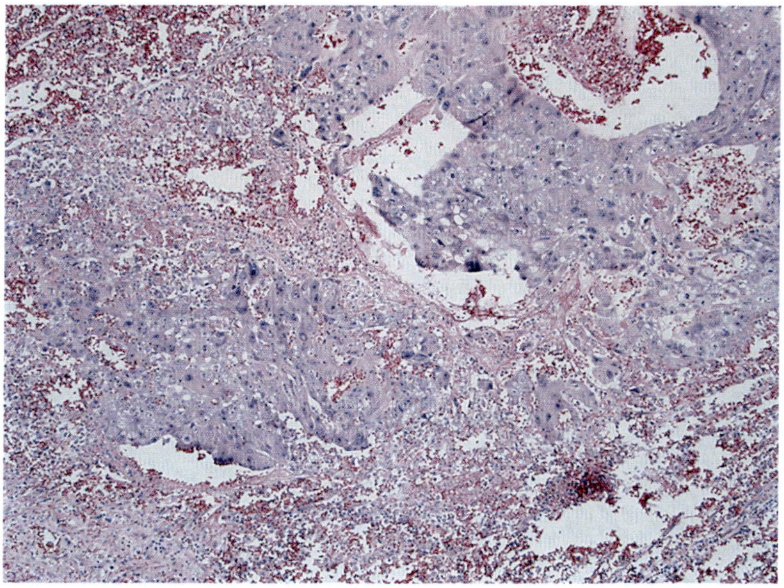

Fig. 8.4 Gestational choriocarcinoma with extensive tumor necrosis

the periphery. At the junction between tumor and myometrium, tumor nests or sheets may surround bundles of smooth muscle. Lymphovascular invasion with tumor thrombi is generally abundant. Chorionic villi are not present in a fully developed choriocarcinoma. Lymphocytic infiltration at various degrees may be present as well.

The background endometrium is usually associated with some degrees of decidual reaction and Aria-Stella reaction. Ectopic decidua may be seen in the cervix, ovary, and peritoneum. Bilateral ovarian enlargement by theca-lutein cysts is commonly seen in over 50% of the cases.

In Situ or Intraplacental Choriocarcinoma

In situ or intraplacental choriocarcinoma has been documented to occur in a full-term placenta [44, 57–64]. Most reported patients had pregnancy history and clinical evidence of metastatic disease [60]. In those who presented initially with metastatic choriocarcinoma, revisit to the corresponding placentas often revealed an intraplacental primary lesion. The involved term placentas had lesions resembling hemorrhagic infarcts upon gross inspection [61]. Friable, papillary to solid lesions may also be seen [62]. It is conceivable that many of these in situ lesions, particularly those of less than 1 cm, may be missed without reporting; yet the patient may present with endomyometrial invasive choriocarcinoma sometime after a seemingly "normal pregnancy." Therefore, some investigators recommend a thorough examination of a term placenta with 5 mm interval sectioning of the entire organ [61].

Ancillary Studies

Most gestational choriocarcinomas are diploid [65]. Molecular DNA genotyping of gestational choriocarcinomas may be used to confirm their various gestational origins (term pregnancy, complete, and partial mole). More importantly, it can be used to separate gestational choriocarcinoma from its nongestational counterpart (see differential diagnosis and Chap. 11) [24, 33, 45, 66–72], particularly when the tumor is found at an unusual location [72].

The neoplastic syncytiotrophoblastic cells of choriocarcinoma are diffusely and strongly positive for hCG, hPL, and HSD3B1 [56, 73]. The neoplastic intermediate trophoblastic cells are positive for HLA-G, MUC-4, Mel-CAM (CD146), and hPL. Typically all tumor cells are cytokeratin (AE1/3) and CEA positive and PLAP negative [73, 74]. The neoplastic cells show a high Ki-67 (>90%) labeling, nuclear staining of beta-catenin, and positivity for MUC-4, p63, and cyclin E.

Although rarely used, ultrastructural features of choriocarcinoma are well known with tumor cells characterized by their simplicity with electron lucent cytoplasm, multiple free ribosomes, and aggregates of particulate glycogen. Nuclei have smooth contours and contain a prominent nucleolus. Syncytiotrophoblastic cells have multiple nuclei, highly complex electron dense cytoplasm with multiple organelles and cell membrane structures with thick bundles of tonofilaments. The cell surface is covered by multiple microvilli bordering intracytoplasmic lumens.

Differential Diagnosis

Complete Hydatidiform Mole

Choriocarcinoma should be distinguished from the residual atypical trophoblastic hyperplasia of a complete mole. Absence of molar villi is generally used to separate an invasive mole from a choriocarcinoma. Pathological examination of curettage specimens obtained sometime after evacuation of a complete mole can be problematic when aggregates of atypical trophoblasts are present without chorionic villi. Submitting the remaining tissue and thorough sectioning are important to rule out recurrent mole before a diagnosis of choriocarcinoma is made. However, a diagnostic separation between the two is not absolutely required under the WHO's "gestational trophoblastic neoplasia – GTN" classification, as all patients with GTN will receive chemotherapy [75, 76]. Conceivably, many choriocarcinomas, particular early ones, are treated nowadays without a tissue diagnosis. Therefore, when a diagnostic separation of residual molar proliferation from choriocarcinoma cannot be reached and additional tissue confirmation is not available, a diagnosis of "atypical trophoblast proliferation" is appropriate (see Chap. 9: Persistent Trophoblastic Disease, for additional information) and sufficient for clinical management.

Early Gestational Villous Trophoblast

Early gestational villous trophoblasts may show aggregates of highly proliferative cells of both mononuclear and syncytiotrophoblastic nature. When present in curettage specimens, the associated villi may be not obvious, therefore mimicking choriocarcinoma. However, trophoblastic tissue in an early gestation is limited in amount, and although a certain degree of cytological atypia may exist, marked atypia seen in choriocarcinoma should be not present. In contrast, the finding of voluminous, highly atypical trophoblast with an absence of villous structures strongly suggests the presence of choriocarcinoma.

Exaggerated Placental Site Reaction

Exaggerated placental site reaction may become a differential diagnosis with choriocarcinoma, particularly in limited curettage specimens. However, the lesion occurs almost always in association with chorionic villi of either normal pregnancy or hydatidiform mole. The absence of a mass lesion, absence of marked hemorrhage and necrosis, and a low Ki-67 index should easily separate it from choriocarcinoma. When in doubt, the absence of relevant clinical history of the patient and abnormal serum hCG level are important clues to avoid an over-diagnosis.

Intermediate Trophoblastic Tumors (PSTT and ETT)

It is important to separate an intermediate trophoblastic tumor (PSTT and ETT) from a choriocarcinoma as their clinical managements are markedly different. Unlike choriocarcinoma, PSTT and ETT are not chemosensitive and usually require hysterectomy [77, 78]. Clinical presentation, serum beta-hCG level, and histological findings are important for the differential diagnosis. HCG immunostain may be useful as it is only focally positive in PSTT in contrast to a more diffuse staining in choriocarcinoma [77]. Diffuse human placental lactogen (hPL) immunoreactivity, on the other hand, is more in favor of PSTT [79]. Comprehensive differential diagnoses can be found in Chaps. 6 and 7. It should be noted that an otherwise typical choriocarcinoma may contain minor foci of PSTT or ETT differentiation, and a diagnosis of mixed gestational trophoblastic tumor may be given.

Nongestational Choriocarcinoma

Gestational choriocarcinoma must be separated from its nongestational counterpart of germ cell or somatic cell origins [80–83]. Nongestational choriocarcinoma occurs in children and young adults before their 40s. A choriocarcinoma in nulligravidae is nongestational by default [9]. Most nongestational choriocarcinomas are of germ cell origin, and young patients with the tumor often present with an adnexal mass, lower abdominal pain mimicking an ectopic pregnancy and, rarely, a hemoperitoneum. In children, an elevated hCG may cause isosexual precocity.

In the past, an extrauterine pure choriocarcinoma in a young woman was usually assumed to be of gestational origin in which the index pregnancy was not known, and the patients were treated accordingly. However, this simple approach to the problem should be abandoned. Nongestational choriocarcinomas have a higher malignant potential and more aggressive invasion into adjacent structures than their gestational counterparts. They have a higher capacity to metastasize via lymphatic vessels while gestational choriocarcinomas mostly spread hematogenously. Moreover, nongestational choriocarcinomas are more resistant to traditional chemotherapy for GTD. However, a histological separation of nongestational choriocarcinoma from its gestational counterpart can be very difficult when the tumor is pure in histology, encountered at extrauterine locations, in a postmenopausal woman, and even more so as a metastatic lesion (Fig. 8.5). Tissue DNA

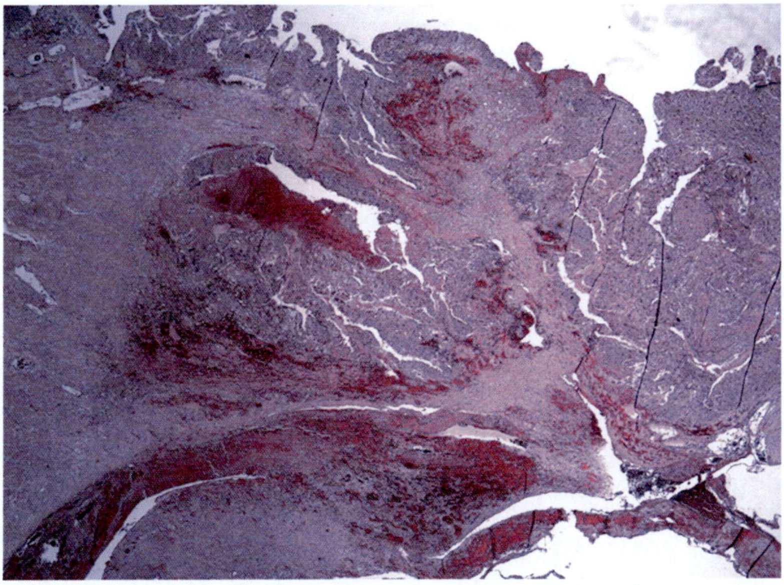

Fig. 8.5 Nongestational choriocarcinoma in a 22-year-old female who presented with a bulky mass involving the broad ligament and mesovarium. The tumor was confirmed nongestational by DNA genotyping

genotyping offers an ultimate separation between the two lesions, see additional discussion in Chap. 11 [72, 84–89].

Poorly Differentiated Uterine Carcinomas

Separation of a choriocarcinoma from a uterine carcinoma is not difficult. Occasionally, however, a poorly differentiated carcinoma may have focal trophoblastic differentiation with syncytiotrophoblastic cells or mononuclear trophoblastic cells. Clinical history of molar pregnancy and high levels of serum hCG are features of gestational choriocarcinoma. Conventional immunohistochemical methods may be used to distinguish a poorly differentiated carcinoma from a choriocarcinoma. Diffuse positivity of hCG, hPL, and inhibin alpha along with the typical biphasic growth pattern attest to the presence of choriocarcinoma. In contrast, a poorly differentiated carcinoma with focal trophoblastic differentiation usually shows trophoblastic marker positivity only in a few syncytiotrophoblastic giant cells [90, 91].

Clinicopathological Correlations

The traditional sequence of events in choriocarcinoma is a prior gestation (normal or abnormal) followed by abnormal vaginal bleeding, then a curettage for diagnosis, and a confirmed diagnosis leading to hysterectomy usually with bilateral salpingo-oophorectomy. The successful introduction of chemotherapy has drastically changed this clinicopathological sequence. An office curettage generally suffices the diagnostic need. The patient receives appropriate chemotherapy thereafter. Even without a definite pathology diagnosis, an interpretation of atypical trophoblastic proliferation usually prompts a similar clinical management of the patient, under the clinical "persistent trophoblastic neoplasia - GTN" category.

Although uterine perforation may occur leading to massive intraabdominal bleeding, hemoperitoneum is more commonly a sequela of ruptured hepatic metastasis [9]. Metastasis is, however, rarely seen nowadays. If not treated or resistant to treatment, choriocarcinoma may metastasize in more than 50% of the cases. Vaginal metastases develop from retrograde spread of tumor cell emboli from the uterus in the paravaginal venous plexus [92], and in some cases, tumor may grow out of the vascular space into the vaginal soft tissue. Lung, liver, brain, kidney, and abdomen are also common organs of distant metastases [9, 77]. An intraplacental choriocarcinoma may present with extrauterine metastasis (brain and lung) [93, 94]. Exceptionally, metastases to the concurrent fetus from an intraplacental choriocarcinoma [58] or transplanted donor organs have been described [28]. Deaths usually occur from pulmonary insufficiency or hemorrhage or complications from irradiation and chemotherapy.

References

1. Stewart CJ. History of gynecological pathology. VIII. John Hammond teacher. Int J Gynecol Pathol. 2000;19(3):284–92.
2. Dallenbach-Hellweg G, Schmidt D. History of gynecological pathology. VI. Jacob Felix Marchand. Int J Gynecol Pathol. 1999;18(3):281–7.
3. Ober WB, Fass RO. The early history of choriocarcinoma. J Hist Med Allied Sci. 1961;16:49–73.
4. Ewing J. Chorioma. Surg Gynecol Obstet. 1910; 10:26.
5. Li MC, Hertz R, Spencer DB. Effect of methotrexate therapy upon choriocarcinoma and choriadenoma. Proc Soc Exp Biol Med. 1956;93:5.
6. Hertz R, Lewis Jr J, Lipsett MB. Five year's experience with the chemotherapy of metastatic choriocarcinoma and related trophoblastic tumors in women. Am J Obstet Gynecol. 1961;82:631–40.
7. Horn LC, Bilek K. Clinicopathologic analysis of gestational trophoblastic disease – report of 158 cases. Gen Diagn Pathol. 1997;143(2–3):173–8.
8. Smith HO, Kohorn E, Cole LA. Choriocarcinoma and gestational trophoblastic disease. Obstet Gynecol Clin North Am. 2005;32(4):661–84.
9. Ober WB, Edgcomb JH, Price Jr EB. The pathology of choriocarcinoma. Ann N Y Acad Sci. 1971; 172(10):299–426.
10. Yingna S, Yang X, Xiuyu Y, Hongzhao S. Clinical characteristics and treatment of gestational trophoblastic tumor with vaginal metastasis. Gynecol Oncol. 2002;84(3):416–9.
11. Lurain JR, Casanova LA, Miller DS, Rademaker AW. Prognostic factors in gestational trophoblastic tumors: a proposed new scoring system based on multivariate analysis. Am J Obstet Gynecol. 1991;164(2):611–6.

12. O'Neill CJ, Houghton F, Clarke J, McCluggage WG. Uterine gestational choriocarcinoma developing after a long latent period in a postmenopausal woman: the value of DNA polymorphism studies. Int J Surg Pathol. 2008;16(2):226–9.
13. Okamoto T, Nomura S, Nakanishi T, Yamada S, Tomoda Y. A case of uterine choriocarcinoma with spontaneous rupture twenty-three years following the antecedent pregnancy. J Obstet Gynaecol Res. 1997; 23(2):189–95.
14. Marcu M, Chefani A, Sajin M. Postmenopausal choriocarcinoma: a case report. Rom J Morphol Embryol. 2005;46(2):145–8.
15. Desai NR, Gupta S, Said R, Desai P, Dai Q. Choriocarcinoma in a 73-year-old woman: a case report and review of the literature. J Med Case Reports. 2010;4(1):379.
16. Bagshawe KD, Golding PR, Orr AH. Choriocarcinoma after hydatidiform mole. Studies related to effectiveness of follow-up practice after hydatidiform mole. Br Med J. 1969;3(5673):733–7.
17. Matsui H, Iizuka Y, Sekiya S. Incidence of invasive mole and choriocarcinoma following partial hydatidiform mole. Int J Gynaecol Obstet. 1996;53(1):63–4.
18. Wong LC, Ma HK. The syndrome of partial mole. Arch Gynecol. 1984;234(3):161–6.
19. Looi LM, Sivanesaratnam V. Malignant evolution with fatal outcome in a patient with partial hydatidiform mole. Aust N Z J Obstet Gynaecol. 1981;21(1): 51–2.
20. Heifetz SA, Czaja J. In situ choriocarcinoma arising in partial hydatidiform mole: implications for the risk of persistent trophoblastic disease. Pediatr Pathol. 1992;12(4):601–11.
21. Medeiros F, Callahan MJ, Elvin JA, Dorfman DM, Berkowitz RS, Quade BJ. Intraplacental choriocarcinoma arising in a second trimester placenta with partial hydatidiform mole. Int J Gynecol Pathol. 2008; 27(2):247–51.
22. Bagshawe KD, Lawler SD, Paradinas FJ, Dent J, Brown P, Boxer GM. Gestational trophoblastic tumours following initial diagnosis of partial hydatidiform mole. Lancet. 1990;335(8697):1074–6.
23. Vejerslev LO, Larsen G, Jacobsen M. Partial hydatidiform mole with subsequent trophoblastic tumor; a case report. Eur J Obstet Gynecol Reprod Biol. 1991; 40(1):73–7.
24. Seckl MJ, Fisher RA, Salerno G, Rees H, Paradinas FJ, Foskett M, et al. Choriocarcinoma and partial hydatidiform moles. Lancet. 2000;356(9223):36–9.
25. Berkowitz RS, Goldstein DP, Bernstein MR. Choriocarcinoma following term gestation. Gynecol Oncol. 1984;17(1):52–7.
26. Detry O, Detroz B, D'Silva M, Pirenne J, Defraigne JO, Meurisse M, et al. Misdiagnosed malignancy in transplanted organs. Transpl Int. 1993;6(1):50–4.
27. Gokel JM, Rjosk HK, Meister P, Stelter WJ, Witte J. Metastatic choriocarcinoma transplanted with cadaver kidney: a case report. Cancer. 1977;39(3):1317–21.
28. Braun-Parvez L, Charlin E, Caillard S, Ducloux D, Wolf P, Rolle F, et al. Gestational choriocarcinoma transmission following multiorgan donation. Am J Transplant. 2010;10(11):2541–6.
29. Marsh Jr JW, Esquivel CO, Makowka L, Todo S, Gordon RD, Tzakis A, et al. Accidental transplantation of malignant tumor from a donor to multiple recipients. Transplantation. 1987;44(3):449–50.
30. Buell JF, Trofe J, Hanaway MJ, Lo A, Rosengard B, Rilo H, et al. Transmission of donor cancer into cardiothoracic transplant recipients. Surgery. 2001; 130(4):660–6; discussion 6–8.
31. Azuma C, Saji F, Nobunaga T, Kamiura S, Kimura T, Tokugawa Y, et al. Studies on the pathogenesis of choriocarcinoma by analysis of restriction fragment length polymorphisms. Cancer Res. 1990;50(3):488–91.
32. Yap KL, Hafez MJ, Mao TL, Kurman RJ, Murphy KM, Shih Ie M. Lack of a y-chromosomal complement in the majority of gestational trophoblastic neoplasms. J Oncol. 2010;2010:364508.
33. Wake N, Tanaka K, Chapman V, Matsui S, Sandberg AA. Chromosome and cellular origin of choriocarcinoma. Cancer Res. 1981;41(8):3137–43.
34. Sheppard DM, Fisher RA, Lawler SD. Karyotypic analysis and chromosome polymorphisms in four choriocarcinoma cell lines. Cancer Genet Cytogenet. 1985;16(3):251–8.
35. Bettio D, Giardino D, Rizzi N, Simoni G. Cytogenetic abnormalities detected by direct analysis in a case of choriocarcinoma. Cancer Genet Cytogenet. 1993; 68(2):149–51.
36. Rodriguez E, Melamed J, Reuter V, Chaganti RS. Chromosomal abnormalities in choriocarcinomas of the female. Cancer Genet Cytogenet. 1995;80(1):9–12.
37. Ahmed MN, Kim K, Haddad B, Berchuck A, Qumsiyeh MB. Comparative genomic hybridization studies in hydatidiform moles and choriocarcinoma: amplification of 7q21-q31 and loss of 8p12-p21 in choriocarcinoma. Cancer Genet Cytogenet. 2000; 116(1):10–5.
38. Asanoma K, Kato H, Inoue T, Matsuda T, Wake N. Analysis of a candidate gene associated with growth suppression of choriocarcinoma and differentiation of trophoblasts. J Reprod Med. 2004;49(8):617–26.
39. Wake N, Arima T, Matsuda T. Involvement of IGF2 and H19 imprinting in choriocarcinoma development. Int J Gynaecol Obstet. 1998;60 Suppl 1:S1–8.
40. Hashimoto K, Azuma C, Koyama M, Ohashi K, Kamiura S, Nobunaga T, et al. Loss of imprinting in choriocarcinoma. Nat Genet. 1995;9(2):109–10.
41. Brewer JI, Mazur MT. Gestational choriocarcinoma. Its origin in the placenta during seemingly normal pregnancy. Am J Surg Pathol. 1981;5(3):267–77.
42. Ollendorff DA, Goldberg JM, Abu-Jawdeh GM, Lurain JR. Markedly elevated maternal serum alpha-fetoprotein associated with a normal fetus and choriocarcinoma of the placenta. Obstet Gynecol. 1990;76(3 Pt 2):494–7.

43. Flam F. Choriocarcinoma in the term placenta: a difficult diagnosis. Eur J Gynaecol Oncol. 1996;17(6): 510–1.
44. Chung C, Kao MS, Gersell D. Incidental placental choriocarcinoma in a term pregnancy: a case report. J Med Case Reports. 2008;2:330.
45. Bower M, Brock C, Fisher RA, Newlands ES, Rustin GJ. Gestational choriocarcinoma. Ann Oncol. 1995; 6(5):503–8.
46. Bentley RC. Pathology of gestational trophoblastic disease. Clin Obstet Gynecol. 2003;46(3):513–22.
47. Kairi-Vassilatou E, Papakonstantinou K, Grapsa D, Kondi-Paphiti A, Hasiakos D. Primary gestational choriocarcinoma of the uterine cervix. Report of a case and review of the literature. Int J Gynecol Cancer. 2007;17(4):921–5.
48. Butler R, Chadha Y, Davies J, Singh M. A case of primary tubal gestational choriocarcinoma. Aust N Z J Obstet Gynaecol. 2010;50(2):200–1.
49. Logani KB, Sharma S, Kohli TP, Khemani M, Prakash N. Gestational choriocarcinoma of the fallopian tube – a case report. Indian J Cancer. 1995;32(4):183–5.
50. Ober WB, Maier RC. Gestational choriocarcinoma of the fallopian tube. Diagn Gynecol Obstet. 1981;3(3): 213–31.
51. Chan DP, Wong WP. Extrauterine gestational choriocarcinoma. Report of two cases. Obstet Gynecol. 1970;35(5):730–3.
52. Maehama T, Uemura S, Higashi M, Kanazawa K, Unten K. A case of primary gestational ovarian choriocarcinoma. Nippon Sanka Fujinka Gakkai Zasshi. 1996;48(6):427–30.
53. Patton Jr GW, Goldstein DP. Gestational choriocarcinoma of the tube and ovary. Surg Gynecol Obstet. 1973;137(4):608–12.
54. Rotas M, Khulpateea N, Binder D. Gestational choriocarcinoma arising from a cornual ectopic pregnancy: a case report and review of the literature. Arch Gynecol Obstet. 2007;276(6):645–7.
55. Veridiano NP, Gal D, Delke I, Rosen Y, Tancer ML. Gestational choriocarcinoma of the ovary. Gynecol Oncol. 1980;10(2):235–40.
56. Mao TL, Kurman RJ, Huang CC, Lin MC, Shih Ie M. Immunohistochemistry of choriocarcinoma: an aid in differential diagnosis and in elucidating pathogenesis. Am J Surg Pathol. 2007;31(11):1726–32.
57. Driscoll SG. Choriocarcinoma: an "incidental finding" in a term placenta. Obstet Gynecol. 1963;21:96–101.
58. Liu J, Guo L. Intraplacental choriocarcinoma in a term placenta with both maternal and infantile metastases: a case report and review of the literature. Gynecol Oncol. 2006;103(3):1147–51.
59. Sebire NJ, Lindsay I, Fisher RA, Seckl MJ. Intraplacental choriocarcinoma: experience from a tertiary referral center and relationship with infantile choriocarcinoma. Fetal Pediatr Pathol. 2005;24(1):21–9.
60. Zanetta G, Maggi R, Colombo M, Bratina G, Mangioni C. Choriocarcinoma coexistent with intrauterine pregnancy: two additional cases and a review of the literature. Int J Gynecol Cancer. 1997;7(1):66–77.
61. Barghorn A, Bannwart F, Stallmach T. Incidental choriocarcinoma confined to a near-term placenta. Virchows Arch. 1998;433(1):89–91.
62. Ganapathi KA, Paczos T, George MD, Goodloe S, Balos LL, Chen F. Incidental finding of placental choriocarcinoma after an uncomplicated term pregnancy: a case report with review of the literature. Int J Gynecol Pathol. 2010;29(5):476–8.
63. Fox H, Laurini RN. Intraplacental choriocarcinoma: a report of two cases. J Clin Pathol. 1988;41(10): 1085–8.
64. Fukunaga M, Ushigome S, Ishikawa E. Choriocarcinoma in situ: a case at an early gestational stage. Histopathology. 1995;27(5):473–6.
65. Fukunaga M, Ushigome S. Malignant trophoblastic tumors: immunohistochemical and flow cytometric comparison of choriocarcinoma and placental site trophoblastic tumors. Hum Pathol. 1993;24(10): 1098–106.
66. Fisher RA, Lawler SD, Povey S, Bagshawe KD. Genetically homozygous choriocarcinoma following pregnancy with hydatidiform mole. Br J Cancer. 1988;58(6):788–92.
67. Chaganti RS, Koduru PR, Chakraborty R, Jones WB. Genetic origin of a trophoblastic choriocarcinoma. Cancer Res. 1990;50(19):6330–3.
68. Osada H, Kawata M, Yamada M, Okumura K, Takamizawa H. Genetic identification of pregnancies responsible for choriocarcinomas after multiple pregnancies by restriction fragment length polymorphism analysis. Am J Obstet Gynecol. 1991;165(3):682–8.
69. Fisher RA, Newlands ES, Jeffreys AJ, Boxer GM, Begent RH, Rustin GJ, et al. Gestational and nongestational trophoblastic tumors distinguished by DNA analysis. Cancer. 1992;69(3):839–45.
70. Suzuki T, Goto S, Nawa A, Kurauchi O, Saito M, Tomoda Y. Identification of the pregnancy responsible for gestational trophoblastic disease by DNA analysis. Obstet Gynecol. 1993;82(4 Pt 1):629–34.
71. Vojtassak J, Repiska V, Zajac V, Konecna B, Korbel M, Danihel L. Origin of choriocarcinoma in previous molar pregnancy proved by DNA analysis. Neoplasma. 1996;43(1):57–9.
72. Fisher RA, Savage PM, MacDermott C, Hook J, Sebire NJ, Lindsay I, et al. The impact of molecular genetic diagnosis on the management of women with hCG-producing malignancies. Gynecol Oncol. 2007;107(3):413–9.
73. Ulbright TM. Germ cell tumors of the gonads: a selective review emphasizing problems in differential diagnosis, newly appreciated, and controversial issues. Mod Pathol. 2005;18 Suppl 2:S61–79.
74. Baker PM, Oliva E. Immunohistochemistry as a tool in the differential diagnosis of ovarian tumors: an update. Int J Gynecol Pathol. 2005;24(1):39–55.
75. Kohorn EI. Negotiating a staging and risk factor scoring system for gestational trophoblastic neoplasia. A progress report. J Reprod Med. 2002;47(6):445–50.
76. Kohorn EI. Gestational trophoblastic neoplasia and evidence-based medicine. J Reprod Med. 2002;47(6): 427–32.

77. Morgan JM, Lurain JR. Gestational trophoblastic neoplasia: an update. Curr Oncol Rep. 2008;10(6): 497–504.
78. Hassadia A, Gillespie A, Tidy J, Everard RGNJ, Wells M, Coleman R, et al. Placental site trophoblastic tumour: clinical features and management. Gynecol Oncol. 2005;99(3):603–7.
79. Shih IM, Kurman RJ. The pathology of intermediate trophoblastic tumors and tumor-like lesions. Int J Gynecol Pathol. 2001;20(1):31–47.
80. Vance RP, Geisinger KR. Pure nongestational choriocarcinoma of the ovary. Report of a case. Cancer. 1985;56(9):2321–5.
81. Kong B, Tian YJ, Zhu WW, Qin YJ. A pure nongestational ovarian choriocarcinoma in a 10-year-old girl: case report and literature review. J Obstet Gynaecol Res. 2009;35(3):574–8.
82. Park SH, Park A, Kim JY, Kwon JH, Koh SB. A case of non-gestational choriocarcinoma arising in the ovary of a postmenopausal woman. J Gynecol Oncol. 2009;20(3):192–4.
83. Ozdemir I, Demirci F, Yucel O, Demirci E, Alper M. Pure ovarian choriocarcinoma: a difficult diagnosis of an unusual tumor presenting with acute abdomen in a 13-year-old girl. Acta Obstet Gynecol Scand. 2004; 83(5):504–5.
84. Zhao J, Xiang Y, Wan XR, Feng FZ, Cui QC, Yang XY. Molecular genetic analyses of choriocarcinoma. Placenta. 2009;30(9):816–20.
85. Lorigan PC, Grierson AJ, Goepel JR, Coleman RE, Goyns MH. Gestational choriocarcinoma of the ovary diagnosed by analysis of tumour DNA. Cancer Lett. 1996;104(1):27–30.
86. Shigematsu T, Kamura T, Arima T, Wake N, Nakano H. DNA polymorphism analysis of a pure non-gestational choriocarcinoma of the ovary: case report. Eur J Gynaecol Oncol. 2000;21(2):153–4.
87. Tsujioka H, Hamada H, Miyakawa T, Hachisuga T, Kawarabayashi T. A pure nongestational choriocarcinoma of the ovary diagnosed with DNA polymorphism analysis. Gynecol Oncol. 2003;89(3): 540–2.
88. Yamamoto E, Ino K, Yamamoto T, Sumigama S, Nawa A, Nomura S, et al. A pure nongestational choriocarcinoma of the ovary diagnosed with short tandem repeat analysis: case report and review of the literature. Int J Gynecol Cancer. 2007;17(1):254–8.
89. Koo HL, Choi J, Kim KR, Kim JH. Pure nongestational choriocarcinoma of the ovary diagnosed by DNA polymorphism analysis. Pathol Int. 2006; 56(10):613–6.
90. Kalhor N, Ramirez PT, Deavers MT, Malpica A, Silva EG. Immunohistochemical studies of trophoblastic tumors. Am J Surg Pathol. 2009;33(4):633–8.
91. Singer G, Kurman RJ, McMaster MT, Shih Ie M. HLA-G immunoreactivity is specific for intermediate trophoblast in gestational trophoblastic disease and can serve as a useful marker in differential diagnosis. Am J Surg Pathol. 2002;26(7):914–20.
92. Acosta-Sison H. The relative frequency of various anatomic sites as the point of first metastasis in 32 cases of chorionepithelioma. Am J Obstet Gynecol. 1958;75(5):1149–52.
93. Tsukamoto N, Kashimura Y, Sano M, Saito T, Kanda S, Taki I. Choriocarcinoma occurring within the normal placenta with breast metastasis. Gynecol Oncol. 1981;11(3):348–63.
94. Kodama S, Yoshiya N, Honma S, Yasuda M, Ikarashi H, Tanaka K. Choriocarcinoma in a term placenta with pulmonary metastasis. Asia Oceania J Obstet Gynaecol. 1994;20(4):367–73.

9 Persistent Trophoblastic Neoplasia

Pei Hui

Keywords
Persistent trophoblastic neoplasia • Differential diagnosis

Introduction

In 2002, FIGO introduced the term "persistent trophoblastic neoplasia" or gestational trophoblastic neoplasia (GTN) to include persistent mole, invasive mole, metastatic mole, choriocarcinoma, and trophoblastic tumors under one clinical term for management purposes [1], because all patients with such a diagnosis require chemotherapy [2]. The criteria include serial hCG level that does not return to normal after evacuation (4 or more hCG levels that show a plateau for more than 3 weeks; an increase of 10% or more in three or more measurements for at least 2 weeks, or persistence of detectable hCG 6 months after evacuation; evidence of metastasis; and a tissue diagnosis of gestational choriocarcinoma). This is a rather important development resulting in a clinical treatment decision based on clinical and serum hCG marker evaluation without a need of tissue diagnosis. Therefore, precise histological diagnosis of GTN has become uncertain in some patients.

P. Hui, MD, PhD (✉)
Department of Pathology,
Yale University School of Medicine, 310 Cedar Street,
254B New Haven, CT 06520-8023, USA
e-mail: pei.hui@yale.edu

Pathology

Persistent Mole

Persistent mole generally represents incompletely evacuated molar tissue that continues to grow and causes a persistent or increased elevation of serum hCG. Persistent complete mole occurs in 17–20% of the cases after the initial evacuation [3]. Although persistent disease after a partial mole is well documented [4–6], misclassification as a complete mole likely explains some cases of postmolar disease after the initial evacuation [6–10]. Follow-up uterine curettage generally removes additional molar tissue.

Invasive Mole Including Metastatic Mole

Invasive mole is an aggressive trophoblastic lesion with myometrial and/or vascular invasion. It is the most common pathological entity under PTN. It is seen in about 10–15% of patients after treatment

P. Hui (ed.), *Gestational Trophoblastic Disease: Diagnostic and Molecular Genetic Pathology*, Current Clinical Pathology, DOI 10.1007/978-1-61779-394-3_9,

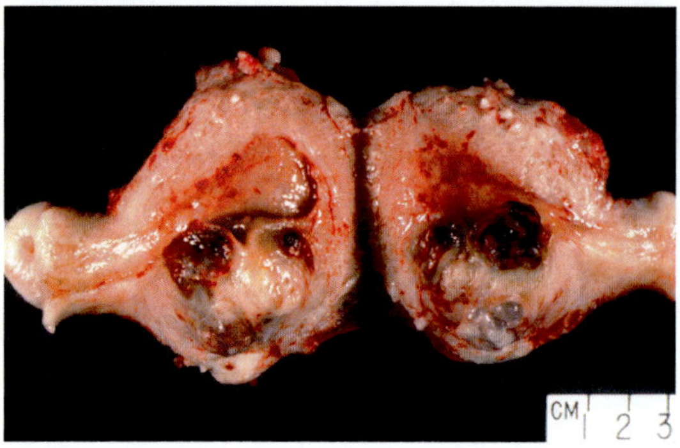

Fig. 9.1 Hysterectomy specimen of invasive complete mole. Note the gross invasiveness of the lesion (Courtesy of Dr. Peter Schwartz, Yale University)

of a complete hydatidiform mole [11] and in 3–4% after a partial mole [9, 12, 13]. Patients generally present with bleeding and persistent elevation of serum beta-hCG after the primary evacuation. Imaging studies may identify an invasive lesion involving uterine myometrium. Metastatic mole likely represents a passive deportation of molar villous tissue upon vascular invasion and can be seen in about 10% of complete moles in the past [14–16]. Cough, difficulty breathing or chest pain, headache, and seizure may signify the presence of metastatic mole, although metastatic choriocarcinoma is also possible.

Grossly, invasive mole appears as an invading hemorrhagic lesion extending from the endometrial surface into the myometrium (Fig. 9.1). Hydropic molar villi may be seen grossly. The lesion is usually limited to the uterus, but transmural invasion with uterine perforation or involving the broad ligament is possible. Invasive mole can only be diagnosed by a histological evidence of direct invasion of molar tissue into the myometrium without intervening decidualized endometrium (Fig. 9.2). Such microscopic confirmation generally requires a hysterectomy specimen. Invasive complete moles generally have diffuse hydropic changes and trophoblastic hyperplasia similar to those of a noninvasive complete mole. Sometimes, the specimen may contain predominantly hyperplastic trophoblasts with marked cytological atypia, simulating choriocarcinoma, and only careful search after submitting additional tissue samples will reveal the presence of chorionic villous structures (Fig. 9.3). Such a lesion may be considered as an emerging choriocarcinoma or an on-going transformation into choriocarcinoma (Fig. 9.3). Distant spread (metastatic mole) commonly involves the lungs, vagina, vulva, and broad ligament in about 20–40% of the cases [17]. Again, a demonstration of the molar villi is also required for the diagnosis of metastatic mole.

In the presence of characteristic clinical, imaging, and serological findings, histological confirmation of the diagnosis of invasive mole is seldom pursued nowadays. In fact, a patient with persistent trophoblastic neoplasia is presumed to have an invasive mole until proven otherwise, and a diagnosis of persistent trophoblastic neoplasia is adequate for further patient management [18, 19]. Hysterectomy for invasive mole may be required if the patient is considered to be at risk for uterine perforation, but this occurs in only a minority of the cases.

The differential diagnoses of invasive mole include gestational choriocarcinoma and placenta increta or percreta. Increase or plateau of hCG may be present in both invasive mole and choriocarcinoma. Both lesions are invasive by imaging studies. Adequate tissue sampling or hysterectomy usually separates an invasive mole from a choriocarcinoma by the presence of chorionic villi. When a curettage specimen is scant and without villous element, a diagnosis of atypical trophoblast proliferation is usually sufficient for clinical management of the patient (Fig. 9.4). The presence of nonhydropic villi, and absence of trophoblastic hyperplasia are features of placenta increta or percreta.

Gestational Trophoblastic Tumors

Gestational trophoblastic tumors may develop following a molar pregnancy, including gestational choriocarcinoma, placental site trophoblastic tumor (PSTT), and epithelioid trophoblast tumor (ETT).

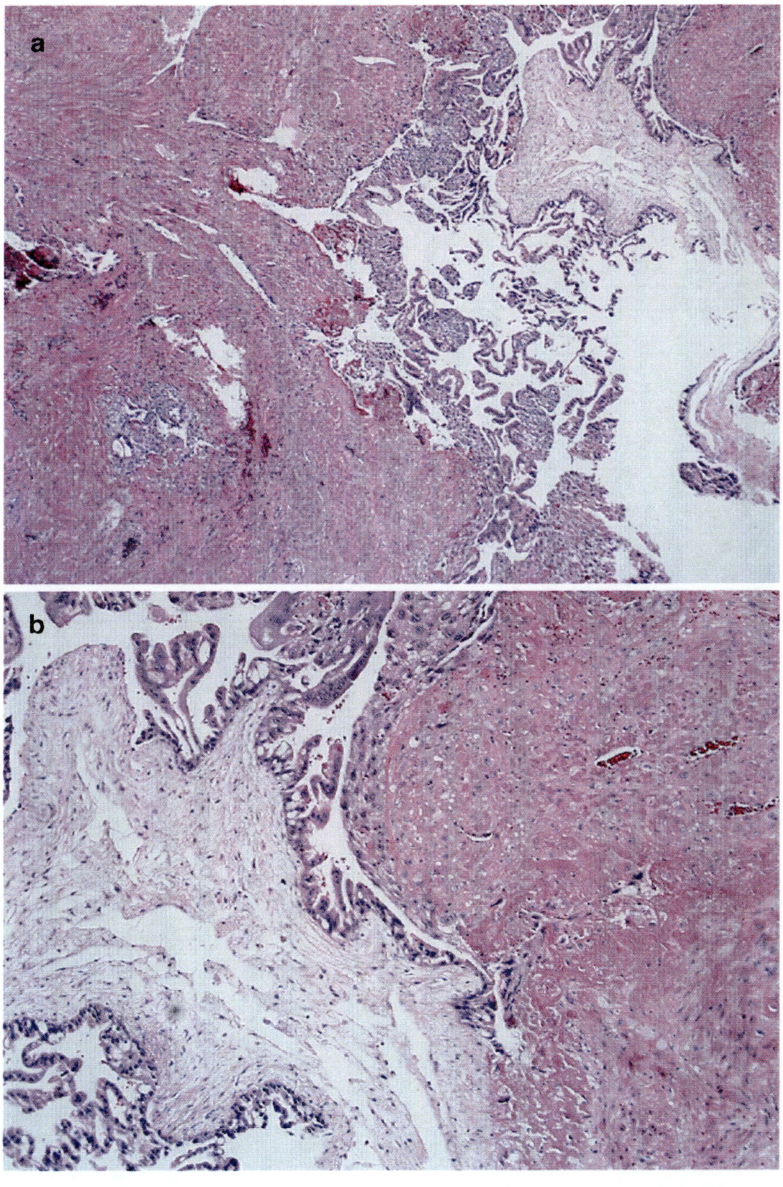

Fig. 9.2 Hysterectomy specimen of invasive complete mole. Note the presence of molar villous structure that directly invades uterine myometrium without intervening decidua ((**a**) low magnification; (**b**) high magnification)

Over 50% of gestational choriocarcinomas arise from a molar gestation (see Chaps. 8 and 12, Fig. 12.2). Such malignant transformation is generally detectable by the molar surveillance program. A marked elevation of serum hCG may correspond to a developing choriocarcinoma, and the patient is treated with chemotherapy, frequently without tissue documentation. Persistent or invasive complete mole may have histological evidence of transformation into gestational choriocarcinoma (Fig. 9.5). In contrast, PSTT and ETT mostly develop long after a pregnancy or a molar episode is over, sometimes after many years. Therefore, patients with these tumors

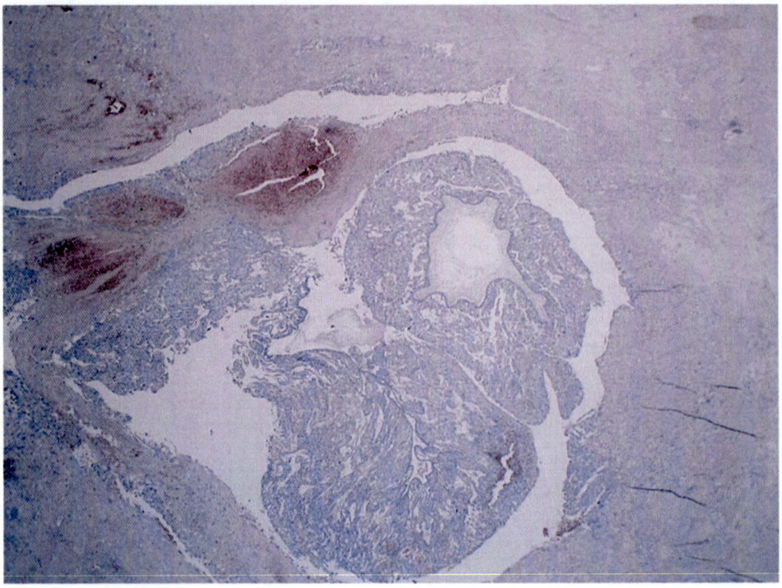

Fig. 9.3 Invasive complete mole with exuberant hyperplasia of the trophoblasts. Note the presence of rare molar villous structure

generally present with "missed abortion" because of mild elevation of serum hCG. A uterine curettage is then performed for an ultimate diagnosis of a trophoblastic tumor (see Chaps. 7 and 8).

The risk factors for choriocarcinoma and other gestational trophoblastic tumors after evacuation of a hydatidiform mole include the patient's age, ethnic group, and prior history of molar gestation. Detailed discussion of the epidemiology and risk factors is given in Chap. 1.

Prognosis

Chemotherapy is highly effective in the treatment of GTN (both invasive and metastatic) with a cure rate of 80–100% depending on the extent of the disease [20]. Even with a wide spread disease, most patients can be cured. Comprehensive discussions of the clinical management and prognosis of PTN can be found in Chap. 12.

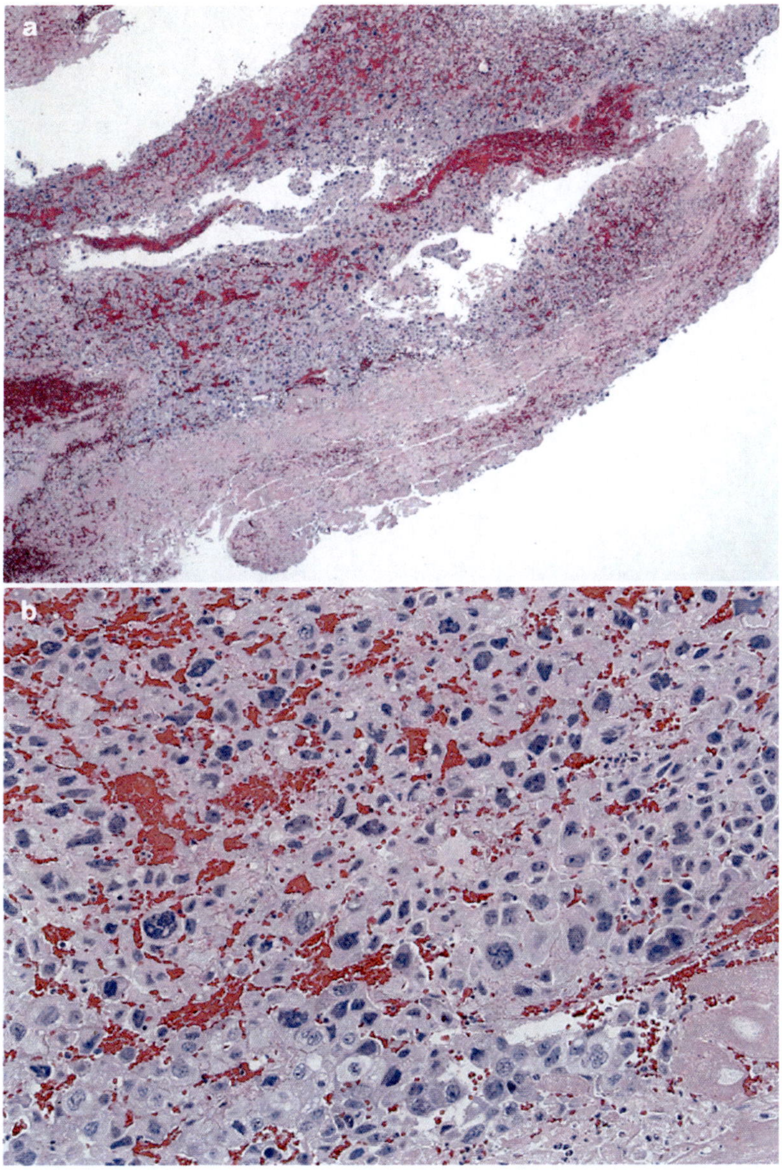

Fig. 9.4 Atypical trophoblast proliferation diagnosed in a curettage specimen. Without analyzing the entire lesional tissue, it is impossible to separate invasive mole from choriocarcinoma in such a case ((**a**) low magnification; (**b**) high magnification)

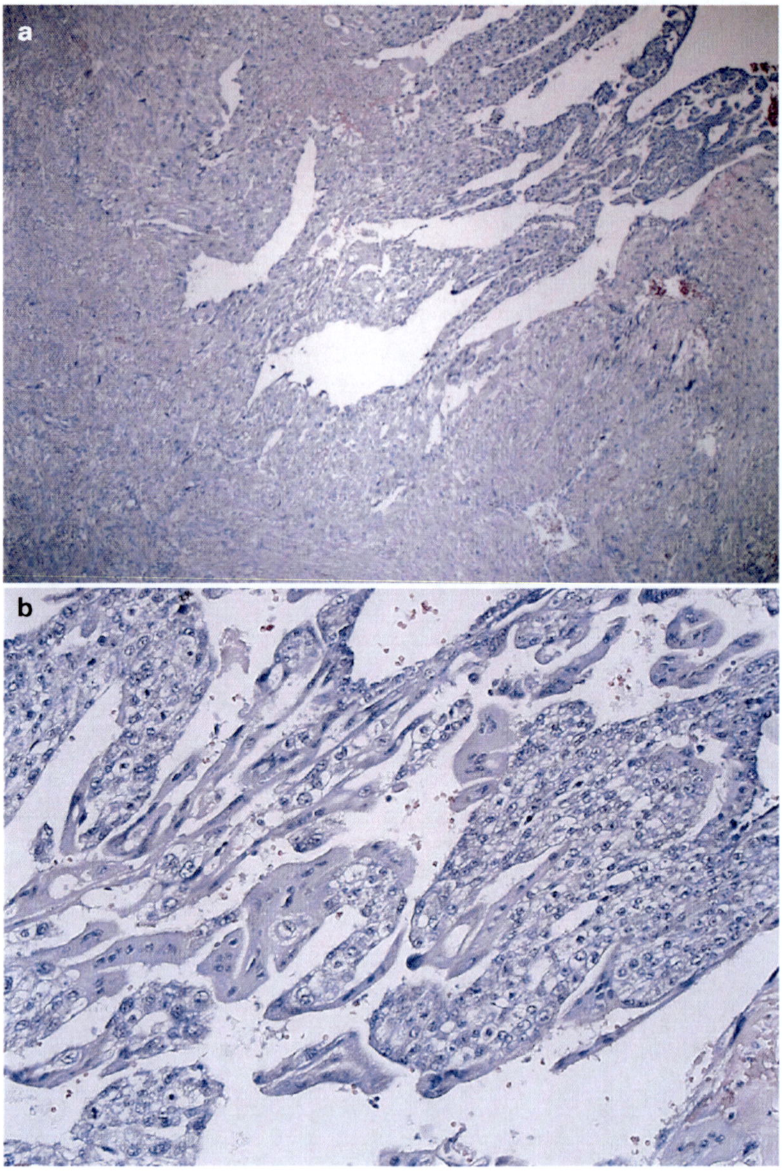

Fig. 9.5 Possible emerging gestational choriocarcinoma arising from an invasive complete mole ((**a**) low magnification; (**b**) high magnification). This is the same case shown in Fig. 9.3, but in a different area of the lesion.

References

1. Kohorn EI. The new FIGO 2000 staging and risk factor scoring system for gestational trophoblastic disease: description and critical assessment. Int J Gynecol Cancer. 2001;11(1):73–7.
2. Berkowitz RS, Goldstein DP. Clinical practice. Molar pregnancy. N Engl J Med. 2009;360(16): 1639–45.
3. Seckl MJ, Fisher RA, Salerno G, Rees H, Paradinas FJ, Foskett M, et al. Choriocarcinoma and partial hydatidiform moles. Lancet. 2000;356(9223):36–9.
4. Menczer J, Girtler O, Zajdel L, Glezerman M. Metastatic trophoblastic disease following partial hydatidiform mole: case report and literature review. Gynecol Oncol. 1999;74(2):304–7.
5. Medeiros F, Callahan MJ, Elvin JA, Dorfman DM, Berkowitz RS, Quade BJ. Intraplacental choriocarcinoma arising in a second trimester placenta with

partial hydatidiform mole. Int J Gynecol Pathol. 2008;27(2):247–51.
6. Hancock BW, Nazir K, Everard JE. Persistent gestational trophoblastic neoplasia after partial hydatidiform mole incidence and outcome. J Reprod Med. 2006;51(10):764–6.
7. Rice LW, Berkowitz RS, Lage JM, Goldstein DP, Bernstein MR. Persistent gestational trophoblastic tumor after partial hydatidiform mole. Gynecol Oncol. 1990;36(3):358–62.
8. Bagshawe KD, Lawler SD, Paradinas FJ, Dent J, Brown P, Boxer GM. Gestational trophoblastic tumours following initial diagnosis of partial hydatidiform mole. Lancet. 1990;335(8697):1074–6.
9. Goto S, Yamada A, Ishizuka T, Tomoda Y. Development of postmolar trophoblastic disease after partial molar pregnancy. Gynecol Oncol. 1993;48(2):165–70.
10. Matsui H, Iizuka Y, Sekiya S. Incidence of invasive mole and choriocarcinoma following partial hydatidiform mole. Int J Gynaecol Obstet. 1996;53(1):63–4.
11. Elston CW. The histopathology of trophoblastic tumours. J Clin Pathol Suppl (R Coll Pathol). 1976;10:111–31.
12. Mandal D, Nandi N, Dey RP, Biswas RR, Bhattacharya AK, Biswas SC. Partial invasive molar pregnancy – 2 case reports. Al Ameen J Med Sci. 2010;3(1):91–3.
13. Szulman AE, Ma HK, Wong LC, Hsu C. Residual trophoblastic disease in association with partial hydatidiform mole. Obstet Gynecol. 1981;57(3):392–4.
14. Bagshawe KD, Garnett ES. Radiological changes in the lungs of patients with trophoblastic tumours. Br J Radiol. 1963;36:673–9.
15. Thiele RA, De Alvarez RR. Metastasizing benign trophoblastic tumors. Am J Obstet Gynecol. 1962;84:1395–406.
16. Meyer JS. Benign pulmonary metastasis from hydatidiform mole. Report of a case. Obstet Gynecol. 1966;28(6):826–9.
17. Driscoll SG. Gestational trophoblastic neoplasia: surgical pathologic considerations with clinical emphasis. Clin Obstet Gynecol. 1984;27(1):160–71.
18. Smith DB, Holden L, Newlands ES, Bagshawe KD. Correlation between clinical staging (FIGO) and prognostic groups with gestational trophoblastic disease. Br J Obstet Gynaecol. 1993;100(2):157–60.
19. Smith DB, O'Reilly SM, Newlands ES. Current approaches to diagnosis and treatment of gestational trophoblastic disease. Curr Opin Obstet Gynecol. 1993;5(1):84–91.
20. Berkowitz RS, Goldstein DP. Chorionic tumors. N Engl J Med. 1996;335(23):1740–8.

10 Tumor-Like Trophoblastic Conditions

Pei Hui

Keywords
PSN • EPS • Differential diagnosis

Introduction

Two well-defined reactive conditions of intermediate trophoblast are placental site nodule (PSN) and exaggerated placental site (EPS) reaction (see Table 1.1 from Chap. 1). PSN is a proliferative lesion of the intermediate trophoblast at the chorionic laeve whereas EPS is a reactive process consisting of the intermediate trophoblast at the implantation site. Clinicopathologically, both lesions are incidental findings and are associated with either a prior pregnancy or a concurrent gestation. They are microscopic and generally not detectable by imaging studies. Histologically and immunohistochemically, PSN and EPS have histological and cytological features simulating their neoplastic counterparts, that is, epithelioid trophoblastic tumor (ETT) and placental site trophoblastic tumor (PSTT), respectively [1]. Recognition by pathologists of both lesions is important as they may simulate trophoblastic tumors and even non-trophoblastic neoplasms, such as squamous cell carcinoma.

P. Hui, MD, PhD (✉)
Department of Pathology,
Yale University School of Medicine, 310 Cedar Street,
254B New Haven, CT 06520-8023, USA
e-mail: pei.hui@yale.edu

Placental Site Nodule/Plaque

Clinical Features

The term placental site nodule was originally used by Carinelli in a study of 17 cases of the condition in an abstract publication [2]. The official use of the name of placental site nodule or plaque was introduced by Young and Lee [3, 4], although the lesion was documented under various names much earlier [5, 6]. PSN occurs in patients 18–49 years of age (average 31.5–34.5 years) and usually is encountered in endometrial curettage specimens of patients with menorrhagia or irregular uterine bleeding. Many cases, however, are found as an incidental finding in a curettage or hysterectomy specimen [3, 7–9]. PSN is not uncommonly found in the cervix [3, 7]. Other rare sites of involvement include fallopian tube [3, 7, 10, 11] and ovary [12], all of which are related to a prior ectopic pregnancy. The interval from the prior pregnancy to the diagnosis ranges from 2 to 96 months (average 21–36 months) [3, 7, 9].

P. Hui (ed.), *Gestational Trophoblastic Disease: Diagnostic and Molecular Genetic Pathology*, Current Clinical Pathology, DOI 10.1007/978-1-61779-394-3_10,

Pathogenesis

PSN has morphological and immunohistochemical features of intermediate trophoblast at the chorionic laeve (Chap. 2, Fig. 2.6) [7]. It is generally considered to be a remnant of persistent placental tissue [3, 9].

Pathology

The lesion is nodular and embedded within the endometrial or cervical mucosa. The size of the lesion ranges from 4 to 10 mm in maximum dimension [9]. Plaque-like lesions may reach a larger size up to 2.5 cm [3]. The lesion has a solid cut surface with color ranging from tan-yellow to hemorrhagic.

Microscopically, PSN consists of single to multiple, well-circumscribed, oval nodules or plaques, with variable cellularity (Fig. 10.1). The extracellular matrix is abundant and hyalinized. The hyalinization is generally uniform in most cases but some cases may show zonal distribution that is more pronounced toward the center of the lesion with a more cellular periphery (Fig. 10.2a, b). Some cases may show irregular to poorly defined margins, however. The lesional trophoblastic cells are typically haphazardly distributed in singles or cords. The cells have sharp to ill-defined cell borders, abundant amphophilic, eosinophilic, or clear cytoplasm (Fig. 10.3a). Most are mononuclear, but multinucleation is not uncommon (Fig. 10.3b). Nuclear pleomorphism and even bizarre nuclei with nuclear pseudoinclusions can be seen. The nuclear membrane is irregular or folded. The chromatin is pale granular, vesicular, or coarse, and scattered hyperchromatic nuclei are common, often with a degenerative appearance (Fig. 10.3c). Nucleoli are small to inconspicuous, but some may be enlarged and prominent. Mitotic figures are absent or rare. Inflammatory cells of both acute and chronic nature are present in the majority of the cases. Rare cases may show necrosis at the center of the hyalinization. PSN involving the fallopian tube is a result of remote ectopic gestation with demise of the embryo and persistence of extraembryonic tissue (Fig. 10.4).

Ancillary Studies

Immunohistochemically, PSN consists of intermediate trophoblasts that express human placental lactogen (hPL) in 78% of the cases and human chorionic gonadotropin (hCG) in 42% of the cases, although their expression is weak and focal. There is strong staining for placental alkaline phosphatase (PLAP) (100%), cytokeratins (CAM5.2, AE1/3, and 34βE12; 96%), and epithelial membrane antigen (EMA) (84%) [1, 9]. Vimentin is strongly positive in most of the cases as well. However, vimentin-positive cells within the lesions are fewer in number and in a different distribution than those expressing PLAP, CK, and EMA [9]. HLA-G is also positive. Ki-67 staining for proliferative index is less than 8% [7]. Ultrastructural study showed the presence of keratin intermediate filaments that were interpreted as Mallory's bodies in a previous study [13].

Differential Diagnosis

Differential diagnoses of PSN include hyalinized decidua, EPS, ETT, and invasive squamous cell carcinoma.

PSN is separated from ETT by its microscopic size, mucosal location, sharp border, extensive hyalinization, and few mitoses. PSN should have a very low level of Ki-67 labeling (<10%) and weak cyclin E expression in comparison with ETT, which has >10% Ki-67 and diffuse strong staining of cyclin E [14]. Table 10.1 summarizes the histological and immunohistochemical features of PSN in comparison with ETT.

Hyalinized decidua contains decidual cells that have pale to somewhat basophilic cytoplasm, distinct cell border, small but uniform cells. They are negative for cytokeratin, PLAP, hPL, hCG, and HLA-G. Hyalinized squamous cell carcinoma may be confused with PSN. However, the invasive mass lesion, dysplastic tumor cells with focal keratin formation, marked cytological atypia and mitoses are features of squamous cell carcinoma. EPS reaction differs from PSN in that the former is poorly circumscribed and infiltrative, involving underlying myometrial smooth muscle and associated with a concurrent pregnancy or a hydatidiform mole.

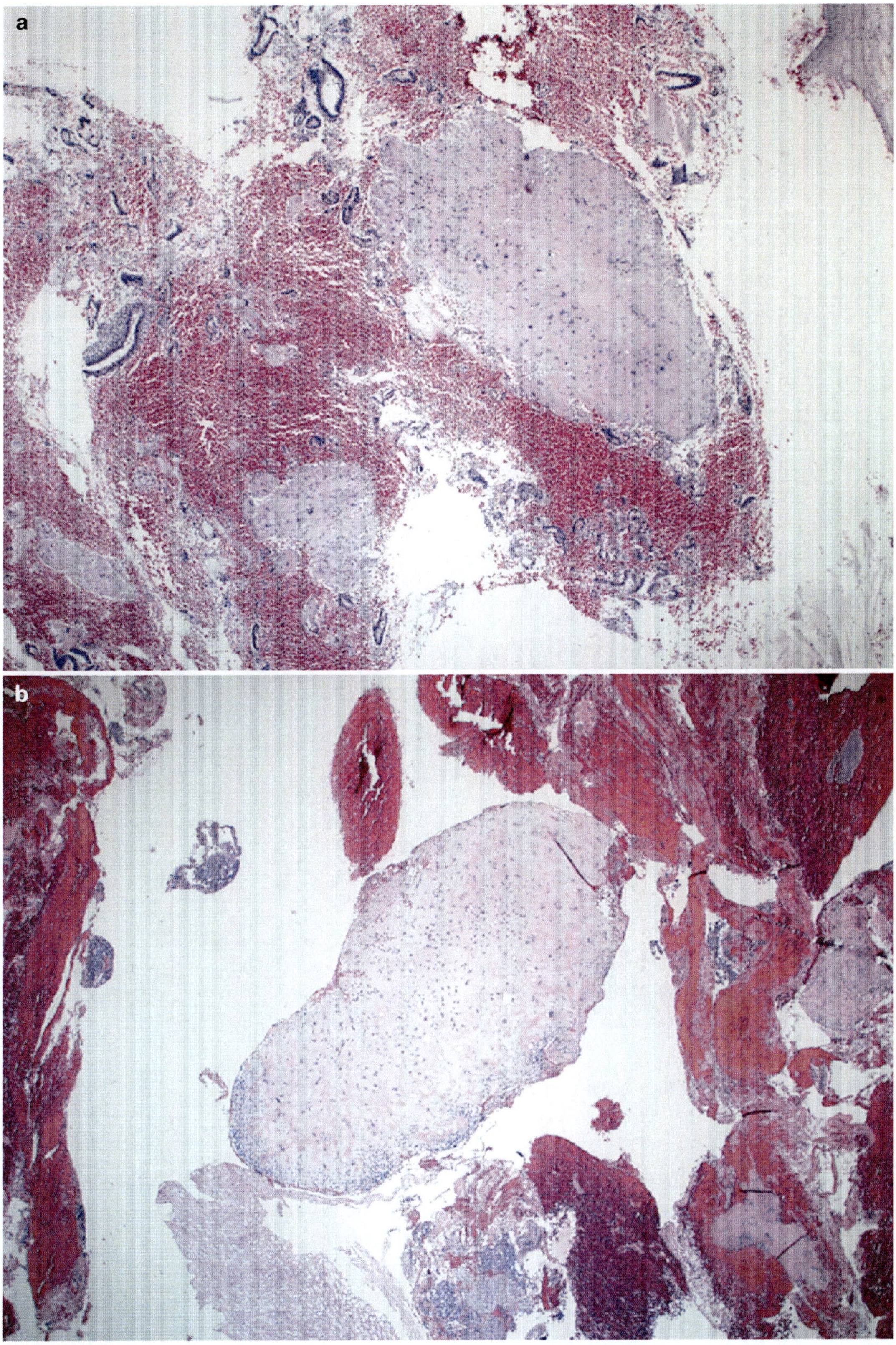

Fig. 10.1 PSN consists of single or multiple, well-circumscribed, oval nodules or plaques with variable cellularity. The lesion is generally admixed with background normal endometrium or cervical mucosa (**a** and **b**)

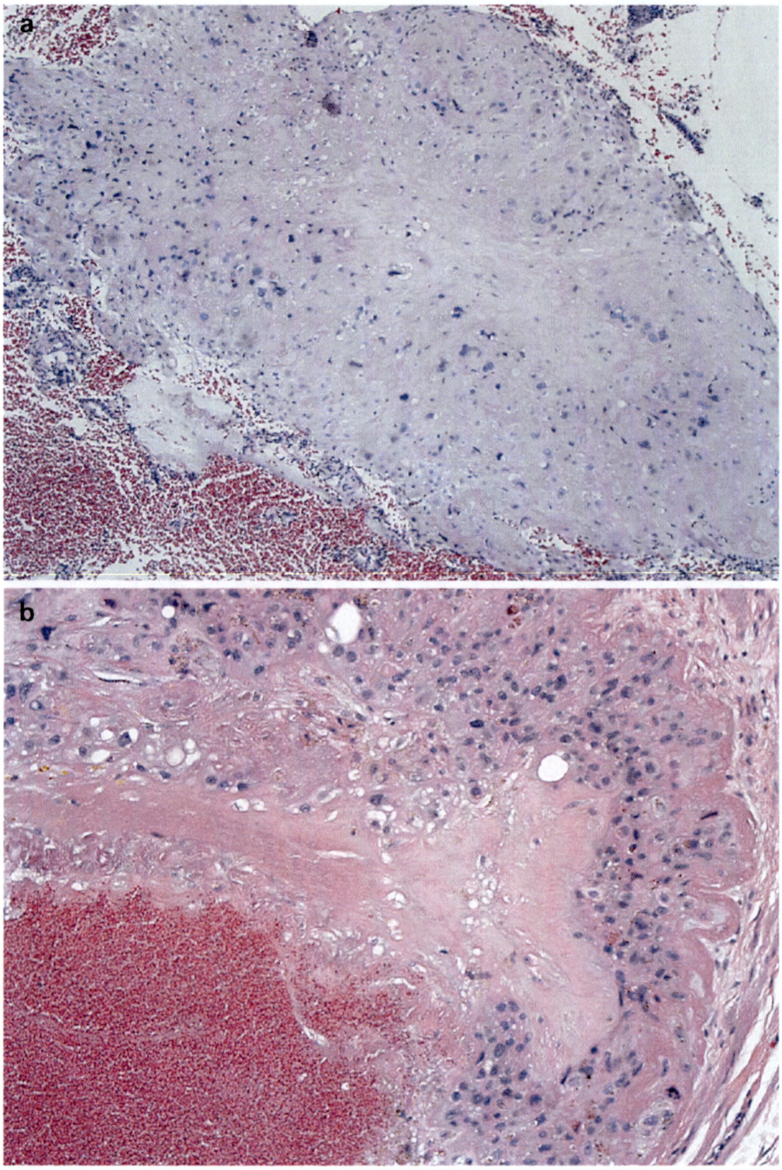

Fig. 10.2 PSN with stromal hyalinization. Note the zonal distribution of hyalinization that is more pronounced toward the center of the lesion with a more cellular periphery (**a**, **b**)

Clinicopathological Correlations

All patients with PSN who have been reported with follow-up data have had a benign clinical course with no recurrence. Atypical PSN was described in a few studies and has been suggested as a possible precursor lesion to ETT [14, 15]. Atypical PNS shows morphologic features that place it in an intermediate position between typical PSN and ETT. A PSN transformed into a malignant ETT was recently documented in a 20-year-old patient, who presented with vaginal bleeding and elevated hCG. The curettage specimen showed a invasive ETT arising in an atypical PSN. After the curettage, her serum hCG continued climbing and she rapidly devel-

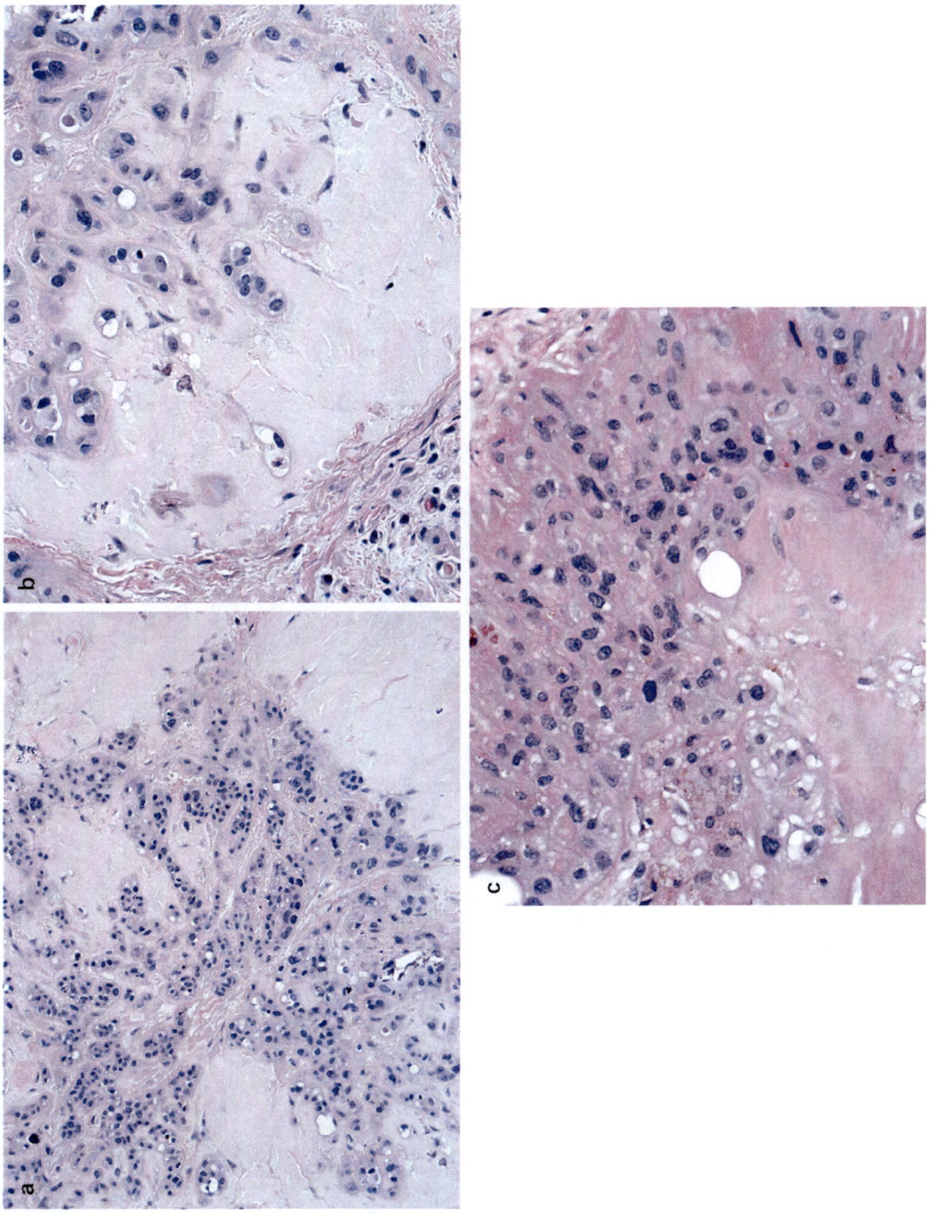

Fig. 10.3 Cytological features of PSN. The lesional cells are typically haphazardly dispersed in forms of singles or cords (**a**). The cellular components of PSN are mostly mononuclear, but multinucleation is common (**b**). Nuclear pleomorphism and even bizarre nuclei with pseudonuclear inclusions can be seen (**c**)

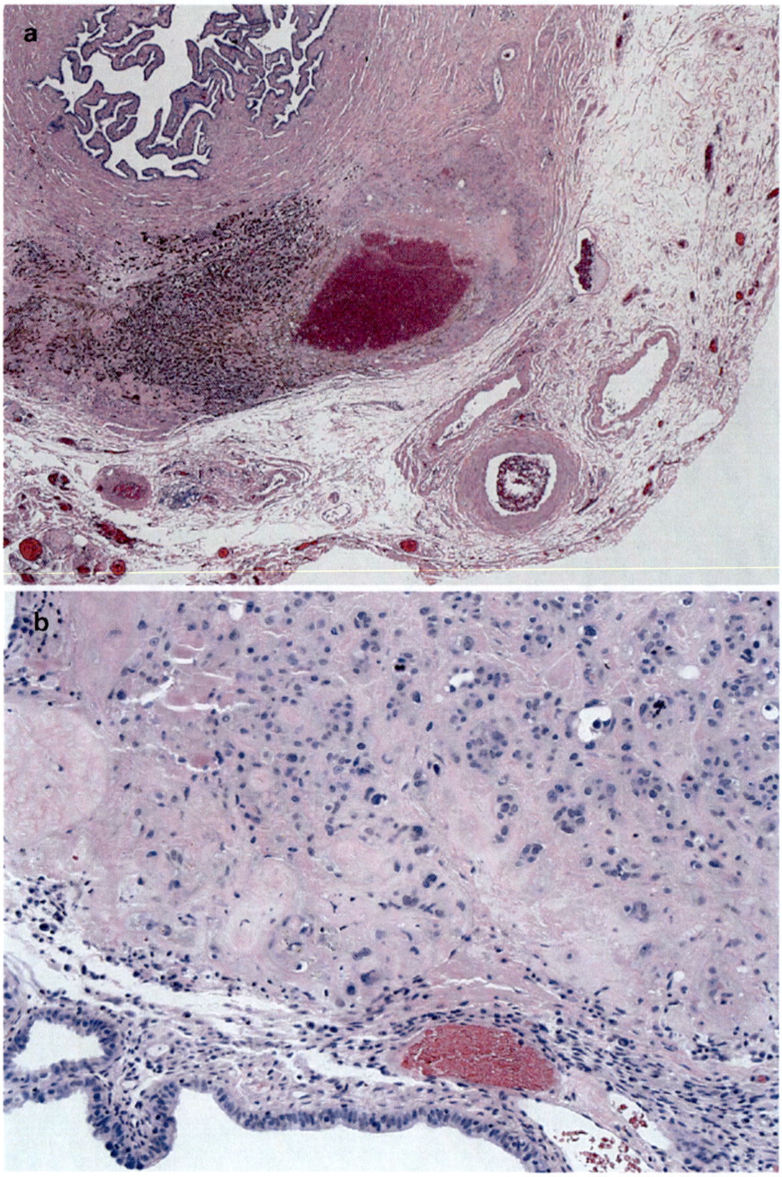

Fig. 10.4 PSN involving the fallopian tube as result of a remote ectopic gestation following the demise of the embryo. Note the presence of old hemorrhage

oped pulmonary metastatic lesions [16]. The patient responded to the subsequent five courses of EMACO treatment, followed by staging surgery and postoperative consolidation chemotherapy. Hysterectomy and staging specimens showed necrotic mass lesions involving uterine cavity and pelvic lymph nodes [16]. The patient was well after 47 months of follow-up.

Exaggerated Placental Site Reaction

Clinical Features

The earliest description of the lesion was made by Ewing in 1910 as syncytial endometritis [17]. The term was frequently used in discussions with other trophoblastic lesions, particularly gestational

Table 10.1 Differential diagnosis between PSN and ETT (contributed by Dr. Katja Gwin, University of Chicago)

	PSN	ETT
Clinical	Incidental	Bleeding, elevated hCG, etc.
Gross	No mass lesion	Invasive mass lesion
Cytology	Uniform and nonatypical	Atypical and pleomorphic
Growth pattern	singles, cords or nests	Sheet, large nests and cords
Hemorrhage	Absent	May be present
Necrosis/fibrinoid debris	Absent	Present
Stromal hyalinization	Extensive	Focal
Mitosis	Absent or very rare	Present
Cyclin E	Negative	Positive
Ki-67	<8%	>10%

choriocarcinoma due to some overlapping pathological features [18–21] in the past, and confusion with its neoplastic counterpart – PSTT in recent times [22, 23]. Indeed, it has been proposed that EPS may be a precursor lesion of PSTT [24]. The term EPS was accepted by the World Health Organization because it is not an inflammatory process and the constituent cells are not syncytial trophoblast [25]. Occurring in women of the reproductive age, EPS is a benign condition consisting of an increased number of intermediate trophoblastic cells that infiltrate the underlying endomyometrium at the implantation site [25]. EPS reaction may occur following normal or ectopic pregnancy, abortion, or hydatidiform mole. The estimated incidence of EPS is 1.6% among first-trimester spontaneous and elective abortions [1].

Pathogenesis

EPS likely represents the upper end of the normal implantation site change, not a pathological process [1, 26]. In fact, a distinction between normal implantation site and EPS is quite arbitrary, and reliable quantitative criteria have not been established. Since sometimes it can be histologically alarming, WHO recognizes its existence as a histological alteration that needs to be separated from neoplastic trophoblastic tumors, particularly PSTT [27].

Pathology

EPS reaction is generally not visible on gross examination. The lesion is also poorly defined microscopically due to its infiltrative border. EPS involves the endometrium and superficial myometrium and consists of implantation site intermediate trophoblast. These cells are pleomorphic and large with abundant eosinophilic cytoplasm, growing largely in a mononuclear cell fashion. Variable numbers of multinucleated intermediate trophoblasts are characteristically present and generally distributed evenly within the lesion (Fig. 10.5a, b). The cells are arranged singly, or in cords and nests to small confluent sheets. They may show marked cytological atypia (Fig. 10.6a, b). The trophoblastic infiltration of EPS is characteristic: individual smooth muscle cells are separated by intermediate trophoblast, remarkably simulating that seen in PSTT. However, despite the exuberant infiltration by the intermediate trophoblast, the architecture of the endomyometrium is not altered (Fig. 10.7). Tissue necrosis and hemorrhage are generally not associated with EPS. However, focal degenerative changes may be seen in the form of fibrin or hyalinization (Fig. 10.8). Recapitulating the biology of the implantation site trophoblast, the cells of EPS typically invade and replace the walls of blood vessels. The associated decidua may demonstrate degenerative regression or necrosis. Depending on the type of gestational conditions, chorionic villi are usually present. In a missed

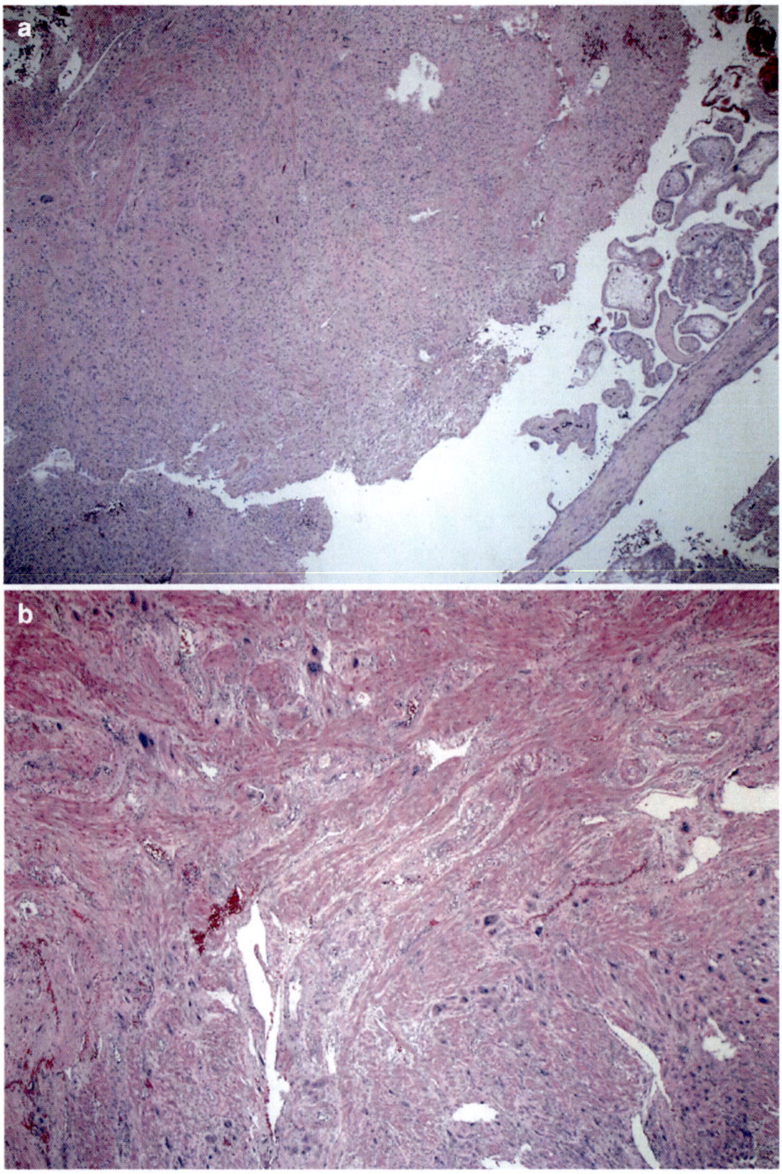

Fig. 10.5 EPS involves the endometrium and superficial myometrium. Note the variable amount of multinucleated intermediate trophoblasts (low power view; high power view)

abortion, hyalinized vasculature and fibrotic villi may be present.

Ancillary Studies

EPS shares a similar immunohistochemical profile with that of intermediate trophoblast at the implantation site and the tumor cells of PSTT: strong immunoreactivity to cytokeratin, hPL, CD 146 (Mel-CAM), HLA-G, E-cadherin, but negative for EMA, and Ber-EP4 [1, 28, 29]. Ki-67 proliferative index of EPS is very low (<1%).

Differential Diagnosis

The most challenging differential diagnosis is the separation of EPS from PSTT (Table 10.2). The pathologist may be frequently alarmed by the remarkable number of intermediate trophoblast and the infiltrative histology in EPS, and a

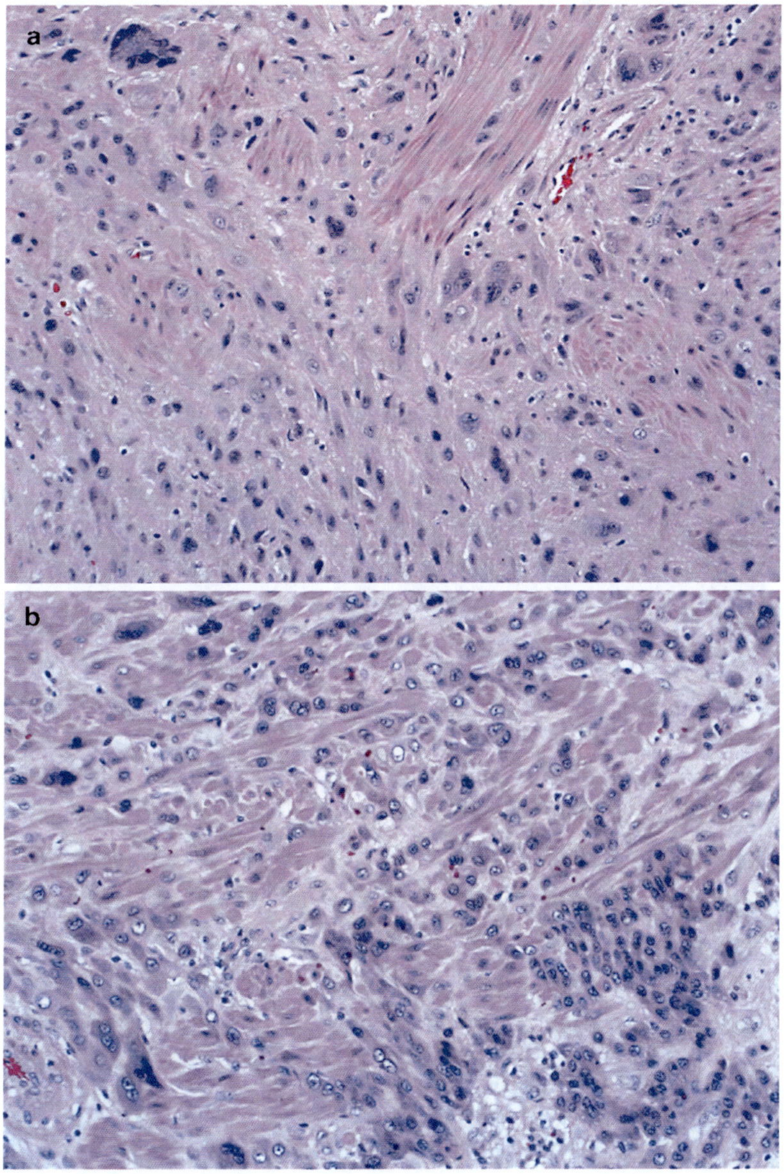

Fig. 10.6 Cytological features of EPS. Note the presence of intermediate trophoblastic cells in singles, cords to small confluent sheet (**a**) and the presence of multinucleation and cytological atypia (**b**)

suspicion for PSTT is frequently raised. Even clinically an EPS may be mistaken as PSTT [30]. Clinical and histological features in favor of a diagnosis of EPS include concurrent pregnancy, absence of a mass lesion, presence of chorionic villi, and the presence of evenly distributed multinucleated trophoblast. Mitotic activity is very low or absent in EPS in contrast to the presence of frequent mitoses in PSTT. In a difficult case, Ki-67 immunostaining can be very helpful in separating EPS from PSTT, as a low level of the labeling (<1%) is characteristic for the former. PSTT is a space-occupying lesion involving myometrium, and usually presents months or years after a full-term pregnancy or an abortion. Patients may have uterine bleeding or amenorrhea along with a mild elevation of serum hCG. Histologically, most of the neoplastic cells of PSTT are mononuclear, and multinucleated cells are usually present in a

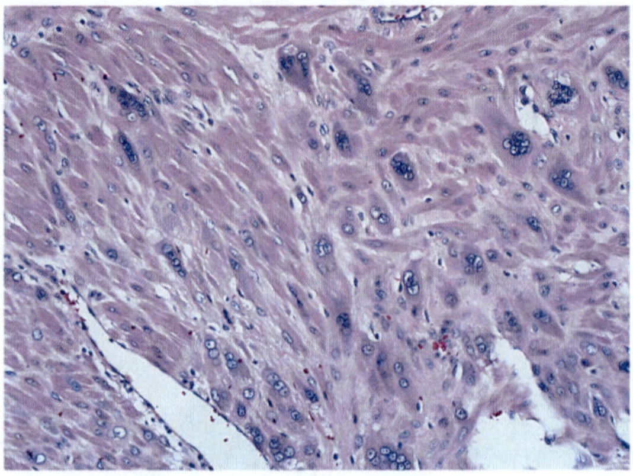

Fig. 10.7 EPS with characteristic infiltrative growth involving myometrial smooth muscle

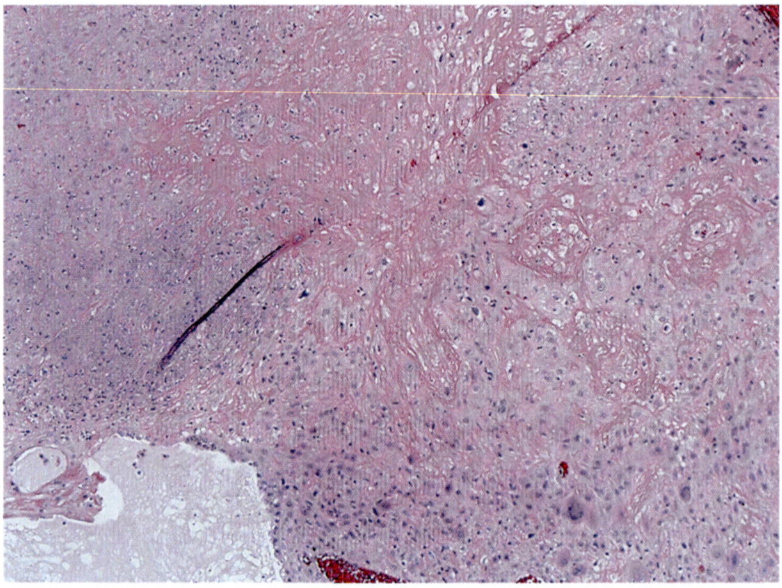

Fig. 10.8 EPS with focal degenerative changes in the format of fibrin deposition or hyalinization

Table 10.2 Differential diagnosis between EPS and PSTT

	EPS	PSTT
Clinical	Concurrent gestation or molar pregnancy	Amenorrhea, vaginal bleeding, elevated hCG
Gross	No mass lesion	Invasive mass lesion
Cytology	Mononuclear intermediate trophoblasts, generally without atypia	Atypical mononuclear intermediate trophoblasts
Growth pattern	Infiltrative with many evenly distributed multinucleated trophoblasts	Confluent sheets with infiltrative periphery with occasional multinucleated trophoblasts
Mitosis	Absent	Present
Chorionic villi	Present	Absent
Ki-67	<1%	>10%

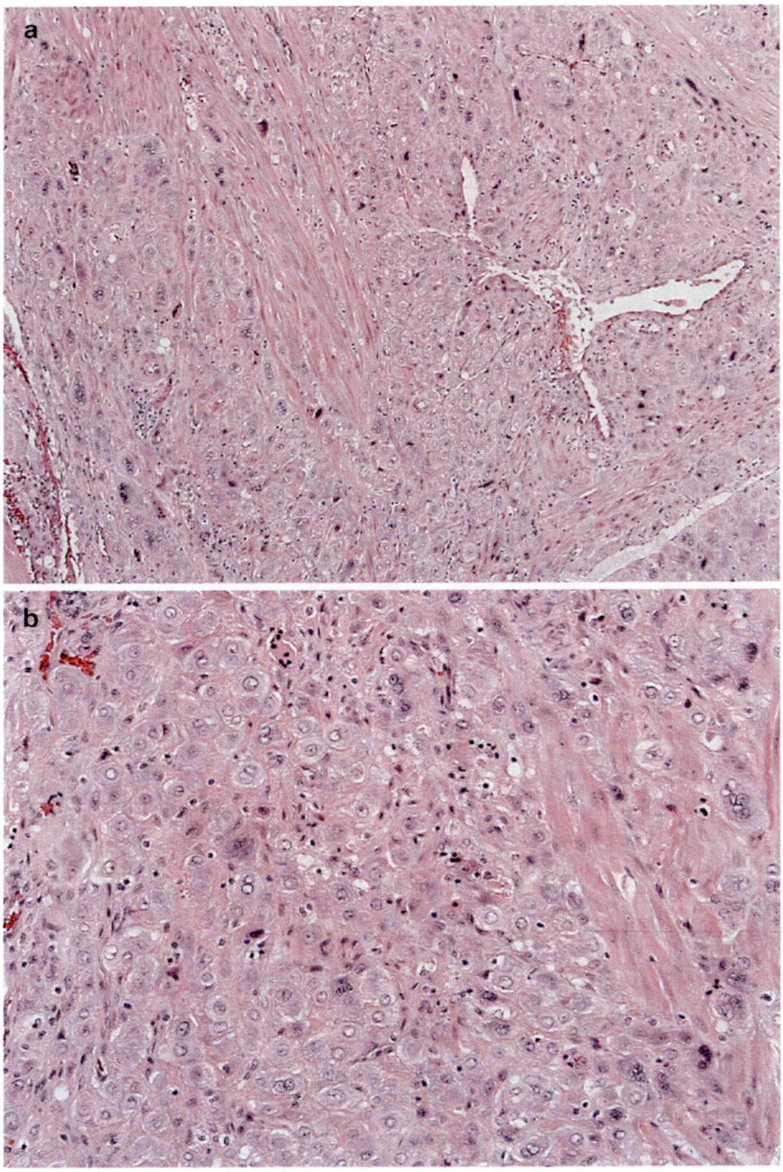

Fig. 10.9 Atypical EPS. Note the presence of more extensive intermediate trophoblastic infiltration (**a**) and moderate to marked cytological atypia (**b**), simulating a PSTT

scattered fashion. Ki-67 immunostaining typically demonstrates a higher level of the labeling (>5 or 14% ± 6.9%) [31]. In curettage specimens, based on which a diagnostic separation of EPS from PSTT cannot be decided [30], imaging studies or close follow-up of the patient with serum hCG monitoring should be recommended. Rare cases of EPS may show more extensive trophoblastic proliferation and infiltration into the underlying myometrium along with moderate to marked cytological atypia, even the presence of mitoses (Fig. 10.9), simulating a PSTT. Such EPS may be interpreted as atypical EPS reaction, and additional studies are required to ascertain the biology of such intermediate lesions.

Rarely, EPS may mimic choriocarcinoma [21]. Diagnostic features separating a choriocarcinoma from an EPS include absence of bilamellar growth pattern, no necrosis or hemorrhage, absence of mitosis, and minimal to zero Ki-67 activity [32, 33].

Clinicopathological Correlations

EPS is a benign process and simple curettage results in a cure. It has been suggested that EPS is a non-neoplastic counterpart of PSTT. EPS and PSTT share many cytological and histological features, and indeed, separation of the two can be difficult in some cases at the microscopic level [1]. Immunophenotypically, EPS and PSTT also share similar profiles to that of the intermediate trophoblastic cells: strong immunoreactivity to cytokeratin, hPL, CD 146 (Mel-CAM), HLA-G, E-cadherin and negative for EMA, and Ber-EP4 [1, 28, 29]. Therefore, it has been speculated that EPS may be a precursor lesion to PSTT, although a recent study failed to support such a hypothesis [34].

Conventional EPS without an association of molar pregnancy has no increased risk for persistent trophoblastic disease. However, EPS in association with complete mole may have a different biology, because of its inherited androgenetic nature. Some authors believe that an EPS should not be diagnosed in association with hydatidiform mole [35]. In complete mole, the implantation site may have even more exuberant trophoblastic proliferation. The trophoblasts may show significant cytological atypia as well. Mitotic activity and increased Ki-67 labeling are generally enhanced, compared with no mitosis and minimal Ki-67 staining in a conventional EPS. As near 50% of gestational choriocarcinomas develop following primary evacuation of complete mole, it can be speculated that choriocarcinoma may develop from a malignant transformation of EPS in assocation with complete mole. In fact, EPS may greatly mimic choriocarcinoma in a curettage specimen in some rare cases [21].

References

1. Shih IM, Kurman RJ. The pathology of intermediate trophoblastic tumors and tumor-like lesions. Int J Gynecol Pathol. 2001;20(1):31–47.
2. Carinelli SG, Vendola N, Benzi G. Placental site nodules. A report of 17 cases (abstract). Pathol Res Pract. 1989;185:30.
3. Young RH, Kurman RJ, Scully RE. Placental site nodules and plaques. A clinicopathologic analysis of 20 cases. Am J Surg Pathol. 1990;14(11):1001–9.
4. Lee KC, Chan JK. Placental site nodule. Histopathology. 1990;16(2):193–5.
5. Williams JW. Regeneration of the uterine mucosa after delivery, with special reference to the placental site. Am J Obstet Gynecol. 1931;22:664–96.
6. Swan RW, Woodruff JD. Retained products of conception. Histologic viability of placental polyps. Obstet Gynecol. 1969;34(4):506–14.
7. Shih IM, Seidman JD, Kurman RJ. Placental site nodule and characterization of distinctive types of intermediate trophoblast. Hum Pathol. 1999;30(6): 687–94.
8. Santos LD, Fernando SS, Yong JL, Killingsworth MC, Wu XJ, Kennerson AR. Placental site nodules and plaques: a clinicopathological and immunohistochemical study of 25 cases with ultrastructural findings. Pathology. 1999;31(4):328–36.
9. Huettner PC, Gersell DJ. Placental site nodule: a clinicopathologic study of 38 cases. Int J Gynecol Pathol. 1994;13(3):191–8.
10. Nayar R, Snell J, Silverberg SG, Lage JM. Placental site nodule occurring in a fallopian tube. Hum Pathol. 1996;27(11):1243–5.
11. Campello TR, Fittipaldi H, O'Valle F, Carvia RE, Nogales FF. Extrauterine (tubal) placental site nodule. Histopathology. 1998;32(6):562–5.
12. Al-Hussaini M, Lioe TF, McCluggage WG. Placental site nodule of the ovary. Histopathology. 2002;41(5): 471–2.
13. Tsang WY, Chum NP, Tang SK, Tse CC, Chan JK. Mallory's bodies in placental site nodule. Arch Pathol Lab Med. 1993;117(5):547–50.
14. Mao TL, Seidman JD, Kurman RJ, Shih Ie M. Cyclin E and p16 immunoreactivity in epithelioid trophoblastic tumor–an aid in differential diagnosis. Am J Surg Pathol. 2006;30(9):1105–10.
15. Mao TL, Kurman RJ, Jeng YM, Huang W, Shih Ie M. HSD3B1 as a novel trophoblast-associated marker that assists in the differential diagnosis of trophoblastic tumors and tumorlike lesions. Am J Surg Pathol. 2008;32(2):236–42.
16. Tsai HW, Lin CP, Chou CY, Li CF, Chow NH, Shih IM, et al. Placental site nodule transformed into a malignant epithelioid trophoblastic tumour with pelvic lymph node and lung metastasis. Histopathology. 2008;53(5):601–4.
17. Ewing J. Chorioma. Surg Gynecol Obstet. 1910; 10:26.

18. Taylor ES, Droegemueller W. Choriocarcinoma, chorioadenoma destruens, and syncytial endometritis. Am J Obstet Gynecol. 1962;83:958–68.
19. Acosta-Sison H. Is syncytial endometritis (syncytioma) always benign? J Philipp Med Assoc. 1963; 39:720–4.
20. Villasanta U. A re-evaluation of trophoblastic diseases: syncytial endometritis, hydatidiform mole (benign and malignant) and choriocarcinoma. Indian Pract. 1966;19(5):329–34.
21. Nigam S, Dass R. Exaggerated placental site reaction mimicking choriocarcinoma. Acta Obstet Gynecol Scand. 2003;82(6):587–8.
22. Micheletti G. A case of deep chorial infiltration of the myometrium (syncytial endometritis) as probable cause of uterine dyskinesia. Riv Ostet Ginecol Prat. 1960;42:829–35.
23. Kurman RJ, Scully RE, Norris HJ. Trophoblastic pseudotumor of the uterus: an exaggerated form of "syncytial endometritis" simulating a malignant tumor. Cancer. 1976;38(3):1214–26.
24. Chen X, Shi Y, Xie X. The clinical and pathological characteristics of exaggerated placental site. Zhonghua Fu Chan Ke Za Zhi. 1998;33(6):352–4.
25. Young RH, Kurman RJ, Scully RE. Proliferations and tumors of intermediate trophoblast of the placental site. Semin Diagn Pathol. 1988;5(2):223–37.
26. Wells M. The pathology of gestational trophoblastic disease: recent advances. Pathology. 2007;39(1):88–96.
27. Tavassoli F, Peter D. World Health Organization: tumours of the breast and female genital organs. Lyon: IARC Press; 2004.
28. Singer G, Kurman RJ, McMaster MT, Shih Ie M. HLA-G immunoreactivity is specific for intermediate trophoblast in gestational trophoblastic disease and can serve as a useful marker in differential diagnosis. Am J Surg Pathol. 2002;26(7):914–20.
29. Shih IM. The role of CD146 (Mel-CAM) in biology and pathology. J Pathol. 1999;189(1):4–11.
30. Yeasmin S, Nakayama K, Katagiri A, Ishikawa M, Iida K, Nakayama N, et al. Exaggerated placental site mimicking placental site trophoblastic tumor: case report and literature review. Eur J Gynaecol Oncol. 2010;31(5):586–9.
31. Shih IM, Kurman RJ. Ki-67 labeling index in the differential diagnosis of exaggerated placental site, placental site trophoblastic tumor, and choriocarcinoma: a double immunohistochemical staining technique using Ki-67 and Mel-CAM antibodies. Hum Pathol. 1998;29(1):27–33.
32. Hui P, Martel M, Parkash V. Gestational trophoblastic diseases: recent advances in histopathologic diagnosis and related genetic aspects. Adv Anat Pathol. 2005;12(3):116–25.
33. Buza N, Hui P. Gestational trophoblastic disease: histopathological diagnosis in the molecular era. Diagn Histopathol. 2010;16(11):526–37.
34. Dotto J, Hui P. Lack of genetic association between exaggerated placental site reaction and placental site trophoblastic tumor. Int J Gynecol Pathol. 2008;27(4): 562–7.
35. Bentley RC. Pathology of gestational trophoblastic disease. Clin Obstet Gynecol. 2003;46(3):513–22.

11 Molecular Diagnosis of Gestational Trophoblastic Disease*

Pei Hui

Key words

Molecular diagnosis of GTD • Tissue genotyping • STR

Introduction

Among gestational trophoblastic disorders, hydatidiform moles are the most common in the daily practice of gynecological pathology and frequently diagnostically challenging. While histological diagnosis of well-developed complete hydatidiform mole is generally reliable (see Chaps. 5 and 6), an early evacuated complete mole often presents with minimal histological abnormalities and is easily mistaken as a hydropic abortus or a normal pregnancy by both clinicians and pathologists [1]. Partial hydatidiform moles have been proven the most diagnostically difficult. At present time and even with available ancillary studies, pathologists cannot reliably classify a partial mole from its many mimics with both under- and over-diagnosis in a significant percentage of the cases. Yet, it is clinically important to distinguish a hydatidiform mole from a non-molar hydropic abortus, primarily because of the associated risk of development of post-molar gestational trophoblastic neoplasia [1–4]. Accurate subclassification of hydatidiform moles is also important as a complete mole has a much higher risk of progression to gestational trophoblastic neoplasia (18–29%) [2] than a partial mole (1.0–5.6%) [2, 4]. On the other hand, over-diagnosis of non-molar pregnancy as partial mole is not without clinical consequence, as all such patients will enter many months of the trophoblastic disease surveillance program, leading to unnecessary treatment and psychological burdens to the patients [2]. While data on complete moles were relatively reliable in the past, traditional epidemiological studies and risk factor assessment have long been suffering from an inaccurate classification of partial moles; therefore, statistical data on partial moles are at best unclear. Thus, reliable diagnosis of molar pregnancy with improved sensitivity and specificity is highly desirable. In difficult cases, the use of ancillary studies such as ploidy analysis and $p57^{KIP2}$ immunohistochemistry may be helpful (see Chapters 4 and 5). However, interpretations of these studies can be difficult with certain diagnostic pitfalls and limitations [5–7].

*This chapter is an update based on Expert Rev. Mol. Diag. 10(8), 1023–1034 (2010) with permission from Expert Reviews Ltd.

P. Hui, MD, PhD (✉)
Department of Pathology,
Yale University School of Medicine, 310 Cedar Street, 254B New Haven, CT 06520-8023, USA
e-mail: pei.hui@yale.edu

P. Hui (ed.), *Gestational Trophoblastic Disease: Diagnostic and Molecular Genetic Pathology*, Current Clinical Pathology, DOI 10.1007/978-1-61779-394-3_11,

It has been well established that the pathogenesis of hydatidiform moles requires specific abnormal genetic compositions present in conception, see Chap. 3 [8]. Such molecular/genetic signatures are considered the "gold standard" for an ultimate diagnosis of hydatidiform moles and were not explored fully for clinical diagnostic applications until very recently [9, 10]. In the past, molecular and genetic evaluations such as DNA ploidy analysis, chromosomal karyotyping, or enumeration by FISH and protein enzyme polymorphism studies have been shown to offer some diagnostic value. However, they all suffer significant limitations in diagnostic sensitivity/specificity and cost-effectiveness [11]. Genotyping by short tandem repeat (STR) polymorphism analysis has been recently validated as a highly accurate and practical method in the diagnosis and subclassification of hydatidiform moles [9, 11–13].

The majority of gestational trophoblastic tumors can be accurately diagnosed by routine histology and immunohistochemistry. However, in rare cases, when a trophoblastic tumor arises or presents at an atypical anatomic location or as a metastatic lesion, a differential diagnosis from a nongestational neoplasm may become very difficult and its gestational nature may not be resolved by conventional histological examination. Since gestational trophoblastic tumors are proliferative lesions arising from the haploid placental trophoblastic cells, molecular detection of the unique paternal genomic elements in the tumor offers an ultimate diagnostic separation of gestational trophoblastic tumors (choriocarcinoma and intermediate trophoblastic tumors) from their maternal mimics (nongestational choriocarcinoma and various carcinomas of the maternal uterus, respectively) [11].

Genetic Basis of Molecular Diagnosis

Molar pregnancies are defined at the genetic level by their specific parental chromosomal complements (Fig. 11.1). The genetic basis for the pathogenesis of hydatidiform moles has been well established in the past 40 years [8, 14–17], as has been extensively discussed in Chap. 2. In contrast to a normal diploid gestation of monogynic and monoandric parental compliment (46, XX or XY), essentially all complete hydatidiform moles have a diandric, paternal-only genome, with either 46, XX diploid karyotype arising from the fertilization of an enucleated egg by one spermatozoon followed by duplication (monospermic or homozygous, 80%), or 46, XX or XY karyotype arising from the fertilization of an enucleated egg by two spermatozoa simultaneously (dispermic or heterozygous, 20%) [12]. Tetraploid complete mole also exists and harbors paternal-only genome. An important exception to the established genetic requirement by the complete mole is the existence of rather rare biparental (monogynic and monoandric genome) complete moles [18, 19]. Biparental complete mole is frequently recurrent with strong familial tendency. Although it has a normal biparental chromosomal compliment, abnormal epigenetic regulation of imprinting genes appears to render silencing of maternal genes leading to an overall gene expression pattern similar to that of a conventional complete mole [20–22]. The morphology and biology of biparental complete mole are however similar to those of the classic diandric complete mole.

Early studies suggested that a complete mole with dispermic/heterozygous genome has more tendency toward malignant transformation than a monospermic/homozygous one [23–26], but disputed by others [27]. However, a recent study has confirmed a more aggressive behavior of a heterozygous complete mole than the one with homozygous genome [28]. Therefore, genotyping of every complete mole offers important prognostic and therapeutic guidance.

The genetic profile of partial hydatidiform moles is triploid with a diandric, monogynic genome arising from the fertilization of a haploid egg by either two spermatozoa (dispermic or heterozygous, 90%) or one spermatozoon with duplication (monospermic or homozygous, 10%) [12]. The resulting conception is triploid with diandric and monogynic haploid genomes, 69, XXX or XXY karyotype. Diploid partial moles were reported in the past but likely represented a misclassification of either a complete mole or a

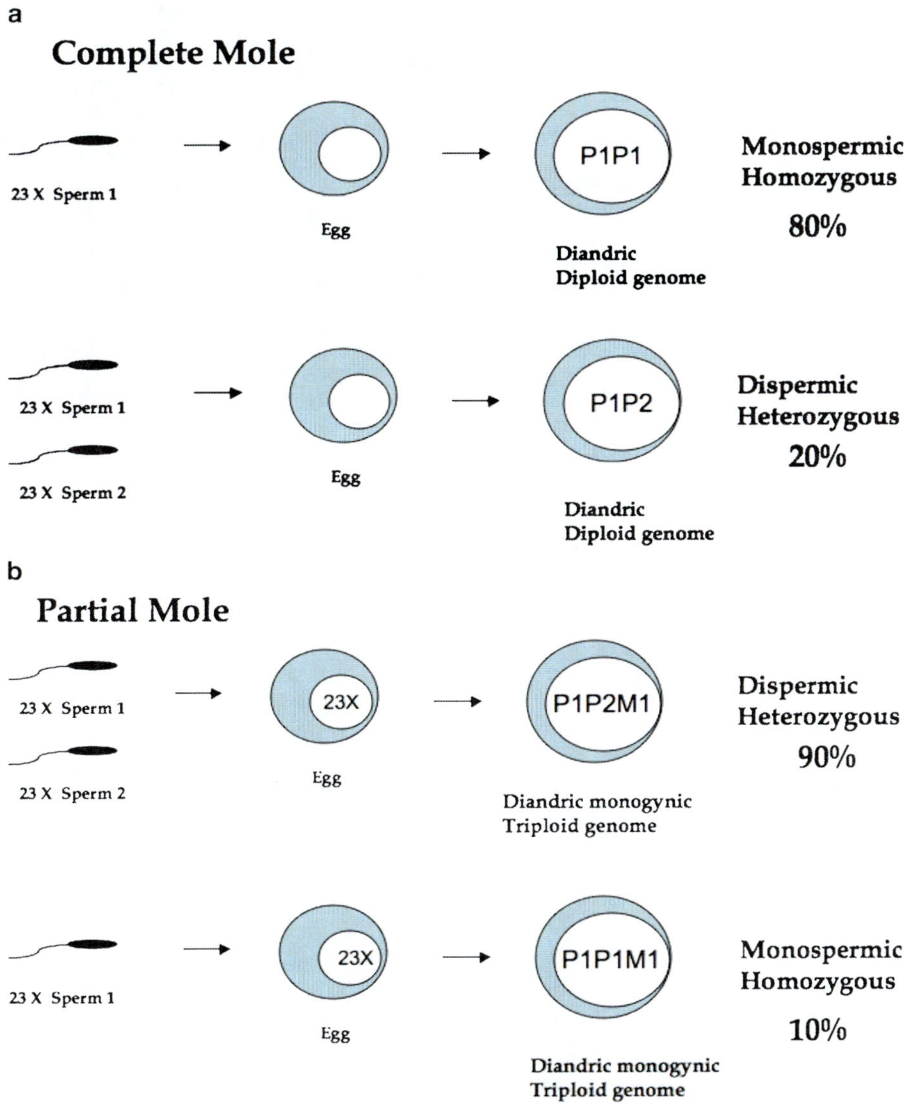

Fig. 11.1 Genetic basis of hydatidiform moles. (**a**) Complete hydatidiform moles have diandric, paternal-only genome, with diploid karyotypes arising either from fertilization of an enucleated egg by one spermatozoon followed by duplication (monospermic or homozygous) or from simultaneous fertilization of an enucleated egg by two spermatozoa (dispermic or heterozygous). (**b**) The genetic profile of partial hydatidiform moles is triploid with a diandric, monogynic genome arising from the fertilization of a haploid egg by either two heterozygous spermatozoa (dispermic or heterozygous) or one spermatozoon with duplication (monospermic or homozygous)

non-molar gestation [29]. It is important to note that one-third of triploid early missed abortions have digynic and monoandric chromosomal composition and are not partial hydatidiform moles on clinical and pathological grounds [3, 30, 31]. Therefore, determination of the parental source of the haploid sets in a triploid conception is important for the diagnosis of partial molar pregnancies.

Gestational trophoblastic tumors are malignant transformations of various trophoblastic cells in the placenta. Therefore, they harbor the paternal haploid genome that is not present in maternal tissue. A demonstration of the paternal genome in such a trophoblastic tumor allows a definitive diagnostic separation from a tumor arising from the maternal source.

Methods of Molecular Diagnosis

A variety of molecular methods targeting the genetic alterations of hydatidiform moles have been explored to improve diagnostic accuracy. These include conventional cytogenetic analysis (karyotyping), DNA ploidy flow cytometry, and chromosomal enumeration by fluorescent in situ hybridization and molecular genotyping. Ploidy analysis is the determination of the number of complete haploid sets of chromosomes present in a particular cell population (23 chromosomes/ haploid sets in a human diploid cell). Flow cytometry is the most common platform for ploidy analysis using tissue specimens [32–35]. DNA ploidy analysis is frequently used for the separation of a partial mole from a complete mole or a diploid non-molar hydropic abortus by a demonstration of triploidy. However, it is not useful in the distinction between a complete mole and a non-molar hydropic abortus. Several studies indicated that only 66% of triploid abortions were true diandric-monogynic partial moles while the remainders were digynic–monoandric non-molar gestations [3, 30, 36]. Therefore, the presence of triploidy by flow cytometry offers helpful, but not diagnostic evidence of partial hydatidiform mole. In addition, ploidy analysis using paraffin-embedded tissue is frequently plagued with technical difficulties and interpretation errors resulting in a significant misclassification of ploidy, and misdiagnosis of hydatidiform mole. This is because the ploidy histograms produced from paraffin-embedded material tend to have increased cellular debris and broader peaks with a high coefficient of variation. Effects of various fixatives and fixation conditions may significantly affect DNA ploidy analysis as well [37].

Conventional karyotyping is the most accurate chromosomal enumeration method that may be used to confirm the presence of triploidy in a partial mole or diploidy in a complete mole. Interphase FISH can be used for the determination of the number of haploid chromosome sets using both fresh and paraffin-embedded tissue samples [38–41]. However, similar to ploidy analysis, chromosomal enumeration has significant limitations in the diagnosis of molar pregnancies in that it cannot specifically ascertain the parental origin of chromosomal contribution to the gestational tissue (Fig. 11.2). Therefore, it cannot distinguish a diploid complete mole from a much more common non-molar hydropic abortus and is unable to separate a true diandric-monogynic partial mole from a digynic–monoandric non-molar gestation. Cytogenetic studies based on analysis of pericentromeric chromosome heteromorphisms can be used to identify the parental source of chromosomes and may specifically diagnose and subtype hydatidiform moles [8, 16] [42–44]. However, similar to conventional karyotyping, it requires fresh chorionic villous samples and in vitro cell culture.

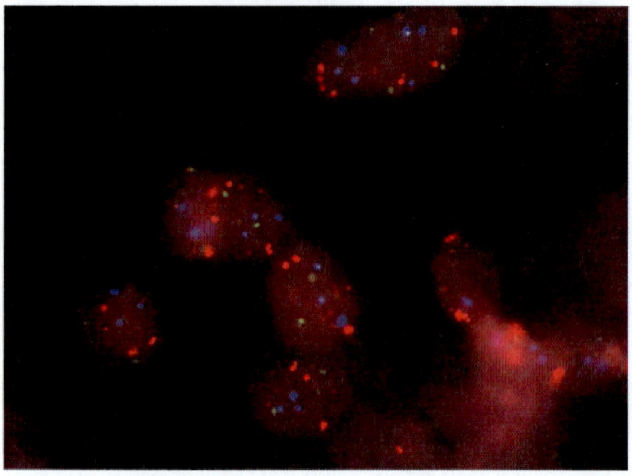

Fig. 11.2 Chromosomal enumeration of a partial hydatidiform mole by FISH. Conventional interphase fluorescence in situ hybridization demonstrates the presence of three hybridization signals of chromosome 3 (large *red* dots), 7 (*green* dots), 17 (*blue* dots), and 9 (small *reddish-gold* dots) probes within nuclei

STR Genotyping Diagnosis of Hydatidiform Moles

Genotyping provides a measurement of the genetic variation between members of a species and, therefore, can be used to identify parental source of genomic haploid set(s) in a hydatidiform mole. Various molecular targets have been explored for the genotypic diagnosis of hydatidiform moles, including DNA restriction fragment length polymorphism, enzyme polymorphism, single-nucleotide polymorphism, and STR polymorphism.

Restriction fragment length polymorphisms (RFLP) was used in the past to diagnose molar gestations by demonstration of the abnormal paternal genome [45, 46] and the maternal mitochondrial DNA [47]. Enzyme polymorphism using tissue culture was also attempted for separation of hydatidiform moles from non-molar abortuses [42, 48]. In addition to the labor intensiveness, RFLP and enzyme polymorphism are limited by analyzing usually only one genetic target and therefore do not provide sufficient resolving power for molar genotyping diagnosis. Single nucleotide polymorphism analysis has been explored recently for diagnostic confirmation of complete moles using the whole genome microarray approach [49]. Recently laboratory and clinical validation of STR genotyping has become the most accurate and reliable method for tissue genotyping and will be the main focus of discussion in this chapter.

STRs are repetitive DNA sequences of 2–7 nucleotides. They are highly prevalent in the noncoding regions of the human genome and genetically stable [50]. A STR polymorphism denotes that a STR locus differs in the number of repeats between individuals. By identification of the number of the STR at specific loci, a genetic profile of an individual or a cell can be ascertained to distinguish one from another. STR polymorphism analysis has become the most proficient method for determining an individual identity in the forensic field. By the same principle, STR polymorphism analysis of gestational tissue in comparison with corresponding maternal tissue offers a genotypic identification of the parental genomic contribution in a hydatidiform mole. There are number of robust commercial STR genotyping kits with various multiplex primer sets, including AmpFlSTR® Identifiler™ PCR Amplification (Applied Biosystem, Inc), AmpFlSTR® Profiler™ PCR Amplification (Applied Biosystem, Inc), and PowerPlex® ©16 System (Promega US, Madison, WI, USA). The AmpFlSTR® Identifiler™ assay is a highly commercialized STR assay that amplifies 15 tetranucleotide STR loci and the amelogenin gender-determining locus in a single multiplex PCR amplification. All 13 of the required loci for the Combined DNA Index System (CODIS) loci are included with two additional loci, D2S1338 and D19S433. The combination of these loci offers a powerful genomic polymorphism analysis (Fig. 11.3) [51]. The amplicons range from 100 to 350 bp making it particularly suitable for the analysis of DNA extracted from paraffin-embedded formalin-fixed tissue samples. This multiplex PCR has a high efficiency of analyzing small amount of template DNA (as little as 1.5–2.5 ng, equivalent to 150–250 diploid cells). As a commercialized test kit, the validity of AmpFlSTR® Identifiler™ has been well established both in forensic practice for human identity testing and in clinical testing for transplant chimerism analysis. The assay resembles a conventional diagnostic molecular procedure, involving manual tissue dissection, DNA extraction, one PCR, and capillary electrophoresis. The cost of AmpFlSTR® Identifiler™ assay kit itself (excluding PCR reagents and those of capillary electrophoresis) is approximately 40 US dollars per case in a diagnostic work-up of molar pregnancy. Moreover, the reagent stability, requirement of expertise and turn-around time fall within the realm of a standard PCR diagnostic test. STR genotyping using AmpFlSTR® Identifiler™ or an equivalent kit has been shown recently to be as an accurate and cost-effective method in the diagnosis and subclassification of hydatidiform moles (see the following).

Previous proof-of-concept studies demonstrated the usefulness of DNA genotyping in distinguishing a hydropic abortion from a hydatidiform mole [52–56]. Using DNA extracted from formalin-fixed, paraffin-embedded tissue samples and PCR amplification of eight polymorphic STR loci, one study analyzed 17 cases of products of conception [53]. The authors identified eight cases of complete moles, of which five had not been previously recognized, and confirmed all five partial mole diagnoses. Another

LOCUS		SIZE (#ALLELE)
D2S1338	VIC	307-359(14)
TPOX (2p23-2per)	NED	222-250(8)
D3S1358	VIC	112-140(8)
FGA (4q28)	PET	215-355(28)
D5S818	PET	134-172(10)
CSF1PI (5q33.3-34)		304-341(10)
D7S820		255-291 (10)
D8S1179		120-170(12)
TH01(11p15.5)	VIC	169-202(10)
vWA (12p12-pter)	NED	145-207(14)
D13S317	VIC	217-245(8)
D16S539	VIC	253-293(9)
D18S51	NED	262-345(23)
D19S433	NED	102-195(15)
D21S11		185-240(24)
Amelogenin	PET	107/113(X/Y)

Fig. 11.3 Microsatellite loci included in the AmpFISTR Genotyping Analysis

study used genotyping to confirm the sensitivity and specificity of p57 immunohistochemistry in the diagnosis of complete mole [57]. However, the clinical application was limited in these early studies likely by technical complexity and/or relatively small number of STR markers. With commercial availability and improved cost-effectiveness of multiplex STR analysis, we recently validated DNA genotyping using the AmpFlSTR Identifiler PCR Amplification system (Applied Biosystems, Inc) for the diagnosis and subtyping of hydatidiform moles [9]. The diagnostic power and clinical applicability of DNA genotyping for routine practice are further confirmed by other studies [10–12, 58].

Interpretation of STR PCR data

STR genotyping for molar pregnancy requires a comparative evaluation of the genetic profiles of gestational tissue, that is, chorionic villi and maternal tissue, that is, gestational endometrium. The key is to identify the paternal allele and its copy number at each STR locus. The first step is to look for informative STR loci, that is, the unique paternal alleles by comparing allelic positions at each STR locus. Although a complete mole should have all alleles derived from the father in either homozygous or heterozygous fashion, shared alleles by the

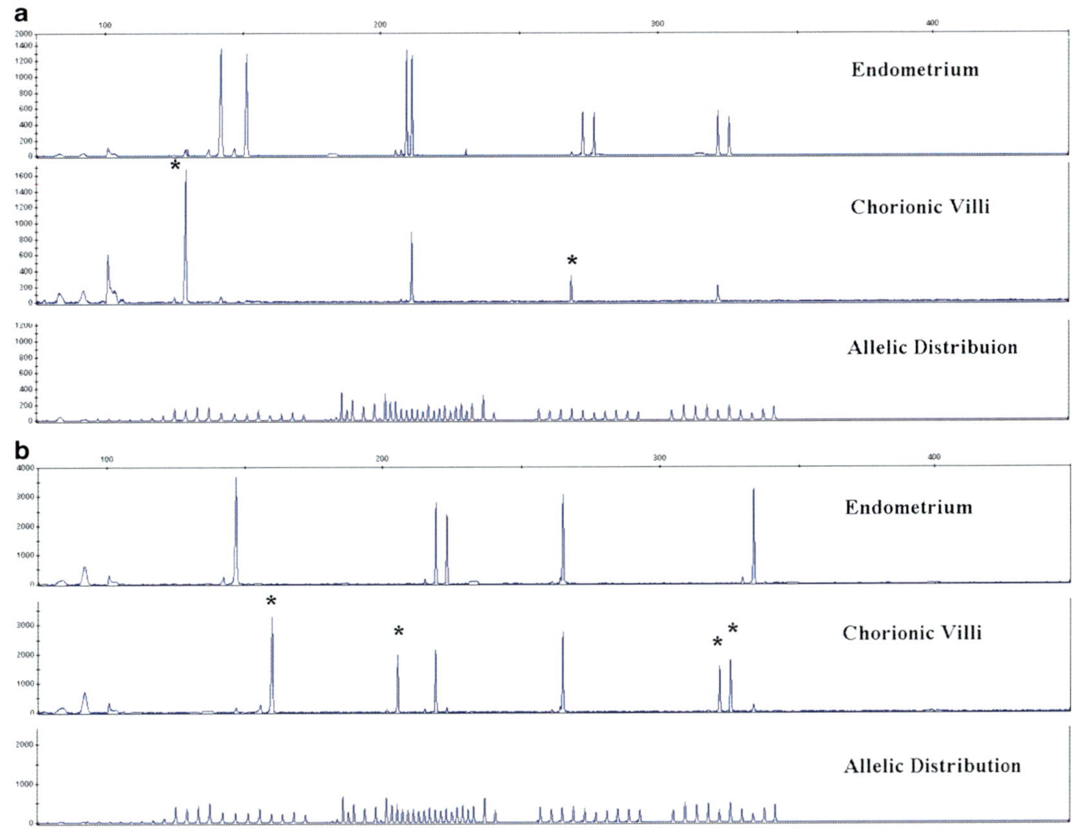

Fig. 11.4 STR genotyping of complete hydatidiform moles (4 of 15 STR loci of AmpFlSTR Identifiler are shown: CSF1PO, D7S820, D8S1179, and D21S11). A homozygous complete mole (**a**) harbors exclusively paternal alleles in the villous tissue at all loci. A heterozygous complete mole (**b**) shows exclusively paternal alleles in the villous tissue at all loci with identifiable two distinct paternal alleles at some loci. The unique paternal alleles are indicated by asterisk

father and the mother are common due to a limited number of alleles at each locus in human. Partial moles and non-molar abortuses share at least one allele with the maternal tissue at all loci, and some paternal alleles may also be shared by the mother. However, given multiple polymorphic loci, the likelihood of identical allele(s) at some but not all STR loci is high, and there should be a sufficient number of informative loci for interpretation. A molecular diagnosis of complete mole is made if the genotypic profile of the villous tissue consists of exclusively paternal alleles of either homozygous (Fig. 11.4a) or heterozygous (Fig. 11.4b) pattern in at least two informative loci. The presence of one maternaland two paternal alleles at each STR locus leads to a diagnosis of partial mole (Fig. 11.5). A dispermic or heterozygous partial mole harbors two unique paternal alleles in addition to one maternal allele in at least two loci (Fig. 11.5a). A monospermic or homozygous partial mole shows one paternal allele with duplicate quantity in addition to one copy of maternal allele at every locus (Fig. 11.5b). Non-molar gestation shows a balanced biallelic profile of both paternal and maternal contributions (Fig. 11.6). It should be noted that genotyping is not affected by the presence of tetraploidy in a complete mole as all such cases contain paternal-only genomes. The most important advantage of genotyping diagnosis over the traditional ploidy and

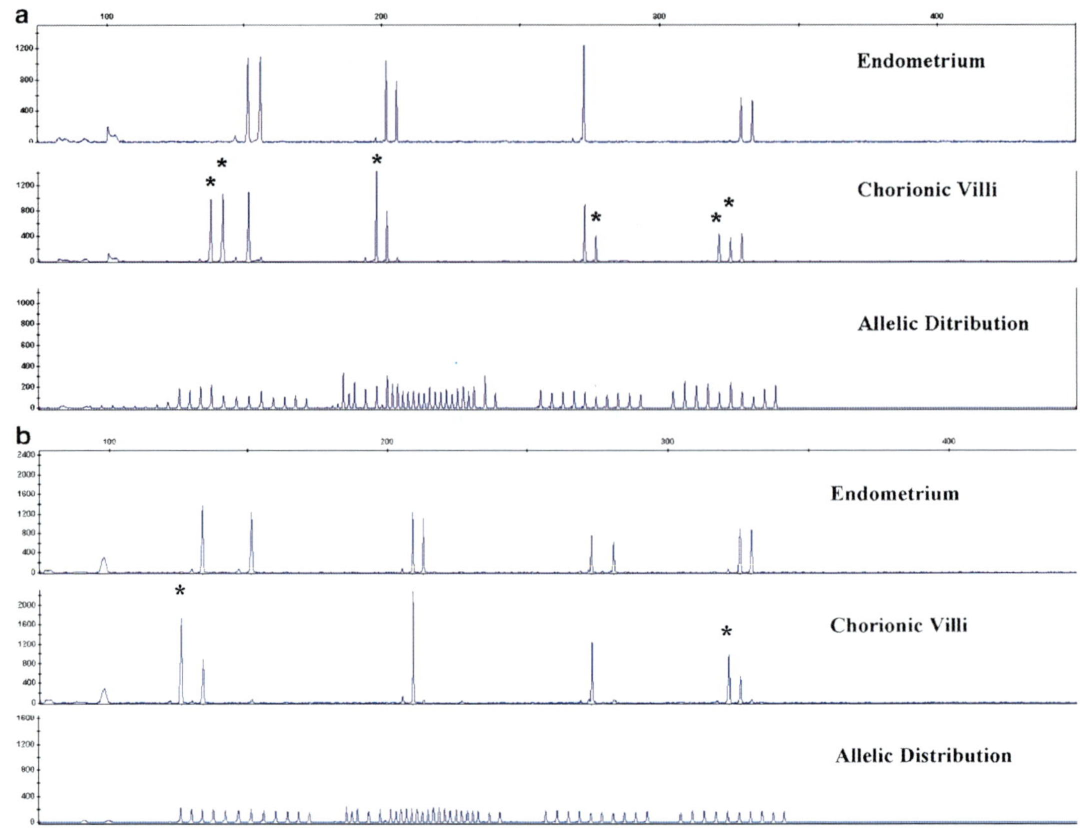

Fig. 11.5 STR genotyping of partial hydatidiform moles (4 of 15 STR loci of AmpFlSTR Identifiler are shown: CSF1PO, D7S820, D8S1179, and D21S11). A heterozygous partial mole (**a**) harbors diandric heterozygous paternal alleles in addition to one maternal allele at every locus. Heterozygosity is evidenced by two distinct paternal alleles at some loci. A homozygous partial mole (**b**) contains diandric homozygous paternal alleles in addition to one maternal allele. Homozygosity is evidenced by one paternal allele with duplicate copy number at all loci. The unique paternal alleles are indicated by asterisk

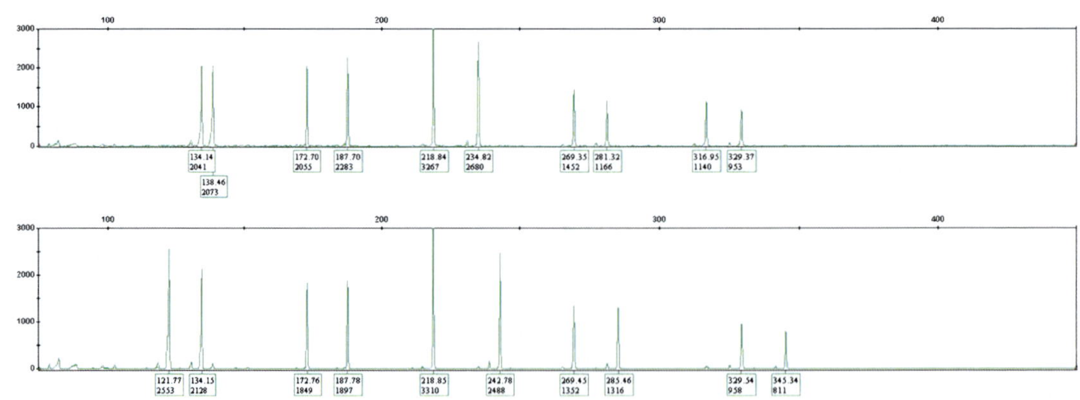

Fig. 11.6 STR genotyping of a non-molar hydropic abortion. A normal balanced parental genome is illustrated (upper panel - maternal endometrium, lower panel - chorionic villi)

karyotyping is its ability to clearly separate a triploid digynic non-molar gestation from a true triploid diandric partial mole. In contrast to the presence of two paternal alleles and one maternal allele at every STR locus, triploid non-molar gestation will have one paternal allele and two maternal alleles at each locus (Fig. 11.7).

As discussed earlier, not all STR loci in a given hydatidiform mole are informative with regard to the presence of identifiable paternal allele(s). This is due to the limited number of alleles in a population. When no unique paternal allele is present at a locus, the copy number/quantitation represented by the height of the PCR product in comparison with the adjacent allele can still be used for haploid assessment. This quantitative information is particularly useful when dealing with triploid partial hydatidiform mole. Analysis of more than one locus ensures an independent confirmation of presence or absence of paternal allele(s) and the copy number. Although quantitative evaluation of copy number of a particular locus by mathematical formula is possible [59, 60], visual inspection of the chromatogram is essentially diagnostic in all cases of molar pregnancy as long as tissue cross-contamination is minimized (see the following). It is also possible to genotype the paternal tissue (the patient's partner) to confirm the informative alleles in the molar tissue. However, this is neither necessary nor practical in most cases.

It is emphasized that there should be concordant genetic alterations at all loci for the diagnosis of hydatidiform moles. Inconsistency at an isolated locus requires careful evaluation of the entire STR profile. In case of a chromosomal aberration leading to a loss or gain of one allele, the analysis of the remaining 14 STR loci easily recognizes such isolated chromosomal aberration, thereby avoiding an interpretation error. For example, rare complete hydatidiform moles have been reported to have a retained maternal chromosome as trisomy [61, 62], which may present as three alleles at the locus. However, the presence of only androgenic alleles in the rest of STR loci points to the correct diagnosis of complete mole.

Target Tissue Selection and Processing

Tissue specimen preparation requires selection and verification of the target tissue for downstream DNA extraction and genotyping. Since genotyping comparison of the villous and the maternal tissue is the key for molar diagnosis, isolation of pure tissue types is important, particularly when dealing with a partial mole. In most tissue samples of product of conception, well-defined areas of chorionic villi and maternal endometrium are easily recognized in serial tissue sections and can be safely dissected from each other into separate test tubes. However, an absolutely pure isolation of villous tissue is generally impossible due to the mixed nature of the specimen unless laser microdissection is used. Maternal blood and endometrial tissue or cells may be intimately admixed with chorionic villous tissue. Initial inspection of the STR genotyping chromatograph should assess the extent of tissue cross-contamination. Minor degrees of contamination generally do not pose interpretation problems for a complete mole as the contaminating allelic products can be visually subtracted. However, tissue cross-contamination may easily jeopardize an interpretation of a partial mole as both the presence of abnormal paternal alleles and the quantitative information of each allele are important, particularly when dealing with a homozygous partial mole. Although mathematical ratio calculation may be used in cases with significant cross-contamination [58], repeat tissue and DNA preparation, particularly using laser microdissection to obtain pure tissue samples, should resolve the problem (Fig. 11.8) [12]. Occasionally, a specimen may contain only gestational tissue without maternal endometrium. A search of the patient file for her prior tissue specimen(s) or request for a new blood or buccal swab sample may be necessary.

Since most cases of genotyping evaluation are performed on formalin-fixed paraffin-embedded tissue samples after a routine histological examination, the types of fixative and the duration of fixation may affect the DNA quality and quantity.

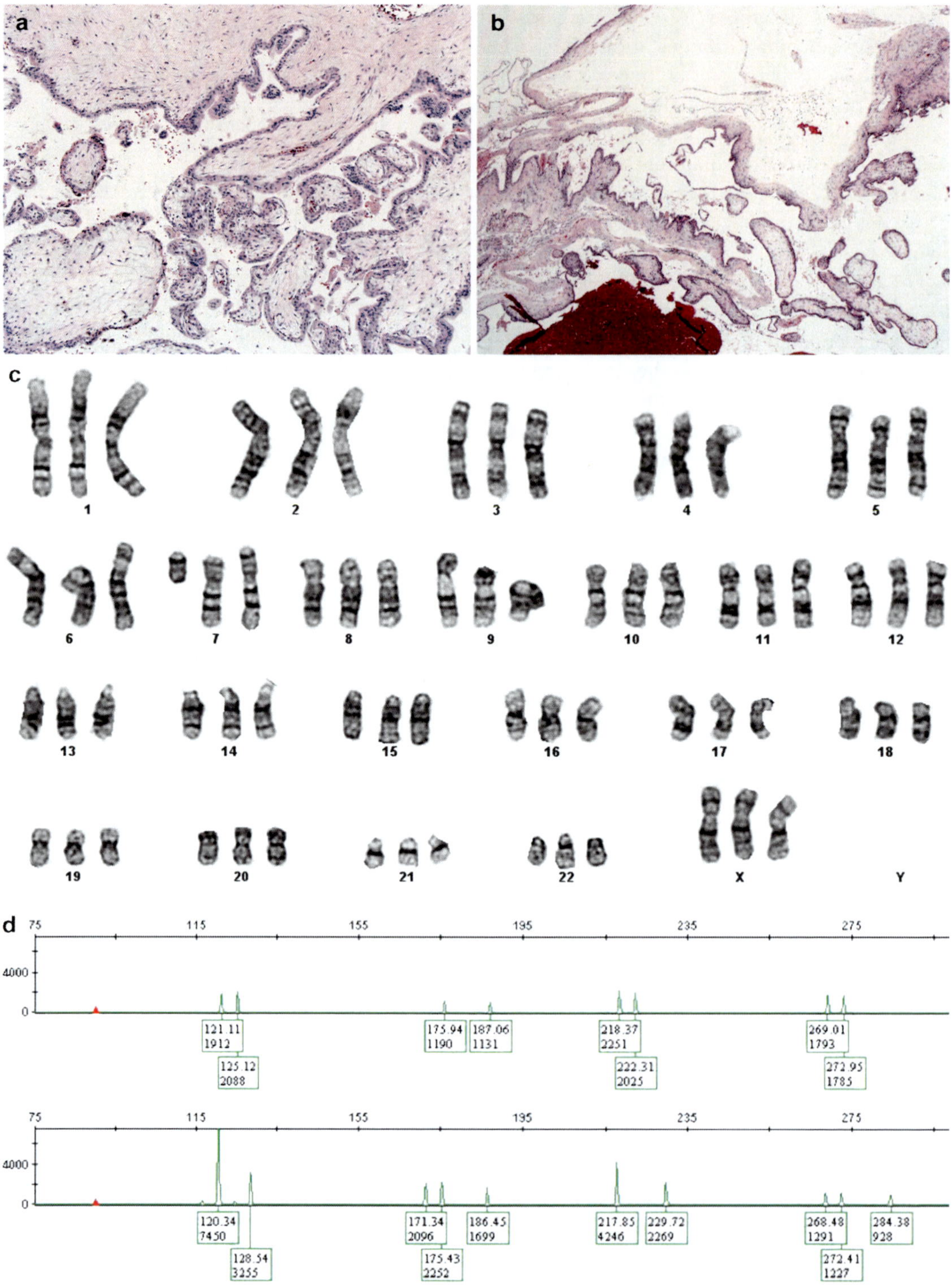

Fig. 11.7 Triploid non-molar gestation. Two representative cases (**a**, **b**) show histological features overlapping with a partial mole. The presence of triploidy is demonstrated by karyotyping analysis of the chorionic villi (**c**) (Courtesy of Dr. Peining Li, Yale University). The nature of a non-molar (digynic–monoandric) triploid gestation can only be revealed by DNA genotyping (**d**). Note, at each of the four STR loci two of the three alleles of the villi (*lower*) match the two maternal alleles of the gestational endometrium (*upper*)

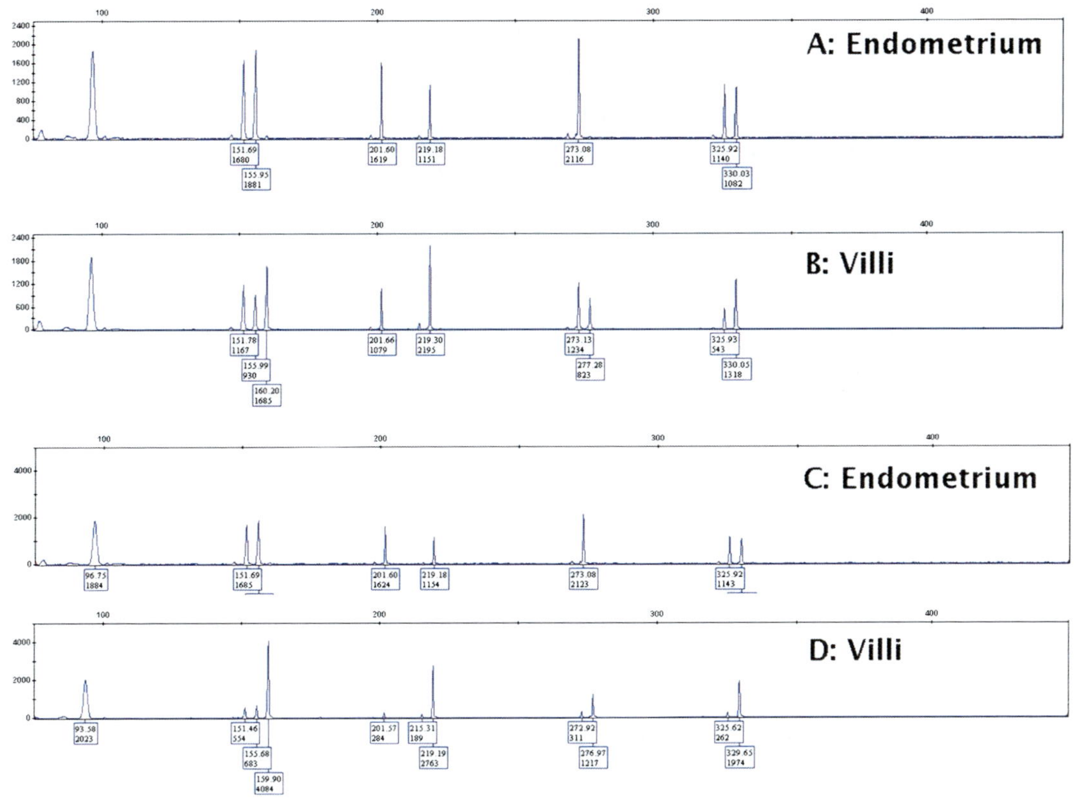

Fig. 11.8 Improved STR analysis by laser microdissection. Normal maternal endometrium shows a balanced biparental allelic pattern at three of the four STR loci (**a**, **c**). Significant cross-contamination by the maternal tissue generates a pseudotriploid allelic pattern in the chorionic villi (**b**). After laser microdissection of pure villous tissue, an allelic pattern of monospermic/homozygous complete mole becomes evident (**d**)

Fixatives containing heavy metals generally retard DNA extraction and/or ruin its quality. Long-term storage of paraffin-embedded tissue may result in severe degradation of DNA leading to uneven amplification, particularly of the larger PCR amplicons. Inefficient PCR amplification can be easily recognized as the amount of the product (peak height) is low. Concurrent amplification of paired maternal tissue from the same specimen may help to recognize the inefficiently amplified loci. Since multiple STR loci are included in the assay, single or a few large uninterpretable amplicons may be overcome by the remaining informative loci. Again, a careful inspection of entire STR chromatograms is essential to identify these problems to avoid an interpretation error.

Diagnostic Pitfalls of STR Genotyping

A potential pitfall for the genotypic diagnosis of hydatidiform mole is the presence of a small subset of complete mole of biparental origin, histologically indistinguishable from the diandric uniparental complete mole [18, 19]. In view of this phenomenon, DNA genotyping is not helpful in such a case as both the paternal and the maternal genomes are present. Clinical investigation, careful histological and immunohistochemical studies are important for the diagnosis. Hydatidiform moles arising from a twin gestation may also potentially complicate the analysis [63–66]. Since uterine curettage generally results in an admixture of gestational

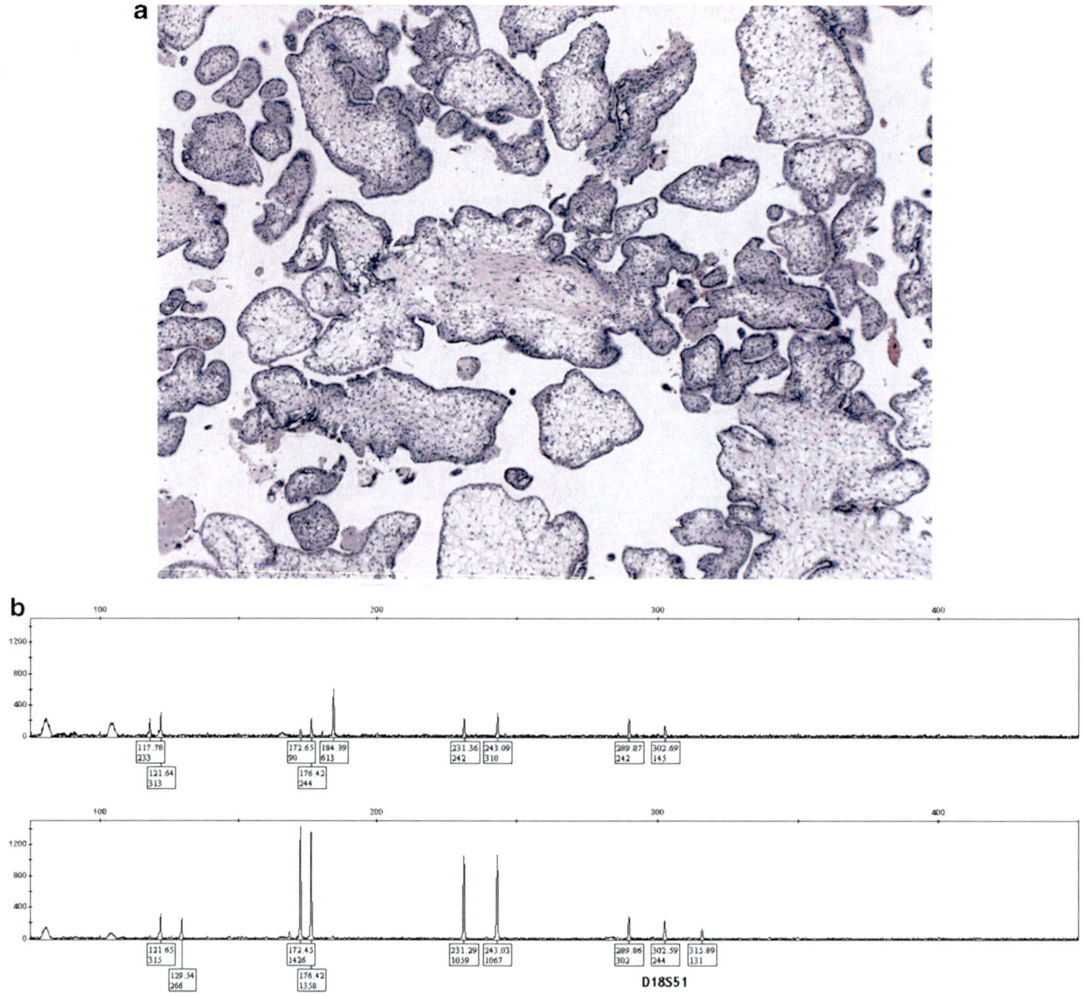

Fig. 11.9 Chorionic villi of Trisomy 18 syndrome. Note the overlapping histological feature with PHM (**a**) and the presence of three alleles at D18S51 locus as the only abnormal finding by DNA genotyping (**b**) lower panel, compared with two alleles in the endometrium in the upper panel

tissues, genetically abnormal molar tissue may be intimately associated with non-molar tissue of the counterpart twin. The genotyping result may be misleading or impossible to interpret depending on the extent of tissue mixing and the type of hydatidiform mole. Clinical information of twin gestation, careful morphological assessment of the tissue followed by isolation of pure hydropic villi, and genotypic comparison with nonhydropic villi may resolve such a difficult situation.

Single allelic gain due to various trisomy syndromes is relatively common among cases undergoing STR genotype work-up of hydatidiform moles, among which trisomy 16, 21, and 18 are frequently encountered [12]. It is worth noting that some of these trisomy syndromes may present villous tissue with morphological changes remarkably overlapping with those of a typical partial mole (Fig. 11.9) [3, 12]. However, a uniform allelic gain at all STR loci easily separates a partial mole from a trisomy syndrome [12]. Rare mosaicism and chimerism in hydatidiform mole may present complex STR profiles that are difficult to interpret [67]. Clinical presentation, careful histological examination, interphase FISH,

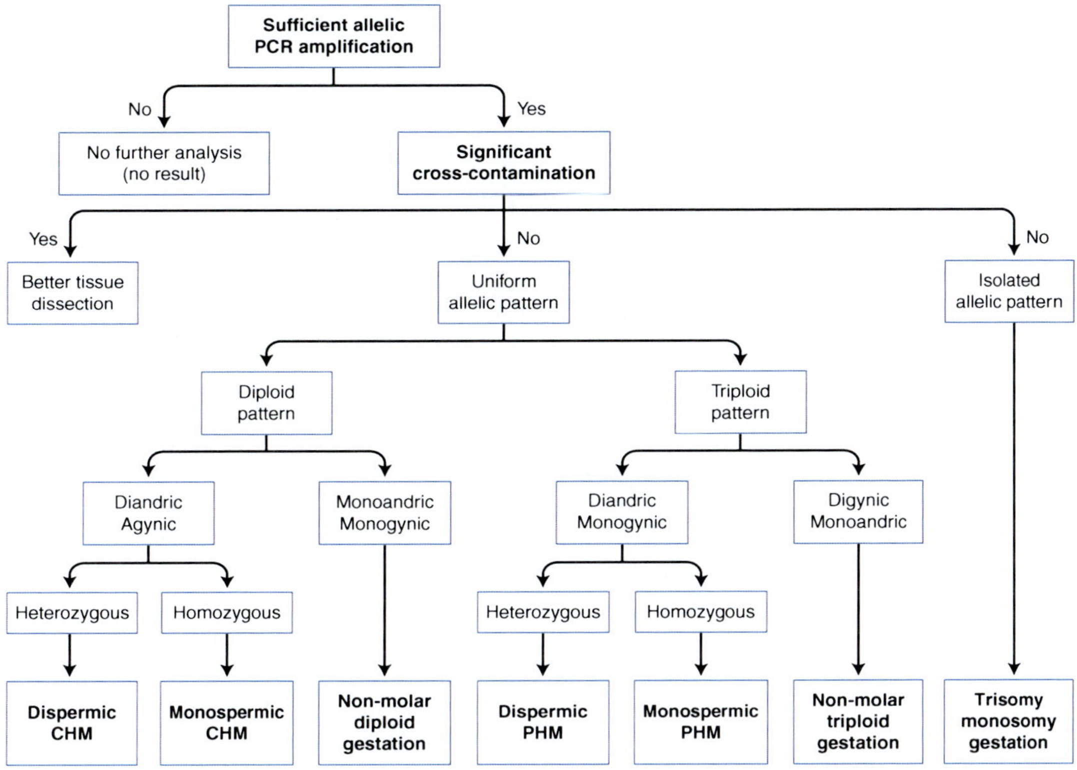

Fig. 11.10 Proposed STR genotyping algorithm for the diagnosis of hydatidiform moles

and immunohistochemistry of p57^{KIP2} may help to identify the villous/cell population of the molar lineage. Occasionally, a missed abortion may have non-molar complex chromosomal alterations involving multiple STR loci. In such a situation, a genotyping report of complex genetic alteration inconsistent with molar gestation is acceptable.

An algorithmic approach is presented in Fig. 11.10 to guide the molecular evaluation for the diagnosis and differential diagnosis of hydatidiform moles.

STR Genotyping Diagnosis of Gestational Trophoblastic Tumors

Most gestational trophoblastic tumors do not pose diagnostic problems when they present as an intrauterine lesion along with appropriate clinical history. However, rare tumors may develop at an unusual location [68]. For example, a trophoblastic tumor may arise from the fallopian tube [69], broad ligament [70], or even peritoneum [71]. Without due suspicion, a nongestational tumor (frequently carcinoma) may be diagnosed. Frequently arising from the endocervix, epithelioid trophoblastic tumor may have remarkable histological and cytological overlaps (Fig. 11.11a) with a keratinizing invasive squamous cell carcinoma, the most common malignancy of the uterine cervix. Clinical history of pregnancy, elevated serum hCG, and immunohistochemical markers are usually helpful in making a correct diagnosis. However, in rare cases, when these traditional means are inconclusive, STR genotyping can provide an ultimate confirmation of the gestational origin of the tumor (Fig. 11.11) [72].

Gestational choriocarcinoma at an unusual site, for example, extrauterine locations, must be

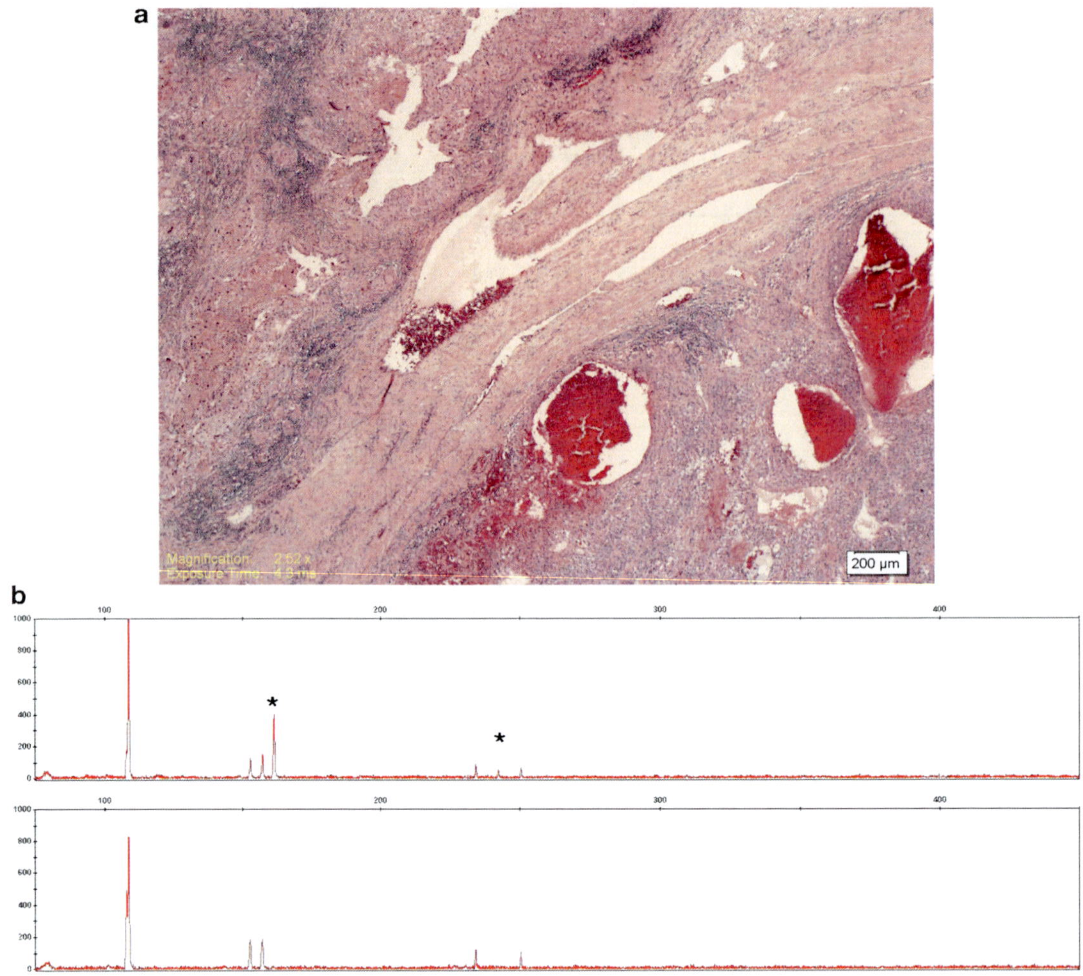

Fig. 11.11 STR genotyping diagnosis of trophoblastic tumor involving unusual anatomic locations. (**a**) Histological features of an epithelioid trophoblastic tumor involving the cervix. The tumor shows a nodular expansile lesion consisting of epithelioid intermediate trophoblastic tumor cells, simulating an invasive squamous cell carcinoma. (**b**) DNA genotyping analysis by AmpFlSTR® Identifiler™ PCR. The tumor cells (*upper panel*) harbor unique paternal alleles at two SRT loci, indicated by asterisk, in addition to the presence of maternal alleles, compared with the allelic pattern of the paired endometrium (*lower panel*)

separated from its nongestational counterpart of germ cell or somatic cell origin, primarily because of the drastically different clinical behaviors and management. Such separation can be very difficult, particularly when the choriocarcinoma presents with pure histology (Fig. 11.12a). Tissue DNA genotyping will definitively separate a gestational choriocarcinoma from its somatic or germ cell mimics by identifying the unique paternal allele(s) in the tumor (Fig. 11.12b) [73].

Prospective

It is important to understand that although hydatidiform moles are evacuated at a much earlier gestational age in modern medicine, their associated risks for post-molar gestational trophoblastic neoplasia have not changed [2]. Pathologists need to have a high index of suspicion for early complete hydatidiform moles, which are easily misinterpreted as hydropic abortions or even

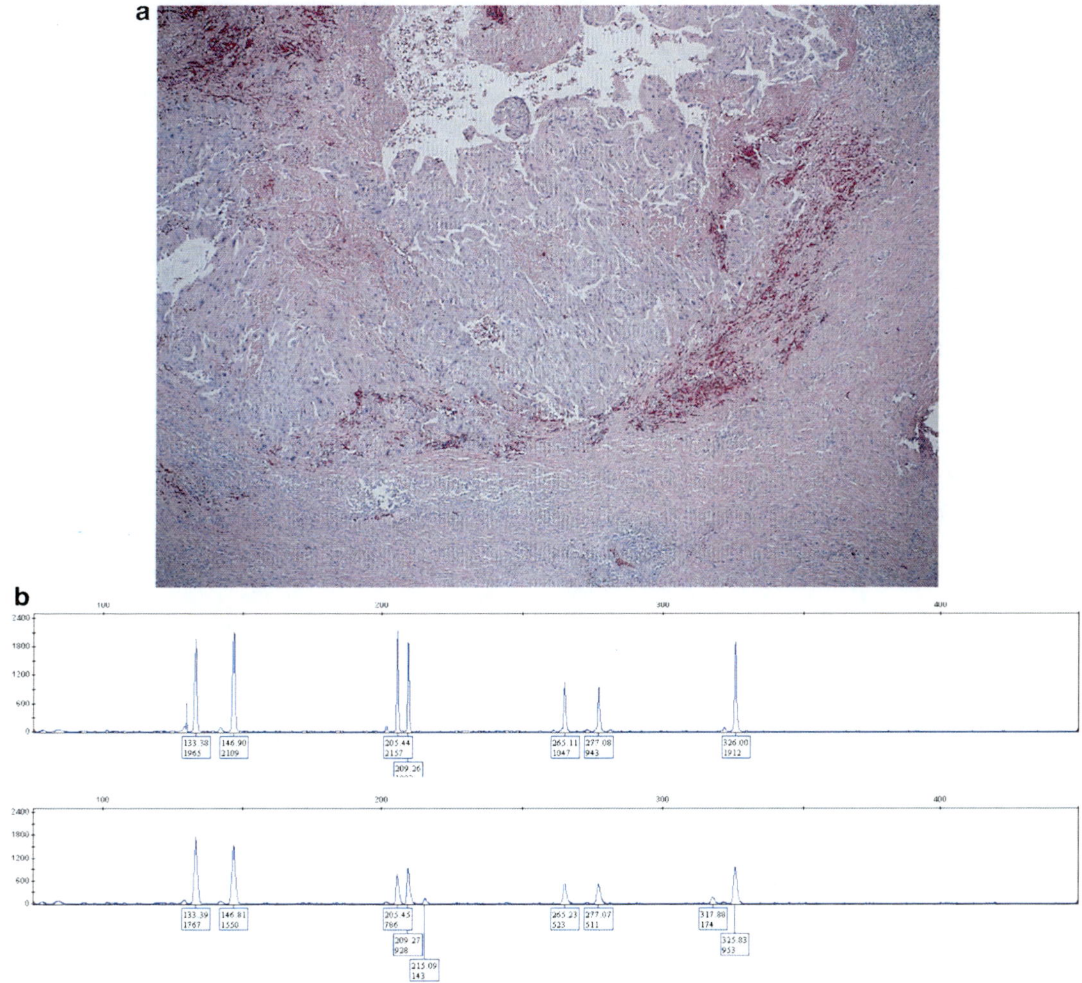

Fig 11.12 STR genotyping diagnosis of nongestational choriocarcinoma. (**a**) Histological features of a pure choriocarcinoma involving extrauterine sites (broad ligament and mesovarium). (**b**) DNA genotyping analysis by AmpFlSTR® Identifiler™ PCR. The tumor cells (*upper*) harbor identical alleles to the normal tissue of the patient (*lower*) at all four SRT loci, confirming a nongestational nature of the tumor

normal pregnancies. When in doubt, ancillary studies including immunohistochemistry and/or STR genotyping should be used to rule out a molar gestation. Recently, it has been confirmed that heterozygous (dispermic) complete moles are more aggressive than the homozygous (monospermic) ones in the development of post-molar gestational trophoblastic neoplasia [24, 25, 28]. Therefore, a precise genotyping of each complete mole may be clinically important for patient management and prognosis. In the presence of current ubiquitous diagnostic problems of partial molar pregnancies, adaptation of more precise diagnostic methods is essential for clinical diagnosis, epidemiology studies, and biological investigations. STR genotyping appears to be the best available method to resolve these issues.

P57^{KIP2} immunohistochemistry and DNA ploidy analysis are likely to remain as ancillary tests in a traditional pathology lab for some time to come. However, as described earlier, there are important confounding issues in the current diagnostic practice by these traditional means. With the increased cost-effectiveness and the diagnostic precision of STR genotyping, a "one-stop shopping" DNA genotyping approach has been advocated [12]. Whether community hospitals will be able to adapt this molecular power in the work-up of hydatidiform mole is depend on how rapidly the entire molecular medicine can be phased into clinical practice. Although a majority of early complete moles may be diagnosed with good accuracy by traditional methods (histological examination, p57^{KIP2} immunostain, and ploidy analysis), it is recommended that most of the partial mole cases should be diagnosed or confirmed by DNA genotyping for patient triage and clinical follow-up. Since an estimated 1/3 of partial mole diagnoses in current practice are in fact non-molar hydropic abortions [3], the money saved by avoiding over-treating non-molar patients should easily offset the overall cost of the molecular testing.

Conclusions

With the advent of closer monitoring of serum hCG and early ultrasound exams, most patients nowadays with hydatidiform moles present in their first trimester before the classic symptoms and ultrasound appearance develop. In the absence of typical clinical and imaging features, the role of the pathologist has become even more crucial in the diagnosis of molar pregnancy. However, histological evaluation continues to suffer significant diagnostic inaccuracy. Unacceptable inter- and intraobserver variability exists, even among expert pathologists. PCR-based STR DNA genotyping provides a powerful discriminatory capability to precisely diagnose and genetically subtype hydatidiform moles. This emerging molecular application is superior to the traditional ploidy flow cytometry and immunohistochemistry. With increasing acquirement of molecular diagnostic capabilities at most medical centers, STR DNA genotyping should become an integral part in the routine diagnostic algorithm of hydatidiform moles and beyond.

References

1. Hui P, Martel M, Parkash V. Gestational trophoblastic diseases: recent advances in histopathologic diagnosis and related genetic aspects. Adv Anat Pathol. 2005; 12(3):116–25.
2. Berkowitz RS, Goldstein DP. Clinical practice. Molar pregnancy. N Engl J Med. 2009;360(16):1639–45.
3. Genest DR. Partial hydatidiform mole: clinicopathological features, differential diagnosis, ploidy and molecular studies, and gold standards for diagnosis. Int J Gynecol Pathol. 2001;20(4):315–22.
4. Feltmate CM, Growdon WB, Wolfberg AJ, Goldstein DP, Genest DR, Chinchilla ME, et al. Clinical characteristics of persistent gestational trophoblastic neoplasia after partial hydatidiform molar pregnancy. J Reprod Med. 2006;51(11):902–6.
5. Fukunaga M, Katabuchi H, Nagasaka T, Mikami Y, Minamiguchi S, Lage JM. Interobserver and intraobserver variability in the diagnosis of hydatidiform mole. Am J Surg Pathol. 2005;29(7):942–7.
6. Howat AJ, Beck S, Fox H, Harris SC, Hill AS, Nicholson CM, et al. Can histopathologists reliably diagnose molar pregnancy? J Clin Pathol. 1993; 46(7):599–602. PMCID: 501384.
7. Javey H, Borazjani G, Behmard S, Langley FA. Discrepancies in the histological diagnosis of hydatidiform mole. Br J Obstet Gynaecol. 1979;86(6): 480–3.
8. Kajii T, Ohama K. Androgenetic origin of hydatidiform mole. Nature. 1977;268(5621):633–4.
9. Bifulco C, Johnson C, Hao L, Kermalli H, Bell S, Hui P. Genotypic analysis of hydatidiform mole: an accurate and practical method of diagnosis. Am J Surg Pathol. 2008;32(3):445–51.
10. McConnell TG, Murphy KM, Hafez M, Vang R, Ronnett BM. Diagnosis and subclassification of hydatidiform moles using p57 immunohistochemistry and molecular genotyping: validation and prospective analysis in routine and consultation practice settings with development of an algorithmic approach. Am J Surg Pathol. 2009;33(6):805–17.
11. Hui P. Molecular diagnosis of gestational trophoblastic disease. Expert Rev Mol Diagn. 2010;10(8): 1023–34.
12. Lipata F, Parkash V, Talmor M, Bell S, Chen S, Maric V, et al. Precise DNA genotyping diagnosis of hydatidiform mole. Obstet Gynecol. 2010;115(4):784–94.
13. Buza N, Hui P. Gestational trophoblastic disease: histopathological diagnosis in the molecular era. Diagnostic histopathology. In Press.
14. Szulman AE, Surti U. The syndromes of hydatidiform mole. I. Cytogenetic and morphologic correlations. Am J Obstet Gynecol. 1978;131(6):665–71.
15. Szulman AE. Syndromes of hydatidiform moles. Partial vs. complete. J Reprod Med. 1984;29(11): 788–91.
16. Jacobs PA, Angell RR, Buchanan IM, Hassold TJ, Matsuyama AM, Manuel B. The origin of human triploids. Ann Hum Genet. 1978;42(1):49–57.

17. Jacobs PA, Szulman AE, Funkhouser J, Matsuura JS, Wilson CC. Human triploidy: relationship between parental origin of the additional haploid complement and development of partial hydatidiform mole. Ann Hum Genet. 1982;46(Pt 3):223–31.
18. Fisher RA, Khatoon R, Paradinas FJ, Roberts AP, Newlands ES. Repetitive complete hydatidiform mole can be biparental in origin and either male or female. Hum Reprod. 2000;15(3):594–8.
19. Helwani MN, Seoud M, Zahed L, Zaatari G, Khalil A, Slim R. A familial case of recurrent hydatidiform molar pregnancies with biparental genomic contribution. Hum Genet. 1999;105(1–2):112–5.
20. Hayward BE, De Vos M, Talati N, Abdollahi MR, Taylor GR, Meyer E, et al. Genetic and epigenetic analysis of recurrent hydatidiform mole. Hum Mutat. 2009;30(5):E629–39.
21. Van den Veyver IB, Al-Hussaini TK. Biparental hydatidiform moles: a maternal effect mutation affecting imprinting in the offspring. Hum Reprod Update. 2006;12(3):233–42.
22. Hodges MD, Rees HC, Seckl MJ, Newlands ES, Fisher RA. Genetic refinement and physical mapping of a biparental complete hydatidiform mole locus on chromosome 19q13.4. J Med Genet. 2003;40(8):e95. PMCID: 1735575.
23. Kajii T, Ferrier A, Niikawa N, Takahara H, Ohama K, Avirachan S. Anatomic and chromosomal anomalies in 639 spontaneous abortuses. Hum Genet. 1980;55(1):87–98.
24. Wake N, Fujino T, Hoshi S, Shinkai N, Sakai K, Kato H, et al. The propensity to malignancy of dispermic heterozygous moles. Placenta. 1987;8(3):319–26.
25. Wake N, Seki T, Fujita H, Okubo H, Sakai K, Okuyama K, et al. Malignant potential of homozygous and heterozygous complete moles. Cancer Res. 1984;44(3):1226–30.
26. Davis JR, Surwit EA, Garay JP, Fortier KJ. Sex assignment in gestational trophoblastic neoplasia. Am J Obstet Gynecol. 1984;148(6):722–5.
27. Fisher RA, Lawler SD. Heterozygous complete hydatidiform moles: do they have a worse prognosis than homozygous complete moles? Lancet. 1984; 2(8393):51.
28. Baasanjav B, Usui H, Kihara M, Kaku H, Nakada E, Tate S, et al. The risk of post-molar gestational trophoblastic neoplasia is higher in heterozygous than in homozygous complete hydatidiform moles. Hum Reprod. 2010;25(5):1183–91.
29. Genest DR, Ruiz RE, Weremowicz S, Berkowitz RS, Goldstein DP, Dorfman DM. Do nontriploid partial hydatidiform moles exist? A histologic and flow cytometric reevaluation of nontriploid specimens. J Reprod Med. 2002;47(5):363–8.
30. Redline RW, Hassold T, Zaragoza MV. Prevalence of the partial molar phenotype in triploidy of maternal and paternal origin. Hum Pathol. 1998;29(5): 505–11.
31. Uchida IA, Freeman VC. Triploidy and chromosomes. Am J Obstet Gynecol. 1985;151(1):65–9.
32. Lage JM, Mark SD, Roberts DJ, Goldstein DP, Bernstein MR, Berkowitz RS. A flow cytometric study of 137 fresh hydropic placentas: correlation between types of hydatidiform moles and nuclear DNA ploidy. Obstet Gynecol. 1992;79(3):403–10.
33. Lage JM, Bagg A. Hydatidiform moles: DNA flow cytometry, image analysis and selected topics in molecular biology. Histopathology. 1996;28(4): 379–82.
34. Lage JM, Popek EJ. The role of DNA flow cytometry in evaluation of partial and complete hydatidiform moles and hydropic abortions. Semin Diagn Pathol. 1993;10(3):267–74.
35. Gschwendtner A, Neher A, Kreczy A, Muller-Holzner E, Volgger B, Mairinger T. DNA ploidy determination of early molar pregnancies by image analysis: comparison to histologic classification. Arch Pathol Lab Med. 1998;122(11):1000–4.
36. Zaragoza MV, Surti U, Redline RW, Millie E, Chakravarti A, Hassold TJ. Parental origin and phenotype of triploidy in spontaneous abortions: predominance of diandry and association with the partial hydatidiform mole. Am J Hum Genet. 2000;66(6): 1807–20. PMCID: 1378061.
37. Esteban JM, Sheibani K, Owens M, Joyce J, Bailey A, Battifora H. Effects of various fixatives and fixation conditions on DNA ploidy analysis. A need for strict internal DNA standards. Am J Clin Pathol. 1991; 95(4):460–6.
38. Cheville JC, Greiner T, Robinson RA, Benda JA. Ploidy analysis by flow cytometry and fluorescence in situ hybridization in hydropic placentas and gestational trophoblastic disease. Hum Pathol. 1995;26(7): 753–7.
39. Yver M, Carles D, Bloch B, Bioulac-Sage P, Martin Negrier ML. Determination of DNA ploidy by fluorescence in situ hybridization (FISH) in hydatidiform moles: evaluation of FISH on isolated nuclei. Hum Pathol. 2004;35(6):752–8.
40. Maggiori MS, Peres LC. Morphological, immunohistochemical and chromosome in situ hybridization in the differential diagnosis of Hydatidiform Mole and Hydropic Abortion. Eur J Obstet Gynecol Reprod Biol. 2007;135(2):170–6.
41. Lescoat D, Jouan H, Loeuillet-Olivo L, Le Calve M. Fluorescent in situ hybridization (FISH) on paraffin-embedded placental tissues as an adjunct for understanding the etiology of early spontaneous abortion. Prenat Diagn. 2005;25(4):314–7.
42. Surti U, Szulman AE, O'Brien S. Complete (classic) hydatidiform mole with 46, XY karyotype of paternal origin. Hum Genet. 1979;51(2):153–5.
43. Ohama K, Kajii T, Okamoto E, Fukuda Y, Imaizumi K, Tsukahara M, et al. Dispermic origin of XY hydatidiform moles. Nature. 1981;292(5823):551–2.
44. Ohama K, Okamoto E, Nomura K, Fujiwara A, Fukuda Y. Genetic studies of hydatidiform mole with 46, XY karyotype (author's transl). Nippon Sanka Fujinka Gakkai Zasshi. 1981;33(10):1664–8.

45. Fisher RA, Povey S, Lawler SD, Martin CA, Abeliovich D. The human chorionic gonadotrophin alpha subunit gene in gestational trophoblastic disease. 1. Restriction fragment length polymorphisms in hydatidiform moles. Dis Markers. 1987;5(4):237–45.
46. Ko TM, Hsieh CY, Ho HN, Hsieh FJ, Lee TY. Restriction fragment length polymorphism analysis to study the genetic origin of complete hydatidiform mole. Am J Obstet Gynecol. 1991;164(3):901–6.
47. Wallace DC, Surti U, Adams CW, Szulman AE. Complete moles have paternal chromosomes but maternal mitochondrial DNA. Hum Genet. 1982; 61(2):145–7.
48. Lawler SD, Pickthall VJ, Fisher RA, Povey S, Evans MW, Szulman AE. Genetic studies of complete and partial hydatidiform moles. Lancet. 1979;2(8142):580.
49. Fan JB, Surti U, Taillon-Miller P, Hsie L, Kennedy GC, Hoffner L, et al. Paternal origins of complete hydatidiform moles proven by whole genome single-nucleotide polymorphism haplotyping. Genomics. 2002;79(1):58–62.
50. Zhivotovsky LA, Bennett L, Bowcock AM, Feldman MW. Human population expansion and microsatellite variation. Mol Biol Evol. 2000;17(5):757–67.
51. Collins PJ, Hennessy LK, Leibelt CS, Roby RK, Reeder DJ, Foxall PA. Developmental validation of a single-tube amplification of the 13 CODIS STR loci, D2S1338, D19S433, and amelogenin: the AmpFlSTR Identifiler PCR Amplification Kit. J Forensic Sci. 2004;49(6):1265–77.
52. Abeln EC, Cornelisse CJ, Dreef EJ, Kuipers-Dijkshoorn NJ, Hogendoorn PC. Molecular identification of a partial hydatidiform mole. Diagn Mol Pathol. 1997;6(1):58–63.
53. Bell KA, Van Deerlin V, Addya K, Clevenger CV, Van Deerlin PG, Leonard DG. Molecular genetic testing from paraffin-embedded tissue distinguishes nonmolar hydropic abortion from hydatidiform mole. Mol Diagn. 1999;4(1):11–9.
54. Lai CY, Chan KY, Khoo US, Ngan HY, Xue WC, Chiu PM, et al. Analysis of gestational trophoblastic disease by genotyping and chromosome in situ hybridization. Mod Pathol. 2004;17(1):40–8.
55. Fukuyama R, Takata M, Kudoh J, Sakai K, Tamura S, Shimizu N. DNA diagnosis of hydatidiform mole using the polymerase chain reaction. Hum Genet. 1991;87(2):216–8.
56. Fisher RA, Newlands ES. Rapid diagnosis and classification of hydatidiform moles with polymerase chain reaction. Am J Obstet Gynecol. 1993;168(2): 563–9.
57. Popiolek DA, Yee H, Mittal K, Chiriboga L, Prinz MK, Caragine TA, et al. Multiplex short tandem repeat DNA analysis confirms the accuracy of p57(KIP2) immunostaining in the diagnosis of complete hydatidiform mole. Hum Pathol. 2006; 37(11):1426–34.
58. Murphy KM, McConnell TG, Hafez MJ, Vang R, Ronnett BM. Molecular genotyping of hydatidiform moles: analytic validation of a multiplex short tandem repeat assay. J Mol Diagn. 2009;11(6):598–605. PMCID: 2765760.
59. Van Deerlin VM, Leonard DG. Bone marrow engraftment analysis after allogeneic bone marrow transplantation. Clin Lab Med. 2000;20(1):197–225.
60. Nollet F, Billiet J, Selleslag D, Criel A. Standardisation of multiplex fluorescent short tandem repeat analysis for chimerism testing. Bone Marrow Transplant. 2001;28(5):511–8.
61. Fisher RA, Nucci MR, Thaker HM, Weremowicz S, Genest DR, Castrillon DH. Complete hydatidiform mole retaining a chromosome 11 of maternal origin: molecular genetic analysis of a case. Mod Pathol. 2004;17(9):1155–60.
62. McConnell TG, Norris-Kirby A, Hagenkord JM, Ronnett BM, Murphy KM. Complete hydatidiform mole with retained maternal chromosomes 6 and 11. Am J Surg Pathol. 2009;33(9):1409–15.
63. Baergen RN, Kelly T, McGinniss MJ, Jones OW, Benirschke K. Complete hydatidiform mole with a coexistent embryo. Hum Pathol. 1996;27(7):731–4.
64. Wax JR, Pinette MG, Chard R, Blackstone J, Do Cartin A. A. Prenatal diagnosis by DNA polymorphism analysis of complete mole with coexisting twin. Am J Obstet Gynecol. 2003;188(4):1105–6.
65. Makrydimas G, Sebire NJ, Thornton SE, Zagorianakou N, Lolis D, Fisher RA. Complete hydatidiform mole and normal live birth: a novel case of confined placental mosaicism: case report. Hum Reprod. 2002;17(9):2459–63.
66. Sebire NJ, Foskett M, Paradinas FJ, Fisher RA, Francis RJ, Short D, et al. Outcome of twin pregnancies with complete hydatidiform mole and healthy co-twin. Lancet. 2002;359(9324):2165–6.
67. Hoffner L, Dunn J, Esposito N, Macpherson T, Surti U. P57KIP2 immunostaining and molecular cytogenetics: combined approach aids in diagnosis of morphologically challenging cases with molar phenotype and in detecting androgenetic cell lines in mosaic/chimeric conceptions. Hum Pathol. 2008;39(1):63–72.
68. Gupta N, Mittal S, Misra R, Vimala N, Das AK. Placental site trophoblastic tumor originating in a tubal ectopic pregnancy. Eur J Obstet Gynecol Reprod Biol. 2006;129(1):92–4.
69. Su YN, Cheng WF, Chen CA, Lin TY, Hsieh FJ, Cheng SP, et al. Pregnancy with primary tubal placental site trophoblastic tumor–A case report and literature review. Gynecol Oncol. 1999;73(2):322–5.
70. Kuo KT, Chen MJ, Lin MC. Epithelioid trophoblastic tumor of the broad ligament: a case report and review of the literature. Am J Surg Pathol. 2004; 28(3):405–9.
71. El Hag IA, Ramesh K, Kollur SM, Salem M. Extrauterine placental site trophoblastic tumour in association with a lithopedion. Histopathology. 2002;41(5):446–9.
72. Xu ML, Yang B, Carcangiu ML, Hui P. Epithelioid trophoblastic tumor: comparative genomic hybridization and diagnostic DNA genotyping. Mod Pathol. 2009;22(2):232–8.
73. Zhao J, Xiang Y, Wan XR, Feng FZ, Cui QC, Yang XY. Molecular genetic analyses of choriocarcinoma. Placenta. 2009;30(9):816–20.

12 Clinical Aspects of Gestational Trophoblastic Disease

Christine E. Richter and Peter E. Schwartz

Keywords
Human chorionic gonadotropin • Methotrexate • EMA-CO • Hydatidiform mole • Choriocarcinoma

Introduction

Gestational trophoblastic disease (GTD) is a rare entity including hydatidiform moles, invasive moles, choriocarcinomas, placental site trophoblastic tumors (PSTTs), and epithelioid trophoblastic tumors (ETTs) [1–3]. All these conditions arise from the placental villous trophoblast [4]. Choriocarcinomas, PSTT, and ETT are also referred to as gestational trophoblastic neoplasia (GTN) because they can be associated with progressive or invasive disease [4].

GTD is primarily a disease of reproductive-aged women [3, 5, 6] and is associated with a prior gestational event [4]. There is a potential association between GTN and hormonal factors since women with menarche after age 12, light menstrual flow and prior oral contraceptive use have an increased risk of GTN in some studies [7, 8].

The cure rate of GTN is >90%, even if widespread disease is present, making it one of the most curable solid tumors [9, 10]. This high cure rate can be attributed to the presence of a sensitive tumor marker (human chorionic gonadotropin, hCG) for the initial detection, management, and early detection of recurrences; the high sensitivity of the tumors to chemotherapy, as well as the treatment and surveillance of patients in specialized centers [4, 6]. The treatment of PSTT and ETT remains more challenging than the other GTD conditions [11].

The incidence of GTD varies with geographic locations with a higher incidence in Asia compared to Europe or North America [4–6, 12]. In all populations, however, the incidence of hydatidiform moles and choriocarcinomas has decreased over the last three decades [4]. Clinical features of the various forms of GTD are presented in Table 12.1.

HCG, the marker for GTD, is a glycoprotein hormone composed of two non-covalently joined subunits, the alpha- and the beta-subunit [13, 14]. HCG is a diverse molecule with three distinct biological variants with different functions: regular hCG, hyperglycosylated hCG, and free beta-subunit of hyperglycosylated hCG [13].

C.E. Richter, MD • P.E. Schwartz, MD (✉)
Division of Gynecologic Oncology,
Department of Obstetrics, Gynecology & Reproductive Sciences, Yale University School of Medicine,
333 Cedar Street, New Haven, CT 06510, USA
e-mail: christine.richter@yale.edu; peter.schwartz@yale.edu

P. Hui (ed.), *Gestational Trophoblastic Disease: Diagnostic and Molecular Genetic Pathology*, Current Clinical Pathology, DOI 10.1007/978-1-61779-394-3_12,

Table 12.1 Clinical features of gestational trophoblastic disease

Gestational trophoblastic disease	Clinical features
Complete hydatidiform mole	15–20% trophoblastic sequelae hCG > 100,000 mIU/mL Medical complications
Partial hydatidiform mole	<5% trophoblastic sequelae hCG < 100,000 mIU/mL Rare medical complications
Invasive mole	15% metastatic (lung/vagina) Usually clinical diagnosis
Choriocarcinoma	Hematogenous spread (lung, brain, liver) Malignant disease
PSTT	Very rare hCG levels less reliable Relatively chemotherapy resistant Mainly surgical treatment
ETT	Very rare Mainly surgical treatments

Modified from Lurain [4]

Regular hCG is produced by the villous syncytiotrophoblast throughout most of the normal pregnancy. It helps maintain efficient placentation via angiogenesis in the myometrial spiral arteries [13]. It is also the predominant hCG variant in cases of complete and partial moles [15].

Hyperglycosylated hCG (hCG-H), a carbohydrate variant of hCG with double-size sugar side chains, is an autocrine factor produced by the extravillous invasive cytotrophoblast cells [13, 16]. HCG-H not only plays a role in implantation during normal pregnancy, but is also detectable in GTD where it seems to promote invasion, growth, and malignancy [13]. The proportion of hCG-H significantly rises as the total hCG rises in patients with GTD [17]. Assaying for hCG-H can help to differentiate invasive from non-invasive hydatidiform moles [13, 15].

The hyperglycosylated free beta-subunit of hCG (hCG free beta) acts as an anti-apoptotic factor in non-trophoblastic malignancies and is produced by PSTTs, a malignancy of non-villous trophoblast. HCG free beta may help distinguish PSTT from choriocarcinoma [15, 18]. In one series of 13 patients with PSTT, 60% of the total hCG immunoreactivity was due to hCG free beta with minimal or no hyperglycosylated hCG found in nine cases and 5–37% hyperglycosylated hCG found in the remaining four patients [18].

There are two conditions that are characterized by a low proportion of hyperglycosylated hCG: quiescent GTD and minimally invasive GTD [18]. Quiescent GTD is considered benign and inactive. It is defined by low persistent hCG levels with no increasing trend over a period of 3 or more months in the absence of disease by clinical evaluation or diagnostic imaging [16]. No hyperglycosylated hCG was identified in 127 of 133 women with quiescent GTD [17]. Minimally invasive GTD is usually slow growing and resistant to chemotherapy [17]. Hyperglycosylated hCG levels range from <1 to 39% in the latter condition [17].

Diagnosis

If there is clinical suspicion for the diagnosis of a GTD, a thorough history and physical exam should be performed [4]. This evaluation should include a complete blood count, coagulation studies, serum chemistries including renal and hepatic function tests, blood type with antibody screening and serum hCG levels [4]. As part of the work-up for metastatic disease, a chest X-ray should be performed [4]. CT scans of the abdomen and pelvis as well as the brain should be obtained if the chest radiograph shows evidence of metastatic disease [19, 20]. The risk of metastases outside of the lung with a normal physical examination and normal chest X-ray is low [4]. If the chest X-ray is normal, some experts recommend a chest CT scan as 40% of patients have pulmonary micrometastases undetectable on chest radiograph but detectable on chest CT scan [4]. These metastases do not affect outcome [19, 20].

When heterophilic antibodies cross-react with hCG assays and cause false-positive results, this is referred to as phantom hCG [21]. A urine pregnancy test can help differentiate a phantom hCG from a true hCG elevation since the large heterophilic antibodies do not cross the renal glomerular boundary and are therefore not detectable in the urine [21].

Hydatidiform Mole

Epidemiology Hydatidiform Moles

Hydatidiform moles are the most common form of GTD [22]. The incidence of GTD shows geographic variations [12, 23, 24]. In North America, Europe, Australia, and New Zealand, the incidence of hydatidiform moles ranges from 0.57 to 1.1/1,000 pregnancies, whereas the incidence in Southeast Asia and Japan has been reported to be as high as 2.0/1,000 pregnancies [4, 12]. Additionally, the incidence of hydatidiform moles is higher in American Indians, Eskimos, African Americans, and Hispanics [4]. The only environmental association that has been established in the etiology of molar pregnancies is an inverse relationship between β-carotene and animal fat dietary intake [25, 26].

Hydatidiform moles occur primarily in the reproductive age group, but molar pregnancies have been described in postmenopausal women [27]. Pregnancies at the extremes of maternal age and a history of a prior molar pregnancy are risk factors for complete hydatidiform moles [4]. The risk for women <21 years of age or >35 years of age of a hydatidiform mole is 1.9 times higher compared to women aged 21–35 [4]. The risk of a prior molar pregnancy increases the risk of a repeat molar pregnancy to 1–2%, 10–20 times that of the general population [28–30]. The risk of a third molar pregnancy after two molar pregnancies is as high as 15–20% [28–30]. Patients who have a hydatidiform mole must be made aware of this risk. Clinicians caring for a patient with a history of a hydatidiform mole should promptly evaluate the patient for a recurrence if she develops symptoms such as irregular vaginal bleeding. There are case reports of partial moles in ectopic pregnancies [31].

Partial vs. Complete Hydatidiform Moles

Based on their histology, karyotype, and natural history, hydatidiform moles can be complete or partial [5]. Partial moles have a triploid genome (usually 69,XXY), a result of the fertilization of a normal egg by two spermatozoa or the fertilization of one spermatozoa with duplication [32–34]. Complete moles are entirely paternal and arise from the fertilization of an empty egg by one spermatozoon with duplication or by the fertilization of an empty egg by two spermatozoa [5, 34–36]. The majority (90%) originate from the duplication of chromosomes after fertilization by a spermatozoa, resulting in a karyotype of 46,XX [35, 36]. The remainder of the complete moles arise from the fertilization by two spermatozoa and show a 46,XY or 46,XX karyotype [35, 36].

Clinical Presentation and Diagnosis of Hydatidiform Moles

The most common presentation of patients with a complete mole is vaginal bleeding in early pregnancy [4]. Partial moles tend to present later in the first or even second trimester since they grow slowly and can present as a missed or incomplete abortion [25, 37]. Today, the classic clinical findings of uterine enlargement, preeclampsia, hyperemesis, hyperthyroidism, and respiratory distress are rare because of the routine use of ultrasonography [38]. On ultrasound, complete moles show a "snowstorm" pattern representing a heterogeneous mass without a fetus present [39]. Ultrasound is associated with high false-positive and false-negative results, and molar pregnancies need to be differentiated from hydropic abortions (Fig. 12.1a, b) [40].

Treatment of Hydatidiform Moles

Patients with a suspected molar pregnancy who desire fertility preservation should undergo a suction dilation and curettage (D&C) (Fig. 12.2a) [41]. When performing the D&C, it is important to delay administering uterotonic agents until tissue is visualized in the suction D&C tubing. Molar tissue embolization to the lungs may otherwise occur. Rhesus-negative patients should

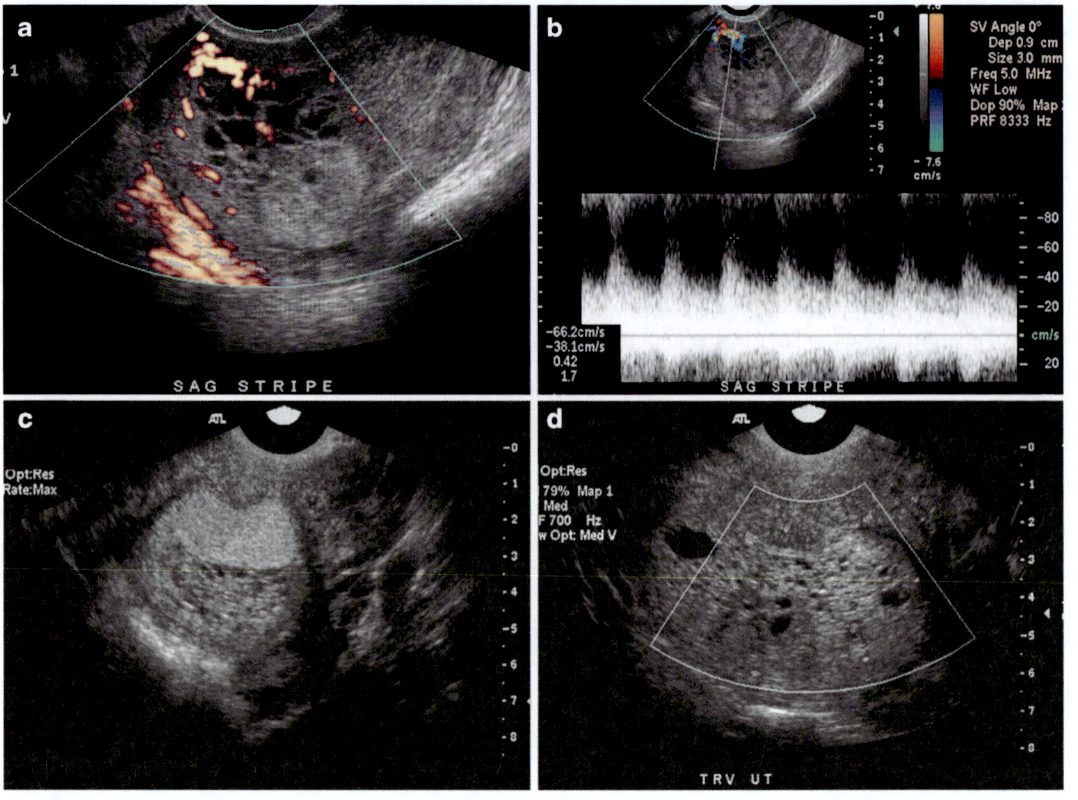

Fig. 12.1 (**a**) A power Doppler sagittal image of the uterus reveals an endometrial mass with numerous cystic areas consistent with the classic appearance of GTN. Note numerous blood vessels. (**b**) A spectral Doppler image demonstrates an increased peak systolic velocity (PSV) and end diastolic velocity (EDV) of patient in Fig. 11.1a with a low resistance index (RI) suggesting trophoblastic arterial flow. (**c**) Gray scale ultrasound image demonstrates an echogenic mass (*asterisk*) within the endometrial canal consistent with placental tissue in this pregnant patient. Note adjacent, more hypoechoic mass with numerous small cystic areas. Findings are most consistent with gestational trophoblastic tissue in a patient with a partial hydatidiform mole. (**d**) Color Doppler image of patient in (**c**) demonstrates a complex mass with numerous small cystic areas distending the endometrial canal. No blood flow is detected

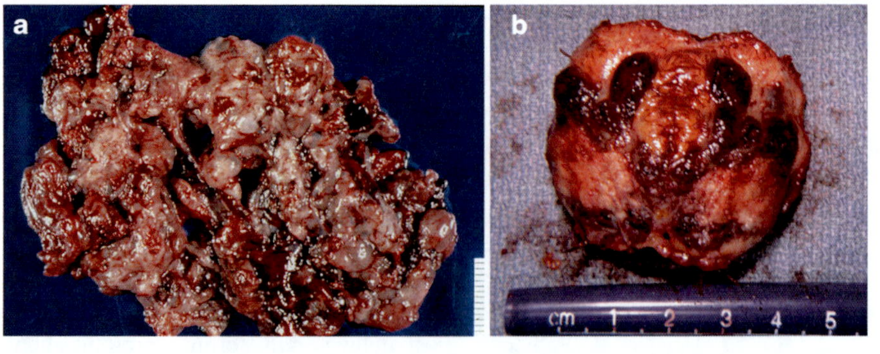

Fig. 12.2 (**a**) A complete hydatidiform mole. Molar tissue was obtained at the time of a D&C. Grossly visible vesicles are present. The patient's β-hCG levels normalized following the D&C. No malignant sequelae occurred in this patient following this procedure. (**b**) A 4 cm mass of choriocarcinoma excised from the patient's pelvis found by diagnostic imaging as a result of persistent hCG elevations despite the use of combination chemotherapy. Extensive hemorrhage is present

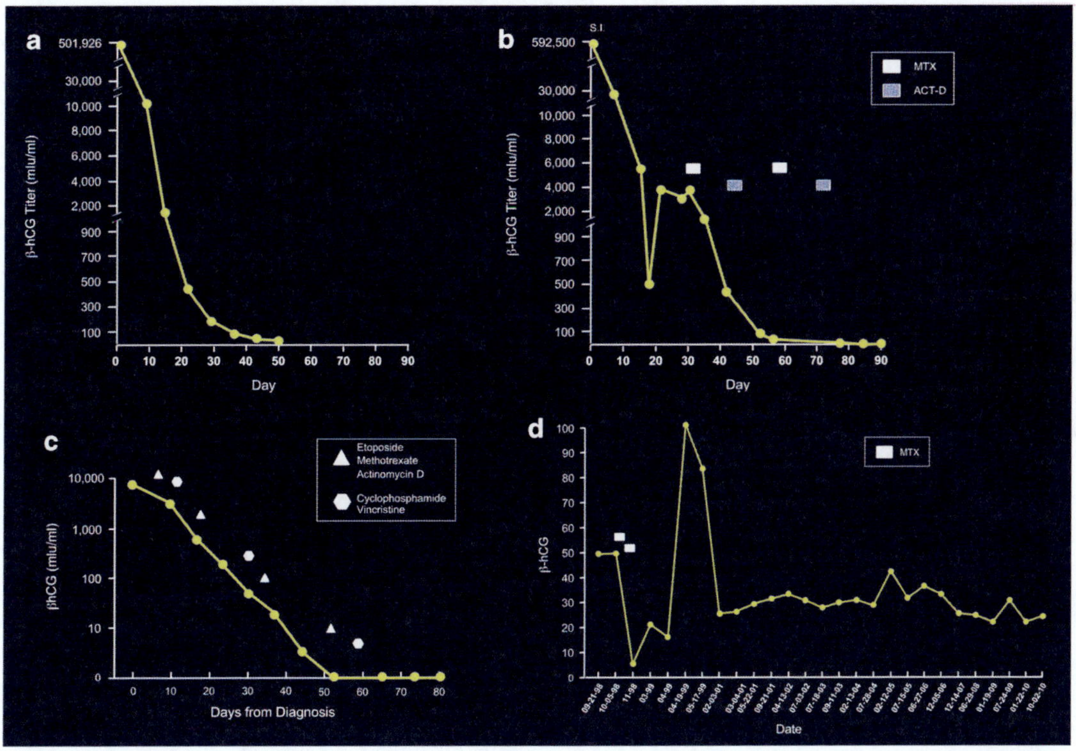

Fig. 12.3 β-hCG curves in different GTD conditions. (**a**) This 22-year-old woman underwent a suction D&C for a complete molar pregnancy. Her β-hCG titers returned to normal without any further intervention. (**b**) A 25-year-old woman underwent a suction D&C for management of a complete molar pregnancy. Her β-hCG titers initially decreased from 592,000 to about 500 mIU/mL and then rose to 4,000 mIU/mL. Diagnostic imaging revealed an isolated pulmonary metastasis. The patient received methotrexate and actinomycin-D in an alternate sequential fashion and rapidly normalized her titers. (**c**) An 18-year-old women was diagnosed to have high-risk metastatic choriocarcinoma. She was treated successfully with EMA-CO chemotherapy and preserved her fertility. (**d**) A 24-year-old nulliparous women presenting with menorrhagia was found to have a positive hCG (20 mIU/mL). An extensive work-up failed to reveal the presence of trophoblastic disease. The patient was given two treatments with methotrexate without any change in the hCG level. The patient was then referred to another institution where the hCG was 100 mIU/mL but the work-up was unremarkable. The patient was referred to Yale where the persistent mildly elevated level of hCG was confirmed, including a high level of urine beta-core fragment of hCG, but no lesions could be identified by diagnostic imaging. She has been followed more than 10 years, has had two full-term pregnancies during the observation period, and continues to have hCG levels in the 20 mIU/mL without receiving additional therapy

be given Rhesus prophylaxis at the time of the procedure [6]. Uterine evacuation leads to cure in about 80% of women with hydatidiform moles (Fig. 12.3a) [42].

In women who have completed childbearing or in cases of life-threatening hemorrhage, a hysterectomy may be indicated [42].

In 1 per 20,000–100,000 pregnancies, a healthy twin can develop along with the hydropic pregnancy [6]. Forty percent of these pregnancies lead to the delivery of a healthy infant [43]. There are no data supporting a higher risk of malignancy with later evacuation of the hydropic tissue [43].

Follow-Up After Hydatidiform Moles

Follow-up after the diagnosis of a molar pregnancy is important as it can result in persistent GTD in 3–4% of the patients with a partial and 20% of the patients with a complete mole

(Fig. 12.3b, c) [22]. Choriocarcinoma has never been reported after a partial mole [4]. Approximately 95% of patients with hydatidiform mole who develop GTN are diagnosed with low-risk GTN [6].

Gestational Trophoblastic Neoplasia

Choriocarcinoma, PSTT, and ETT are included in the group of GTN.

Diagnosis of GTN

At least one of the following factors needs to be present in order to diagnose postmolar GTN [4, 6, 44]:

- hCG plateau for four consecutive values over 3 weeks
- hCG rise of ≥10% for three values over 2 weeks
- hCG persistence 6 months after molar evacuation
- Histopathologic diagnosis of choriocarcinoma
- Presence of metastatic disease

While the majority of GTD are associated with elevations in hyperglycosylated hCG, the proportion of hyperglycosylated hCG levels can be very low in quiescent GTD, which is usually considered as clinically benign (Fig. 12.3d) [15]. Minimally invasive GTD is characterized by a very slow increase in hCG levels [15].

Staging of GTN

The International Federation of Gynecology and Obstetrics (FIGO) adopted a staging system for postmolar GTN in 2002 (Table 12.2) that combines anatomical staging and a modified World Health Organization (WHO) risk factor scoring system [45].

The stage of the disease consists of the FIGO stage in Roman numerals followed by the modified WHO score in Arabic numerals (Tables 11.3 and 12.2) [45]. PSTT and ETT are staged according to the FIGO staging system for GTD [46]. The WHO scoring system cannot be used for PSTT and ETT [46].

Table 12.2 FIGO staging for GTN

Stage	Description
I	Disease confined to uterus
II	Disease extends beyond uterus, but limited to genital structures (adnexal, vagina, broad ligament)
III	Disease extends to lungs with or without genital tract involvement
IV	Disease involves other metastatic sites

Reproduced with permission from Lurain [4]

Clinical Presentation GTN

The symptoms of patients with high-risk disease depend on the location of the metastases and can vary from seizures, headaches, or hemiparesis with brain metastases to hemoptysis, chest pain, and shortness of breath with lung metastases [47]. The work-up of patients with suspected high-risk GTD should include body CT, brain MRI, pelvic MRI, and Doppler ultrasonography [48]. Biopsies of any metastases should be avoided unless the lesions are easily accessible for control of bleeding since the lesions are highly vascularized [6].

With PSTT, most patients present with abnormal vaginal bleeding [11].

Choriocarcinoma

Just like hydatidiform moles, the incidence of choriocarcinomas (Fig. 12.2b) also varies based on the geographic location. In Europe and North America, choriocarcinomas are diagnosed in 1 in 40,000 pregnancies and 1 in 40 hydatidiform moles, while Southeast Asia and Japan show rates of 3.2/40,000 pregnancies, respectively [49]. The risk of choriocarcinoma is increased with a prior complete molar pregnancy (1,000 times more likely than after normal pregnancy), ethnicity, and advanced maternal age [4]. Women with the blood group A and a long-term use of contraceptives also seem to be at higher risk [4].

Choriocarcinoma originates from the villous trophoblast and secretes hCG [50]. It is chemotherapy-sensitive and highly curable [20]. Most young women diagnosed with choriocarcinoma and other

Table 12.3 FIGO scoring system GTN

	Score			
Risk factor	0	1	2	4
Age, years	≤39	>39	–	–
Antecedent pregnancy	Mole	Abortion	Term	–
Pregnancy event to treatment interval, mo	<4	4–6	7–12	>12
Pretreatment hCG, mIU/mL	$<10^3$	10^3–10^4	10^4–10^5	$>10^5$
Largest tumor mass, including uterus, cm	<3	3–4	≥5	–
Site of metastases	–	Spleen, kidney	GI tract	Brain, liver
Number of metastases	–	1–4	5–8	>8
Previous failed chemotherapy	–	–	Single drug	≥2 drugs

Reproduced with permission from Lurain [4]

GTDs can achieve a complete remission while preserving their fertility, even with metastatic disease (Table 12.4) [1, 3, 12, 22, 41].

PSTT

PSTT is extremely rare and originates from the intermediate-type trophoblast [51–54]. In the majority of patients, disease is confined to the uterus [52]. A literature review of 286 PSTT patients revealed that 17 (5.9%) were associated with retroperitoneal lymph node metastases [55]. Hematogenous dissemination to the brain, lung, liver, and conjunctiva has been reported [56]. However, in 10% of the patients with PSTT, metastatic disease is present at presentation [52, 53]. PSTTs secrete human placental lactogen (hPL) and hCG [51, 54].

An age >35 years, a pregnancy interval >24 months, an hCG > 1,000 IU/L, deep myometrial invasion and pathologic characteristics of the PSTT such as a high mitotic index, necrosis, and clear cytoplasm are associated with a worse survival [56].

In PSTT, the tumor load does not always correlate with the hCG levels. PSTT can present years after the last known pregnancy event [57].

ETT

ETT is very rare and is derived from the intermediate trophoblast [46, 58]. Available data are extremely limited, but metastases are reported to occur in 25% and death in 10% of patients diagnosed with ETT [58]. ETT may be found in the uterine cervix, and such lesions need to be distinguished from invasive squamous cell cancers [59].

Treatment of GTN

GTN is the most curable gynecologic malignancy [1] and is based on the stage of the disease according to the FIGO stage and the WHO scoring system [4].

Patients with stage I disease and low-risk metastatic GTN (FIGO stages II and III, WHO risk score <7) are treated with single-agent chemotherapy (Figs. 12.3b and 12.4) [4]. Survival rates for this group of patients approach 100%, and most patients can preserve their fertility [4]. Patients with high-risk metastatic disease (FIGO stage IV and stages II and III, WHO risk score ≥7) are treated with multiagent chemotherapy with or without radiation and surgery [4]. Cure rates for patients with high-risk disease range from 80 to 90% (Figs. 12.3d and 12.4) [4]. Indications for chemotherapy in the management of GTD are presented in Table 12.5.

Quiescent GTD does not require therapy, and minimally invasive GTD tends to be chemotherapy resistant [15].

Treatment of Low-Risk Disease

The data regarding the treatment of patients with GTN after hydatidiform mole with a second dilation and curettage are controversial, with some authors recommending a repeat curettage and

Table 12.4 Pregnancies after diagnosis of GTD

References	Patients	Procedure	Total number of pregnancies (*)	Attempted pregnancies after GTD	Live births after GTD	Preterm deliveries <36 w GA after GTD	Term deliveries after GTD	Recurrences	Deaths
Resection ± chemotherapy									
Behtash et al. [1]	1 CC	Craniotomy + EMA-EP + brain XRT	3	1	1	0	1	0	0
Liszka [103]	1 PSTT	Tumor resection	0	1	0	0	0	0	0
Pfeffer et al. [89]	1 PSTT	Partial hysterectomy + MTX/ EMA-CO/gemcitabine	NR	NR	NR	NR	NR	1	0
Rojas-Espaillat [102]	1 persistent GTD	Tumor resection + EMA-CO	NR	NR	NR	NR	NR	0	0
Machtinger et al. [51]	1 PSTT	Hysteroscopic resection + EMA-CO × 3 courses	NR	NR	NR	NR	NR	0	0
Tsuji et al. [54]	1 PSTT	Tumor resection + EMA-CO	NR	NR	NR	NR	NR	0	0
Case et al. [5]	1 persistent GTD	Tumor resection	2	1	2	0	2	0	0
Leiserowitz and Webb [52]	1 PSTT	Tumor resection	3	1	1	0	1	0	0
Total resection ± chemotherapy	5 PSTT, 2 persistent GTD, 1 CC		8	4	4	0	4	1	0
Chemotherapy									
Numnum et al. [53]	1 PSTT	EMA-EP	1	1	1	0	1	0	0
Goto et al. [3]	62 CC	MTX/MTX + actinomycin ± cyclophosphamide/etoposide/ etoposide + actinomycin	43	NR	36	NR	NR	NR	12
Total chemotherapy	1 PSTT, 62 CC		44	1	37	0	1	0	12
Total	6 PSTT, 2 persistent GTD, 63 CC		52	5	41	0	5	1	12

CC choriocarcinoma; *EMA-EP* etoposide, methotrexate, actinomycin – etoposide, cisplatinum; *XRT* radiation therapy; *EMA-CO* etoposide, methotrexate, actinomycin – cyclophosphamide, vincristine; *NR* not recorded

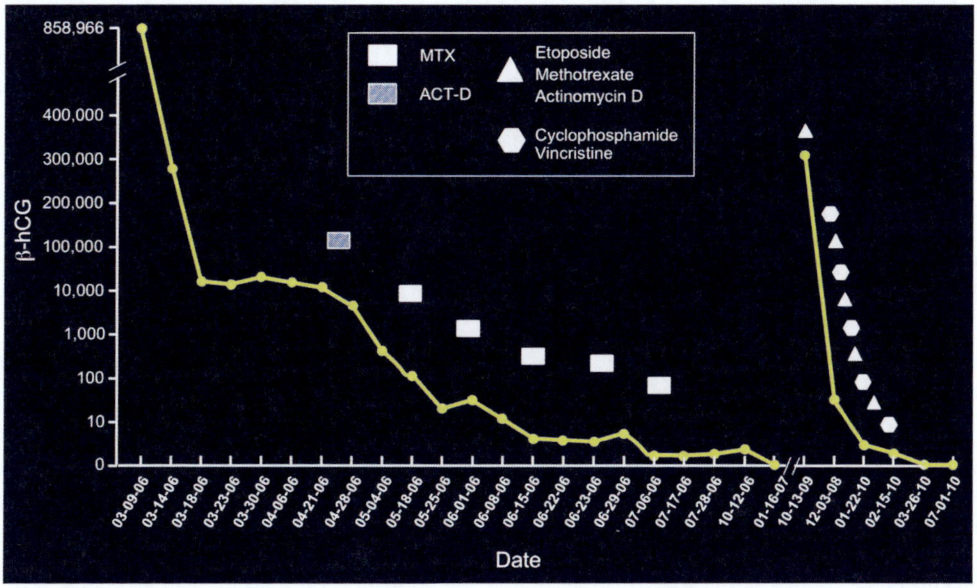

Fig. 12.4 A 32-year-old G4, P0 woman underwent a spontaneous abortion in January 2006. The patient was placed on oral contraceptives. The patient continued to have menometrorrhagia. A β-hCG in March 2006 was 858,966 mIU/mL. The patient underwent a suction D&C and was placed on actinomycin-D after her titers plateaued and then elevated. She developed severe facial acne with the first cycle of actinomycin-D. She was then successfully treated with methotrexate. The patient delivered a healthy child in July 2008. The patient experienced "constant bleeding" thereafter. A β-hCG titer was obtained in October 2009, which was 303,174 mIU/mL. She was then treated with EMA-CO, followed by a hysterectomy

Table 12.5 Indications for chemotherapy

Indications for chemotherapy for GTD
Plateaued or rising hCG concentrations after hydatidiform mole evacuation
Heavy vaginal bleeding or evidence of gastrointestinal or intraperitoneal hemorrhage
Histologic evidence of choriocarcinoma
Evidence of metastases in brain, liver, or gastrointestinal tract, or radiological opacities greater than 2 cm on chest radiograph
Serum hCG concentrations of 20,000 IU/L or more, 4 weeks or more after hydatidiform mole evacuation, because of the risk of uterine perforation
Raised hCG concentrations 6 months after evacuation, even when still decreasing

Modified from Seckl et al. [6]

others recommending chemotherapy [60–63]. Classically, the treatment for patients with low-risk GTN is single-agent methotrexate or actinomycin-D (Table 12.6) [64].

There are multiple different regimens of single-agent methotrexate or actinomycin-D (Table 12.6). Overall, the treatment regimens consisting of weekly IM or intermittent IV injections of methotrexate or the biweekly actinomycin-D injections are associated with a higher response rate [4]. In randomized studies comparing weekly IM methotrexate with biweekly actinomycin-D, however, there was a higher complete response rates with actinomycin-D (69–90 vs. 49–53%) [65–67].

The data regarding an improved efficacy of the 5-day IM methotrexate protocol compared to the 8-day methotrexate–folinic acid protocol for low-risk nonmetastatic disease is conflicting, and the few randomized studies are underpowered [68–70]. Kohorn described a higher remission rate with pulsed actinomycin-D compared to 5-day actinomycin [71].

Bone marrow suppression is associated with the use of methotrexate and with actinomycin-D. Stomatitis is the most common side effect of the treatment [4]. When comparing single-agent methotrexate or actinomycin-D regimens to

Table 12.6 Treatment of low-risk GTN

Chemotherapy regimen	Primary remission rate (%)
MTX 0.4 mg/kg (max 25 mg)/day IV or IM for 5 days, repeat every 14 days	87–93
MTX 30–50 mg/m^2 IM weekly	49–74
MTX 1 mg/kg IM d1, 3, 5, 7; folinic acid 0.1 mg/kg IM d2, 4, 6, 8; repeat every 15–18 days, or as needed	74–90
MTX 100 mg/m^2 IVP, then 200 mg/m^2 in 500 mL D5W over 12 h; folinic acid 15 mg IM or po q 12 h or 4 doses beginning 24 h after start of MTX; repeat every 18 days or as needed	69–90
Act-D 10–13 μg/kg IV qd for 5 days; repeat every 14 days	77–94
Act-D 1.25 mg/m^2 IV every 2 weeks	69–90
Alternating MTX/Act-D regimens 1 and 5	100

Reproduced with permission from Lurain [4]

combination regimens of the two drugs, efficiency remains unchanged, but side effects increase [72]. In general, in the setting of the high cure rates, the patient should be treated with the least toxic regimen first [6]. One advantage of methotrexate when compared to actinomycin is that it does not cause hair loss [73]. Two percent of women develop mouth ulcers, sore eyes, and very rarely serositis [74]. Severe acneiform rashes have been associated with actinomycin-D.

Increased chemotherapy resistance is detected in patients aged >35 years, patients with higher hCG levels >100,000 U/mL, a nonmolar antecedent pregnancy, large vaginal metastases, and a histopathological diagnosis of choriocarcinoma [75–77]. In total, 1–14% of the patients need multiagent chemotherapy after failed single-agent chemotherapy [73]. Based on the experience from three specialized centers in the United States, all patients who failed single-agent chemotherapy resistance were eventually cured (Figs. 12.3b, c and 12.5) [4].

Chemotherapy is continued until hCG values have returned to normal, and at least one course of chemotherapy has been administered after the first normal hCG [4]. Changing chemotherapy to another single agent is indicated if the hCG levels plateau above normal or if toxicity requires a change of agent [73].

Multi-agent chemotherapy is indicated in patients with hCG elevations, development of metastases, or resistance to sequential chemotherapy [78]. In persistent disease, a hysterectomy may be necessary [4].

Treatment of High-Risk Metastatic Disease

Patients with FIGO stage IV and stages II–III with WHO scores ≥7 should be considered high-risk GTN [4]. Because the risk of drug resistance is high and the chance of cure with monotherapy is low, the initial treatment for this group of patients is multiagent chemotherapy (Fig. 12.4) [79].

The primary regimen used today consists of etoposide, high-dose methotrexate with folinic acid, actinomycin-D, cyclophosphamide, and vincristine (EMA-CO) (Table 12.7) [80]. Complete response rates on that regimen range from 71 to 78%, and long-term survival rates range from 85 to 94% [81–87]. Metastases in the lung and the vagina tend to show a good response to chemotherapy [44].

Unlike in low-risk disease, the chemotherapy for high-risk disease is continued for two to three cycles after the first normal hCG level [49]. Reimaging is recommended after completion of treatment to assess the posttreatment disease status for future comparison [6]. There is no role for the removal of residual masses since it does not affect the risk of disease recurrence after treatment [88]. Overall, the recurrence risk is <3% [88]. According to a report from the John Brewer Trophoblastic Disease Center, the mortality rate of patients with high-risk disease ranges from 10 to 20% [44]. The survival of GTN patients with cerebral metastases is 26–44% [1].

Whole brain irradiation (3,000 cGy in 200-cGy fractions) is administered for central nervous

Table 12.7 Chemotherapy for high-risk disease

Day	Drug	Dosing
1	Etoposide	100 mg/m^2 IV over 30 min
	MTX	100 mg/m^2 IVP, then 200 mg/m^2 in 500 mL D5W over 12 h
	Actinomycin-D	0.5 mg IVP
2	Etoposide	100 mg/m^2 IV over 30 min
	Actinomycin-D	0.5 mg IVP
	Folinic acid	25 mg IM or PO every 12 h for 4 doses starting 24 h after start of MTX
8	Cyclophosphamide	600 mg/m^2 IV
	Vincristine	1.0 mg/m^2 IVP

Reproduced with permission from Lurain[4]
IV intravenous; *IVP* intravenous push

system metastases [4]. Alternatively, surgical excision with stereotactic irradiation or intrathecal methotrexate infusions can be offered [4]. The cure rates for patients with brain metastases range from 50 to 80% [4]. Survival depends on the number and size of metastases and their location in the brain [4]. Surgical resection of other metastatic disease may be necessary in about 50% of high-risk patients [4].

Thirty percent of patients only show an incomplete response after the initial multiagent chemotherapy or will relapse [73]. Patients with multiple metastatic sites are at particular risk for initial treatment failure [88]. In this group of patients, salvage chemotherapy with platinum or etoposide or surgical excision may be necessary [4]. These interventions will then cure the majority of resistant patients [4].

Treatment of PSTT and ETT

Compared to the other gestational trophoblastic tumors, PSTT and ETT grow more slowly, metastasize later and are chemotherapy resistant [51, 54]. They also produce less hCG than the other GTDs [89].

Hysterectomy with pelvic lymph node dissection is the treatment of choice for PSTT and ETT since these tumors may demonstrate lymphatic spread [51, 55]. Unless the patient is postmenopausal or has a family history of breast or ovarian cancer, the ovaries can be preserved [6]. In young women who want to preserve fertility, uterus-sparing treatment may be possible in select cases; however, only after careful counseling since multifocal uterine disease has been reported [51, 52, 54, 90]. The mortality rate of patients with PSTT is 10–20% [52, 54].

For patients with PSTT, conservative treatment can only be considered in a patient without evidence of extrauterine spread [52]. Patients >35 years of age with a pregnancy interval >24 months, an hCG > 1,000 IU/L, deep myometrial invasion, extensive necrosis, and the presence of cells with clear cytoplasm are poor candidates for successful conservative treatment. There are no data on fertility preservation in patients with ETT.

The role of adjuvant chemotherapy for PSTT and ETT has not been established [51]. PSTT seems to be more chemotherapy resistant than other GTN [57]. Chemotherapy is indicated in the presence of metastatic disease, deep myometrial invasion, tumor necrosis, and a mitotic count >6/10 high power field and if the interval from the last pregnancy exceeds 2 years [4, 44]. The chemotherapy regimens that are most commonly used are EMA-EP, and paclitaxel/cisplatin alternating with paclitaxel/etoposide (Table 12.8) [11]. Some authors, however, recommend the use of adjuvant chemotherapy even in patients with stage I disease [57]. The chemotherapy should be continued until the hCG levels have been negative for 8 weeks [11].

For patients with nonmetastatic PSTT, the survival is 90–100% compared to a survival of 50–60% in patients with metastatic disease [11, 44, 53, 54, 91]. In a study by Schmid et al. [11], only time from previous pregnancy to first treatment was predictive for survival in patients with PSTT, with significantly better survival if the time interval was <48 months, regardless of the stage of the

Table 12.8 Chemotherapy for PSTT and ETT

Regimen	Drug	Dosing
TP-TE	Paclitaxel	135 mg/m^2 IV over 3 h
	Cisplatin	60 mg/m^2 IV over 3 h
	Alternating with paclitaxel	135 mg/m^2 IV over 3 h
	Etoposide	150 mg/m^2 IV over 3 h every 2×8 weeks
EP-EMA	Etoposide	150 mg/m^2 IV over 3 h
	Cisplatin	60 mg/m^2 IV over 3 h
	Alternating every week with etoposide	100 mg/m^2 IV over 30 min
	Dactinomycin	0.5 mg IV bolus
	Methotrexate	300 mg/m^2 IV over 12 h

Modified from Lurain [4]
IV intravenous

disease. Recurrence of PSTT after chemotherapy has been reported [54]. Immunohistochemical studies have demonstrated the presence of epidermal growth factor receptor (EGFR) and vascular endothelial growth factor (VEGF) to be present PSTT, suggesting a role for molecularly targeted therapy in the treatment of recurrent disease [55].

Treatment Failure GTN

Lurain et al. [90] reviewed the patients with treatment failure from 1979 until 2006 prior to their presentation at the Brewer Trophoblastic Disease Center. The group identified use of single-agent chemotherapy in patients with high-risk disease and inappropriate use of weekly intramuscular methotrexate in patients with metastatic disease, FIGO scores ≥7, and/or non-postmolar choriocarcinoma as the main reasons for treatment failures [90]. With the appropriate secondary chemotherapy, survival of these patients was 100% with low-risk disease and 84% with high-risk disease [92]. This is due to the early detection of disease progression or relapse by rising hCG levels or imaging [93]. HCG has a short half-life of 48 h after complete surgical removal of the lesions [94]. A combination of paclitaxel–etoposide alternating with paclitaxel–cisplatin every 2 weeks seems to be well-tolerated and effective in the setting of drug-resistant disease [95]. A randomized trial comparing paclitaxel–etoposide alternating with paclitaxel–cisplatin and etoposide–cisplatin alternating with EMA has been proposed by the International Society of Trophoblastic Diseases (ISSTD) [95].

Follow-Up GTN

The treatment and surveillance of patients with GTD or neoplasia should take place in specialized centers [80].

After the treatment of GTN, hCG levels should be monitored until their return to normal [96]. After regression to normal, the hCG levels should be monitored weekly on a monthly basis for 12 months [96]. The risk of relapse in the first year after completion of chemotherapy is 3%, and contraception for 1 year is highly recommended [97]. The patients should undergo routine physical exams at intervals of 6–12 months [97]. Most chemotherapy side effects regress in a matter of weeks or months [97].

Many of the patients with GTD and GTN are of reproductive age, and fertility is an important concern. EMA-CO has been shown to advance the age of the onset of menopause by 3 years [1, 3, 98]. The pregnancy rate following treatment is 83% [99]. The data on congenital abnormalities with chemotherapy is conflicting, with some studies reporting no increase in the rate of congenital malformations [99, 100] and others quoting a higher rate of congenital heart abnormalities in the offspring of women previously treated with combination chemotherapy [3].

Effective contraception for 1 year after the completion of treatment and normalization of hCG levels also allows for regular hCG follow-up and the elimination of mature ova that may have been damaged by exposure to cytotoxic drugs [96, 99, 100]. Even if a pregnancy occurs within the first year after completion of treatment, most women have a favorable pregnancy outcome [97]. A pregnancy during the first 12 months after treatment should be monitored by ultrasonography, and hCG levels should be checked 6 and 10 weeks after delivery to ensure that there is no disease recurrence [97].

In subsequent pregnancies, the risk of GTD is 1–2% [97]. In any subsequent pregnancy, a pelvic ultrasound should be performed in the first trimester to confirm the presence of a normal gestation, and the hCG level should be checked 6 weeks after the completion of any pregnancy [4].

The risk of secondary malignancies has not been shown to be increased with methotrexate monotherapy, but Rustin et al. [101] reported a significant increase with etoposide-containing combination chemotherapies.

References

1. Behtash N, Behnamfar F, Hamedi B, Ramzanzadeh F. Term delivery following successful treatment of choriocarcinoma with brain metastases, a case report and review of literature. Arch Gynecol Obstet. 2009;279:579–81.
2. Schorge JO, Goldstein DP, Bernstein MR, Berkowitz RS. Gestational trophoblastic disease. Curr Treat Options Oncol. 2000;1:169–75.
3. Goto S, Ino K, Mitsui T, Kikkawa F, Suzuki T, Nomura S, et al. Survival rates of patients with choriocarcinoma treated with combination chemotherapy without hysterectomy: effects of anticancer agents on subsequent births. Gynecol Oncol. 2004;93:529–35.
4. Lurain JR. Gestational trophoblastic disease II: classification and management of gestational trophoblastic neoplasia. Am J Obstet Gynecol. 2011; 204(1):11–8.
5. Case AM, Wilson S, Colgan TJ, Greenblatt EM. Fertility-sparing surgery, with subsequent pregnancy, in persistent gestational trophoblastic disease. Hum Reprod. 2001;16:360–4.
6. Seckl MJ, Sebire NJ, Berkowitz RS. Gestational trophoblastic disease. Lancet. 2010;376:717–29.
7. Palmer JR, Driscoll SG, Rosenberg L, et al. Oral contraceptive use and risk of gestational trophoblastic tumors. J Natl Cancer Inst. 1999;91:635–40.
8. Buckley JD, Henderson BE, Morrow CP, Hammond CB, Kohorn EI, Austin DF. Case-control study of gestational choriocarcinoma. Cancer Res. 1988;48: 1004–10.
9. Newlands ES, Bagshawe KD, Begent RH, Rustin GJ, Holden L. Results with EMA/CO (etoposide, methotrexate, actinomycin D, cyclophosphamide, vincristine) regimen in high risk gestational trophoblastic tumours. Br J Obstet Gynaecol. 1991;98: 550–7.
10. Kim SJ, Bae SN, Kim JH, et al. Effects of multiagent chemotherapy and independent risk factors in the treatment of high-risk GTT-25 years experiences of KRI-TRD. Int J Gynaecol Obstet. 1998;60:S85–96.
11. Schmid P, Nagai Y, Agarwal R, et al. Prognostic markers and long-term outcome of placental-site trophoblastic tumours: a retrospective observational study. Lancet. 2009;374:48–55.
12. Horowitz NS, Goldstein DP, Berkowitz RS. Management of gestational trophoblastic neoplasia. Semin Oncol. 2009;36:181–9.
13. Cole LA. New discoveries on the biology and detection of human chorionic gonadotropin. Reprod Biol Endocrinol. 2009;7(8):1–37.
14. Swaminathan N, Bahl OP. Dissociation and recombination of the subunits of human chorionic gonadotropin. Biochem Biophys Res Commun. 1970;40: 422–7.
15. Muller CY, Cole LA. The quagmire of hCG and hCG testing in gynecologic oncology. Gynecol Oncol. 2009;112:663–72.
16. Cole LA, Bulter SA, Khanlian SA, et al. Gestational trophoblastic diseases: 2. Hyperglycosylated hCG as a reliable marker of active neoplasia. Gynecol Oncol. 2006;102:151–9.
17. Cole LA, Muller CY. Hyperglycosylated hCG in the management of quiescent and chemorefractory gestational trophoblastic diseases. Gynecol Oncol. 2010;116:3–9.
18. Cole LA, Khanlian SA, Muller CY, Giddings A, Kohorn E, Berkowitz R. Gestational trophoblastic diseases: 3. Human chorionic gonadotropin-free β-subunit, a reliable marker of placental site trophoblastic tumors. Gynecol Oncol. 2006;102:160–4.
19. Ngan HY, Chan FL, Au VW, Cheng DK, Ng TY, Wong LC. Clinical outcome of micrometastasis in the lung in stage IA persistent gestational trophoblastic disease. Gynecol Oncol. 1998;70:192–4.
20. Darby S, Jolley I, Pennington S, Hancock BW. Does chest CT matter in the staging of GTN? Gynecol Oncol. 2009;112:155–60.
21. Cole LA, Khanlian SA. The need for a quantitative urine hGC assay. Clin Biochem. 2009;42:676–83.
22. Thirumagal B, Sinha D, Raghavan R, Bhatti N. Gestational trophoblastic neoplasia: are we compliant with the standards? J Obstet Gynecol. 2009; 29:434–6.
23. Bracken MB. Incidence and aetiology of hydatidiform mole: an epidemiological review. Br J Obstet Gynaecol. 1987;94:1123–35.

24. Palmer JR. Advances in the epidemiology of gestational trophoblastic disease. J Reprod Med. 1994;39: 155–62.
25. Berkowitz RS, Cramer DW, Bernstein MR, Cassells S, Driscoll SG, Goldstein DP. Risk factors for complete molar pregnancy from a case-control study. Am J Obstet Gynecol. 1985;152:1016–20.
26. Parazzini F, La Vecchia C, Mangili G, et al. Dietary factors and risk of trophoblastic disease. Am J Obstet Gynecol. 1988;158:93–9.
27. Abike F, Temizkan O, Payasli A, Avsar F, Karahan N, Baspinar S. Postmenopausal complete hydatidiform mole: a case report. Maturitas. 2008;59:95–8.
28. Bagshawe KD, Dent J, Webb J. Hydatidiform mole in England and Wales 1973–1983. Lancet. 1986; 328:673–7.
29. Garrett LA, Garner EI, Feltmate CM, Goldstein DP, Berkowitz RS. Subsequent pregnancy outcomes in patients with molar pregnancy and persistent gestational trophoblastic neoplasia. J Reprod Med. 2008; 53:481–6.
30. Sebire NJ, Fisher RA, Foskett M, Rees H, Seckl MJ, Newlands ES. Risk of recurrent hydatidiform mole and subsequent pregnancy outcome following complete or partial hydatidiform molar pregnancy. BJOG. 2003;110:22–6.
31. Ghazi GF, Donovan PO. Partial mole in ectopic pregnancy. Gynecol Surg. 2006;3:141–3.
32. Szulman A, Surti U. The syndromes of hydatidiform mole. I. Cytogenetic and morphological correlations. Am J Obstet Gynecol. 1978;113:665–71.
33. Lawler SD, Fisher RA, Dent J. A prospective genetic study of complete and partial hydatidiform moles. Am J Obstet Gynecol. 1991;164:1270–7.
34. Lipata F, Parkash V, Talmor M, Bell S, Chen S, Maric V, et al. Precise DNA genotyping diagnosis of hydatidiform mole. Obstet Gynecol. 2010;115:784–94.
35. Kajii T, Ohama K. Androgenetic origin of hydatidiform mole. Nature. 1977;268:633–4.
36. Fisher RA, Newlands ES. Gestational trophoblastic disease: molecular and genetic studies. J Reprod Med. 1998;43:81–97.
37. Czernobilsky B, Barash A, Lancet M. Partial moles: a clinicopathologic study of 25 cases. Obstet Gynecol. 1982;59:75–7.
38. Hou JL, Wan XR, Xiang Y, Qi QW, Yang XY. Changes of clinical features in hydatidiform mole: analysis of 113 cases. J Reprod Med. 2008;53: 629–33.
39. Santos-Ramos R, Forney JP, Schwartz BE. Sonographic findings and clinical correlations in molar pregnancy. Obstet Gynecol. 1980;56:186–92.
40. Sebire NJ, Fisher RA, Rees HC. Histopathological diagnosis of partial and complete hydatidiform mole in the first trimester of pregnancy. Pediatr Dev Pathol. 2003;6:69–77.
41. Berkowitz RS, Goldstein DP. Current management of gestational trophoblastic diseases. Gynecol Oncol. 2009;1122:654–62.
42. Elias K, Goldstein DP, Berkowitz RS. Complete hydatidiform mole in women older than age 50. J Reprod Med. 2009;55:208–12.
43. Seckl MJ, Dhillon T, Dancey G, et al. Increased gestational age at evacuation of a complete hydatidiform mole: does it correlate with increased risk of requiring chemotherapy? J Reprod Med. 2004;49: 527–30.
44. Khoo SK, Sidhu M, Baartz D, Yip WL, Tripcony L. Persistence and malignant sequelae of gestational trophoblastic disease: clinical presentation, diagnosis, treatment and outcome. Aust N Z J Obstet Gynecol. 2010;50:81–6.
45. Kohorn EI. Negotiating a staging and risk factor scoring system for gestational trophoblastic neoplasia. A progress report. J Reprod Med. 2002;47: 445–50.
46. Behtash N, Zarchi MK. Placental site trophoblastic tumor. J Cancer Res Clin Oncol. 2008;134:1–6.
47. Seckl MJ, Rustin GJS, Newlands ES, Gwyther SJ, Bomanji J. Pulmonary embolism, pulmonary hypertension, and choriocarcinoma. Lancet. 1991;338:1313–5.
48. Newlands ES, Holden L, Seckl M, McNeish I, Strickland S, Rustin GJ. Management of brain metastases in patients with high-risk gestational trophoblastic tumors. J Reprod Med. 2002;47:465–71.
49. Ngan S, Seckl MJ. Gestational trophoblastic neoplasia management: an update. Curr Opin Oncol. 2007;19:486–91.
50. Sebire NJ, Lindsay I. Current issues in the histopathology of gestational trophoblastic tumors. Fetal Pediatr Pathol. 2010;29:30–44.
51. Machtinger R, Gotlieb WH, Korach J, Fridman E, Apter S, Goldenberg M, et al. Placental site trophoblastic tumor: outcome of five cases including fertility preserving management. Gynecol Oncol. 2005; 96:56–61.
52. Leiserowitz GS, Webb MJ. Treatment of placental site trophoblastic tumor with hysterotomy and uterine reconstruction. Obstet Gynecol. 1996;88: 696–9.
53. Numnum TM, Kilgore LC, Conner MG, Strughn JM. Fertility sparing therapy in a patient with placental site trophoblastic tumor: a case report. Gynecol Oncol. 2006;103:1141–3.
54. Tsuji Y, Tsubamoto H, Hori M, Ogasawara T, Koyama K. Case of PSTT treated with chemotherapy followed by open uterine tumor resection to preserve fertility. Gynecol Oncol. 2002;87:303–7.
55. Lan C, Li Y, He J, Liu J. Placental site trophoblastic tumor: lymphatic spread and possible target markers. Gynecol Oncol. 2010;116:430–7.
56. Chatterjee S, Hancock BW, Suvarna SK, et al. Placental site trophoblastic tumor – a rare cause of recurrent spontaneous pneumothoraces and conjunctival metastasis. J R Coll Physicians Edinb. 2009; 39:129–33.
57. Kohorn EI. Long-term outcome of placental-site trophoblastic tumors. Lancet. 2009;374:6–7.

58. Lo C, Low I, Tan AL, Baranyai J. Epithelioid trophoblastic tumor: a case report. Int J Gynecol Cancer. 2006;16:1473–6.
59. Phippen NT, Lowery WJ, Leath III CA, Kost ER. Epithelioid trophoblastic tumor masquerading as invasive squamous cell carcinoma of the cervix after an ectopic pregnancy. Gynecol Oncol. 2010;117:387–8.
60. Pezeshki M, Hancock BW, Silcocks P, et al. The role of repeat uterine evacuation in the management of persistent gestational trophoblastic disease. Gynecol Oncol. 2005;95:423–9.
61. Van Trommel NEM, Massuger LF, Verheijen RH, et al. The curative effect of a second curettage in persistent trophoblastic disease: a retrospective cohort survey. Gynecol Oncol. 2005;99:6–13.
62. Garner EI, Feltmate CM, Goldstein DP, et al. The curative effect of a second curettage in persistant trophoblastic disease: a retrospective cohort survey. Gynecol Oncol. 2005;99:3–5.
63. Savage P, Seckl MJ. The role of repeat uterine evacuation in trophoblast disease. Gynecol Oncol. 2005;99:251–2.
64. Alazzam M, Tidy J, Hancock BW, et al. First line chemotherapy in low risk gestational trophoblastic neoplasia. Cochrane Database Syst Rev. 2009;1: CD007102.
65. Gilani MM, Yarandi F, Eftekhar Z, et al. Comparison of pulse methotrexate and pulse actinomycin D in the treatment of low-risk gestational trophoblastic neoplasia. Aust N Z J Obstet Gynecol. 2005; 45:161–4.
66. Yarandi F, Eftekhar Z, Shojaei H, et al. Pulse methotrexate versus pulse actinomycin D in the treatment of low-risk gestational trophoblastic neoplasia. Int J Gynecol Obstet. 2008;103:33–7.
67. Osborne R, Filiaci M, Schink J, et al. A randomized phase III trial comparing weekly parenteral methotrexate and "pulsed" actinomycin as primary management for low-risk gestational trophoblastic neoplasia: a Gynecologic Oncology Group study. Gynecol Oncol. 2008;108:52.
68. Lertkhachonsuk AA, Israngura N, Wilailak S, et al. Actinomycin D versus methotrexate-folinic acid as the treatment of stage I, low-risk gestational trophoblastic neoplasia: a randomized controlled trial. Int J Gynecol Cancer. 2009;19:985–8.
69. Wong LC, Choo YC, Ma HK. Methotrexate with citrovorum factor rescue in gestational trophoblastic disease. Am J Obstet Gynecol. 1985;152:59–62.
70. Gleeson NC, Finan MA, Fiorica JV, et al. Nonmetastatic gestational trophoblastic disease: weekly methotrexate compared with 8-day methotrexate-folinic acid. Eur J Gynecol Oncol. 1993; 14:461–5.
71. Kohorn EI. Decision making for chemotherapy administration in patients with low-risk gestational trophoblastic disease. Int J Gynecol Cancer. 1996; 6:279–85.
72. Abrao RA, de Andrade JM, Tiezzi DG, et al. Treatment for low-risk gestational trophoblastic disease: comparison of single-agent methotrexate, dactinomycin and combination regimens. Gynecol Oncol. 2008;108:149–53.
73. Berkowitz RS, Goldstein DP, Bernstein MR. Ten year's experience with methotrexate and folinic acid as primary therapy for gestational trophoblastic disease. Gynecol Oncol. 1986;112:353–7.
74. McNeish IKA, Strickland S, Holden L, et al. Low risk persistent gestational trophoblastic disease: outcome following initial treatment with low-dose methotrexate and folinic acid, 1992–2000. J Clin Oncol. 2002;20:1838–44.
75. DuBeshter B, Berkowitz RS, Goldstein DP. Management of low-risk gestational trophoblastic tumors. J Reprod Med. 1991;36:36–9.
76. Soper JT, Clarke-Pearson DL, Berchuk A, et al. Five-day methotrexate for women with metastatic gestational trophoblastic disease. Gynecol Oncol. 1994;54:76–9.
77. Roberts JP, Lurain JR. Treatment of low-risk metastatic gestational trophoblastic tumors with single-agent chemotherapy. Am J Obstet Gynecol. 1996; 174:1917–24.
78. McGrath S, Short D, Harvey R. The management and outcome of women with post-hydatidiform mole "low-risk" gestational trophoblastic neoplasia, but hCG levels in excess of 100 000 IU L^{-1}. Br J Cancer. 2010;102:810–4.
79. Bagshawe KD. Treatment of trophoblastic tumours. Recent results. Cancer Res. 1977;62:192–9.
80. Newlands ES, Mulholland PJ, Holden L, Seckl MJ, Rustin GJS. Etoposide and cisplatin/etoposide, methotrexate, and actinomycin D (EMA) chemotherapy for patients with high-risk gestational trophoblastic tumor refractory to EMA/cyclophosphamide and vincristine chemotherapy and patients presenting with metastatic placental site trophoblastic tumors. J Clin Oncol. 2000;18:854–9.
81. Bolis G, Bonazzi C, Landoni F, et al. EMA/CO regimen in high-risk gestational trophoblastic tumor (GTT). Gynecol Oncol. 1988;31:439–44.
82. Bower M, Newlands ES, Holden L, et al. EMA/CO for high-risk gestational trophoblastic disease: results from a cohort of 272 patients. J Clin Oncol. 1997;15:2636–43.
83. Matsui H, Suzuka K, Iitsuka Y, et al. Combination therapy with methotrexate, etoposide and actinomycin D for high-risk gestational trophoblastic tumors. Gynecol Oncol. 2000;78:28–31.
84. Escobar PF, Lurain JR, Singh DK, et al. Treatment of high-risk gestational trophoblastic neoplasia with etoposide, methotrexate, actinomycin D, cyclophosphamide, and vincristine chemotherapy. Gynecol Oncol. 2003;91:552–7.
85. Lurain JR, Singh DK, Schink JC, et al. Primary treatment of metastatic high-risk gestational tropho-

blastic neoplasia with EMA-CO chemotherapy. J Reprod Med. 2006;51:767–72.
86. Turan T, Karacay O, Tulunay G, et al. Results with EMA/CO (etoposide, methotrexate, actinomycin D, cyclophosphamide, vincristine) chemotherapy in gestational trophoblastic neoplasia. Int J Gynecol Cancer. 2006;16:1432–8.
87. Lu WG, Ye F, Shen YM, et al. EMA-CO chemotherapy for high-risk gestational trophoblastic neoplasia: a clinical analysis of 54 patients. Int J Gynecol Cancer. 2008;18:357–62.
88. Yang J, Xiang Y, Wan X, Yang X. The prognosis of gestational trophoblastic neoplasia patient with residual lung tumor after completing treatment. Gynecol Oncol. 2006;103:479–82.
89. Pfeffer PE, Sebire N, Lindsay I, et al. Fertility-sparing partial hysterectomy for placental-site tumor. Lancet Oncol. 2007;8:744–6.
90. Lurain JR, Hoekstra AV, Schink JC. Results of treatment of patients with gestational trophoblastic neoplasia referred to the Brewer Trophoblastic Disease Center after failure of treatment elsewhere (1979–2006). J Reprod Med. 2008;53:535–40.
91. Baergen RB, Rutgers JL, Young RH, Osann K, Scully RE. Placental site trophoblastic tumor: a study of 55 cases and review of the literature emphasizing factors of prognostic significance. Gynecol Oncol. 2006;100:511–20.
92. Powles T, Savage PM, Stebbing J, et al. A comparison of patients with relapsed and chemo-refractory gestational trophoblastic neoplasia. Br J Cancer. 2007;96:732–7.
93. Newlands EY. The management of recurrent and drug-resistant gestational trophoblastic neoplasia (GTN). Best Pract Res Clin Obstet Gynaecol. 2003;17:905–23.
94. Wang J, Short D, Sebire NJ, et al. Salvage chemotherapy of relapsed or high-risk gestational trophoblastic neoplasia (GTN) with paclitaxel/cisplatin alternating with paclitaxel/etoposide (TP/TE). Ann Oncol. 2008;19:1578–83.
95. Woolas RP, Bower M, Newlands ES, et al. Influence of chemotherapy for gestational trophoblastic disease on subsequent pregnancy outcome. Br J Obstet Gynecol. 1998;105:1032–5.
96. Blagden SP, Foskett MA, Fisher RA, et al. The effect of early pregnancy following chemotherapy on disease relapse and foetal outcome in women treated for gestational trophoblastic tumours. Br J Cancer. 2002;86:26–30.
97. Bower M, Rustin GJS, Newlands ES, et al. Chemotherapy for gestational trophoblastic tumors hastens menopause by 3 years. Eur J Cancer. 1998;34:1204–7.
98. Rustin GJS, Booth M, Dent J, et al. Pregnancy after cytotoxic chemotherapy for gestational trophoblastic tumors. Br Med J. 1984;288:103–6.
99. Matsui H, Iitsuka Y, Suzuka K, et al. Early pregnancy outcomes after chemotherapy for gestational trophoblastic tumor. J Reprod Med. 2004;49:531–4.
100. Garrett LA, Garner EI, Feltmate CM, et al. Subsequent pregnancy outcomes in patients with molar pregnancy and persistent gestational trophoblastic neoplasia. J Reprod Med. 2008;53:481–6.
101. Rustin GJS, Newlands ES, Lutz JM, et al. Combination but not single agent methotrexate chemotherapy for gestational trophoblastic tumors (GTT) increases the incidence of second tumors. J Clin Oncol. 1996;14:2769–73.
102. Rojas-Espaillat L, Houck KL, Hernandez E, Berkowitz RS. Fertility-sparing surgery for persistent gestational trophoblastic neoplasia in the myometrium: a case report. J Reprod Med. 2007;52(5):431–4.
103. Liszka L, Wilk M, Wodolazski A, Palen P, Sikora J. Successful treatment of placental site trophoblastic tumor in twin pregnancy without hysterectomy. Tumori. 2009;95(1):108–11.

Appendix

P. Hui (ed.), *Gestational Trophoblastic Disease: Diagnostic and Molecular Genetic Pathology*, Current Clinical Pathology, DOI 10.1007/978-1-61779-394-3,

Gestational Trophoblastic Tumors Staging Form

Clinical *Extent of disease before any treatment*	Stage Category Definitions		Pathologic *Extent of disease through completion of definitive surgery*
❑ y clinical – staging completed after neoadjuvant therapy but before subsequent surgery	Tumor Size: ______	Laterality: ☐ left ☐ right ☐ bilateral	❑ y pathologic – staging completed after neoadjuvant therapy AND subsequent surgery

Primary Tumor (T)

TNM Category (Clinical)	FIGO Stage	Definition	TNM Category (Pathologic)	FIGO Stage
❑ TX		Primary tumor cannot be assessed	❑ TX	
❑ T0		No evidence of primary tumor	❑ T0	
❑ T1	I	Tumor confined to uterus	❑ T1	I
❑ T2	II	Tumor extends to other genital structures (ovary, tube, vagina, broad ligaments) by metastasis or direct extension	❑ T2	II

Regional Lymph Nodes (N)

There is no regional nodal designation in the staging of these tumors. Nodal metastases should be classified as metastatic (M1) disease.

Distant Metastasis (M)

TNM Category (Clinical)	FIGO Stage	Definition	TNM Category (Pathologic)	FIGO Stage
❑ M0		No distant metastasis (no pathologic M0; use clinical M to complete stage group)		
❑ M1		Distant metastasis	❑ M1	
❑ M1a	III	Lung metastasis	❑ M1a	III
❑ M1b	IV	All other distant metastasis	❑ M1b	IV

Anatomic Stage • Prognostic Groups

Clinical

Group	T	N	M	Risk Score
❑ I	T1		M0	Unknown
❑ IA	T1		M0	Low risk
❑ IB	T1		M0	High risk
❑ II	T2		M0	Unknown
❑ IIA	T2		M0	Low risk
❑ IIB	T2		M0	High risk
❑ III	Any T		M1a	Unknown
❑ IIIA	Any T		M1a	Low risk
❑ IIIB	Any T		M1a	High risk
❑ IV	Any T		M1b	Unknown
❑ IVA	Any T		M1b	Low risk
❑ IVB	Any T		M1b	High risk

❑ Stage unknown

Pathologic

Group	T	N	M	Risk Score
❑ I	T1		M0	Unknown
❑ IA	T1		M0	Low risk
❑ IB	T1		M0	High risk
❑ II	T2		M0	Unknown
❑ IIA	T2		M0	Low risk
❑ IIB	T2		M0	High risk
❑ III	Any T		M1a	Unknown
❑ IIIA	Any T		M1a	Low risk
❑ IIIB	Any T		M1a	High risk
❑ IV	Any T		M1b	Unknown
❑ IVA	Any T		M1b	Low risk
❑ IVB	Any T		M1b	High risk

❑ Stage unknown

Hospital Name/Address	Patient Name/Information

(continued on next page)

GESTATIONAL TROPHOBLASTIC TUMORS STAGING FORM

PROGNOSTIC FACTORS (SITE-SPECIFIC FACTORS)

REQUIRED FOR STAGING: Prognostic Risk Scoring Index

	Risk Score			
Prognostic Factor	*0*	*1*	*2*	*4*
Age	<40	≥40		
antecedent pregnancy	Hydatidiform mole	Abortion	Term pregnancy	
Interval months from index pregnancy	<4	4–6	7–12	>12
Pretreatment hCG (IU/ml)	$<10^3$	10^3-10^4	10^4-10^5	$>10^5$
Largest tumor size, including uterus	<3 cm	3–5 cm	>5 cm	
Site of metastases	Lung	Spleen, kidney	Gastrointestinal tract	Brain, liver
Number of metastases identified		1–4	5–8	>8
Previous failed chemotherapy			Single drug	Two or more drugs
Total score				

Low risk is a score of 6 or less. High risk is a score of 7 or greater.

CLINICALLY SIGNIFICANT:

FIGO stage: ______

Histologic Grade (G) *(also known as overall grade)*

Grading system	***Grade***
❑ 2 grade system	❑ Grade I or 1
❑ 3 grade system	❑ Grade II or 2
❑ 4 grade system	❑ Grade III or 3
❑ No 2, 3, or 4 grade system is available	❑ Grade IV or 4

ADDITIONAL DESCRIPTORS

Lymphatic Vessel Invasion (L) and Venous Invasion (V) have been combined into Lymph-Vascular Invasion (LVI) for collection by cancer registrars. The College of American Pathologists' (CAP) Checklist should be used as the primary source. Other sources may be used in the absence of a Checklist. Priority is given to positive results.

❑ Lymph-Vascular Invasion Not Present (absent)/Not Identified
❑ Lymph-Vascular Invasion Present/Identified
❑ Not Applicable
❑ Unknown/Indeterminate

General Notes:
For identification of special cases of TNM or pTNM classifications, the "m" suffix and "y," "r," and "a" prefixes are used. Although they do not affect the stage grouping, they indicate cases needing separate analysis.

m suffix indicates the presence of multiple primary tumors in a single site and is recorded in parentheses: pT(m)NM.

y prefix indicates those cases in which classification is performed during or following initial multimodality therapy. The cTNM or pTNM category is identified by a "y" prefix. The ycTNM or ypTNM categorizes the extent of tumor actually present at the time of that examination. The "y" categorization is not an estimate of tumor prior to multimodality therapy.

r prefix indicates a recurrent tumor when staged after a disease-free interval, and is identified by the "r" prefix: rTNM.

a prefix designates the stage determined at autopsy: aTNM.

surgical margins is data field recorded by registrars describing the surgical margins of the resected primary site specimen as determined only by the pathology report.

neoadjuvant treatment is radiation therapy or systemic therapy (consisting of chemotherapy, hormone therapy, or immunotherapy) administered prior to a definitive surgical procedure. If the surgical procedure is not performed, the administered therapy no longer meets the definition of neoadjuvant therapy.

Residual Tumor (R)

The absence or presence of residual tumor after treatment. In some cases treated with surgery and/or with neoadjuvant therapy there will be residual tumor at the primary site after treatment because of incomplete resection or local and regional disease that extends beyond the limit of ability of resection.

❑ RX Presence of residual tumor cannot be assessed
❑ R0 No residual tumor
❑ R1 Microscopic residual tumor
❑ R2 Macroscopic residual tumor

HOSPITAL NAME/ADDRESS	PATIENT NAME/INFORMATION

(continued from previous page)

Gestational Trophoblastic Tumors Staging Form

❑ Clinical stage was used in treatment planning (describe): ______________________________

❑ National guidelines were used in treatment planning ❑ NCCN ❑ Other (describe): ______________

____

____

Physician signature Date/Time

Hospital Name/Address	Patient Name/Information

(continued on next page)

Gestational Trophoblastic Tumors Staging Form

Illustration

Indicate on diagram primary tumor and regional nodes involved.

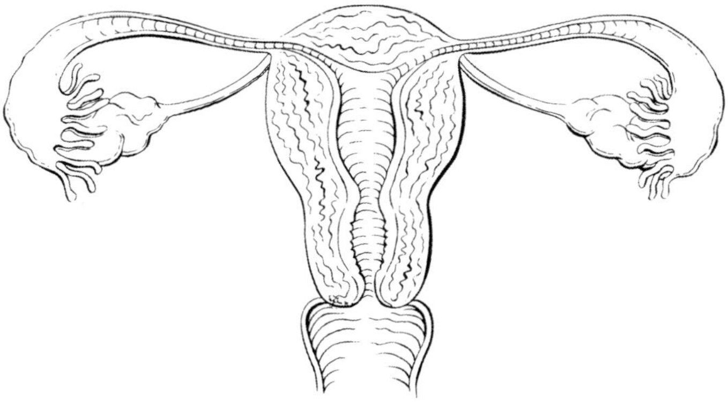

Hospital Name/Address	Patient Name/Information

(continued from previous page)

Index

Printed by Publishers' Graphics LLC
MO20120927-214-284